Sensitive Skin Syndrome
Second Edition

Sensitive Skin Syndrome
Second Edition

Edited by
Golara Honari
Rosa M. Andersen
Howard Maibach

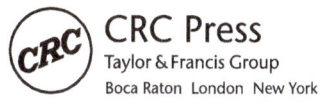

CRC Press
Taylor & Francis Group
Boca Raton London New York

CRC Press is an imprint of the
Taylor & Francis Group, an **informa** business

CRC Press
Taylor & Francis Group
6000 Broken Sound Parkway NW, Suite 300
Boca Raton, FL 33487-2742

Printed on acid-free paper in the UK by Ashford Colour Press Ltd.
Version Date: 20161119

International Standard Book Number-13: 978-1-4987-3734-0 (Hardback)

Library of Congress Cataloging-in-Publication Data

Names: Honari, Golara, editor. | Andersen, Rosa M. editor. | Maibach, Howard I., editor.
Title: Sensitive skin syndrome / [edited by] Golara Honari, Rosa M. Andersen, Howard I. Maibach.
Description: Second edition. | Boca Raton, FL : CRC Press/Taylor & Francis Group, [2017] | Includes bibliographical references and index.
Identifiers: LCCN 2016043692| ISBN 9781498737340 (hardback : alk. paper) | ISBN 9781498737357 (ebook)
Subjects: | MESH: Dermatitis, Contact--diagnosis | Dermatitis, Contact--therapy | Skin Care--methods
Classification: LCC RL244 | NLM WR 175 | DDC 616.5/1--dc23
LC record available at https://lccn.loc.gov/2016043692

Visit the Taylor & Francis Web site at
http://www.taylorandfrancis.com

and the CRC Press Web site at
http://www.crcpress.com

Contents

Section I   Introduction and Background

Section II   Pathophysiology of Sensitive Skin

Section III   Investigative Methods

Preface

Sensitive skin is a prevalent clinical condition that dermatologists should be prepared to recognize, understand, and manage. Affected individuals mostly report unpleasant sensations of itching, burning, and stinging with exposure to various skin care products and/or environmental factors. In some western counties, as high as 50% of women and a 33% of men report various degrees of skin sensitivity affecting their quality of life.

New developments and research over the past few years have shed light on some aspects of underlying pathomechanisms, yet there is much to be learned. Correct clinical categorization of patients is key for clinical management and focused research. Currently, the diagnosis is clinical and based on constellation of symptoms, suggesting the diagnosis of sensitive skin syndrome; however, patients may, in fact, be affected with more than one syndrome/condition. Work of astute clinicians and directed research can further elucidate involved mechanisms and provide management solutions.

We hope that this book provides a comprehensive overview on the main physiological basis of skin reactivity, as well as underlying pathomechanisms associated with sensitive skin and management options.

We sincerely thank all the authors, editors, and publisher, in particular, Mr. Robert Peden, Ms. Adel Rosario, and Ms. Judith Simon for their generous contributions. We also thank our readers in advance and appreciate any comments, corrections, and suggestions for future editions of this book.

Golara Honari
Rosa M. Andersen
Howard Maibach

Contributors

Rosa M. Andersen
Department of Dermatology
University of California at San Francisco
San Francisco, California
and
National Allergy Research Centre
Department of Dermato-Allergology
Gentofte University Hospital
University of Copenhagen
Copenhagen, Denmark

David A. Basketter
DABMEB Consultancy Ltd
Sharnbrook, United Kingdom

Enzo Berardesca
San Gallicano Dermatological Institute
IRCCS
Rome, Italy

Heike Buntrock
Department of Cosmetic Science
Division of Biochemistry and Molecular Biology
and
Division of Chemistry
Department of Cosmetic Science
University of Hamburg
Hamburg, Germany

Jin Ho Chung
Department of Dermatology
Seoul National University College of Medicine
and
Laboratory of Cutaneous Aging Research
Biomedical Research Institute
Seoul National University Hospital
and
Institute of Human–Environment Interface
    Biology
Seoul National University
Seoul, Republic of Korea

Denise Falcone
Department of Dermatology
Radboud University Medical Center
Nijmegen, the Netherlands

Miranda A. Farage
The Procter & Gamble Company
Cincinnati, Ohio

Elena González-Guerra
Department of Dermatology
Hospital Clínico San Carlos
Madrid, Spain

Aurora Guerra-Tapia
Department of Dermatology
Hospital 12 de Octubre
and
Department of Medicine
Universidad Complutense
Madrid, Spain

Golara Honari
Department of Dermatology
Stanford School of Medicine
Stanford, California

Arun C. Inamadar
Department of Dermatology
Sri BM Patil Medical College Hospital &
    Research Center
BLDE University
Karnataka, India

Roland Jourdain
L'Oréal Research and Innovation
Aulnay-sous-Bois, France

Martina Kerscher
Department of Cosmetic Science
Division of Biochemistry and Molecular Biology
and
Division of Chemistry
Department of Cosmetic Science
University of Hamburg
Hamburg, Germany

Eun Ju Kim
Department of Dermatology
Seoul National University College of Medicine
and
Laboratory of Cutaneous Aging Research
Biomedical Research Institute
Seoul National University Hospital
and
Institute of Human–Environment Interface
    Biology
Seoul National University
Seoul, Republic of Korea

Dong Hun Lee
Department of Dermatology
Seoul National University College of Medicine
and
Laboratory of Cutaneous Aging Research
Biomedical Research Institute
Seoul National University Hospital
and
Institute of Human–Environment Interface
    Biology
Seoul National University
Seoul, Republic of Korea

Howard Maibach
Department of Dermatology
University of California
School of Medicine
San Francisco, California

Lidia Maroñas-Jiménez
Department of Dermatology
Hospital 12 de Octubre
Madrid, Spain

Ian McDonald
Department of Dermatology and UCD Charles
    Institute of Translational Dermatology
University College Dublin
Dublin, Ireland

Francis McGlone
School of Natural Sciences & Psychology
Liverpool John Moores University
and
Institute of Psychology
Health & Society University of Liverpool
Liverpool, United Kingdom

Laurent Misery
Laboratory of NeuroSciences of Brest
Faculty of Medicine
University of Brest
and
Department of Dermatology
University Hospital of Brest
Brest, France

Aparna Palit
Department of Dermatology
Sri BM Patil Medical College Hospital &
    Research Center
BLDE University
Karnataka, India

Gérald E. Piérard
Laboratory of Skin Bioengineering and Imaging
Department of Dermatopathology
University Hospital of Liège
Liège, Belgium

Helen Rea
Department of Dermatology and UCD Charles
    Institute of Translational Dermatology
University College Dublin
Dublin, Ireland

David Reilly
Life Sciences Group
Unilever Research & Development
Colworth, United Kingdom

Renée J. H. Richters
Department of Dermatology
Radboud University Medical Center
Nijmegen, the Netherlands

Luís M. Rodrigues
Universidade Lusófona (CBIOS—Research
    Center for Biosciences and Health
    Technologies)
and
Department of Pharmacological Sciences
Universidade de Lisboa—School of Pharmacy
Lisboa, Portugal

Catarina Rosado
Universidade Lusófona (CBIOS—Research
    Center for Biosciences and Health
    Technologies)
Lisboa, Portugal

Sparsha Saxena
Department of Dermatology
University of California San Francisco
San Francisco, California

Martin Schmelz
Department of Anesthesiology and Intensive Care
    Medicine
Medical Faculty Mannheim
Heidelberg University
Mannheim, Germany

Henrique Silva
Universidade Lusófona (CBIOS—Research
    Center for Biosciences and Health
    Technologies)
and
Department of Pharmacological Sciences
Universidade de Lisboa—School of Pharmacy
Lisboa, Portugal

Martin Steinhoff
Department of Dermatology and UCD Charles
    Institute of Translational Dermatology
University College Dublin
Dublin, Ireland
and
Department of Dermatology
University of San Diego
San Diego, California
and
Department of Neurosciences
University of California
Davis, California

Charles Taïeb
Department of Public Health
Hôpital Necker-Enfants Malades
and
European Market Maintenance Assessment
Paris, France

Natallia E. Uzunbajakava
Philips Research
Philips Electronics B.V.
Eindhoven, the Netherlands

Piet E. J. van Erp
Department of Dermatology
Radboud University Medical Center
Nijmegen, the Netherlands

Peter C. M. van de Kerkhof
Department of Dermatology
Radboud University Medical Center
Nijmegen, the Netherlands

Section I

Introduction and Background

1

What Is Sensitive Skin?

**Renée J. H. Richters, Natallia E. Uzunbajakava,
Piet E. J. van Erp, and Peter C. M. van de Kerkhof**

Sensitive Skin in Context

Previously, sensitive skin has rarely been described in scientific literature, and a physiological cause and recognition as a medical entity was questioned by biomedical researchers. Only a few research groups focused on objective approaches to identifying the key mechanisms underlying sensitive skin (1–10). In 1947, Bernstein already described that cleansing of sensitive skin requires extra care (11). Maibach et al. already investigated skin irritation in 1989, in order to elucidate the mechanisms of irritation and to define more predictive screening assays (12). In the latter study, it was shown that some irritants could discriminate between subjects with hand eczema and those with normal skin, while other irritants could not.

In the past two decades, this skeptical view on sensitive skin was subject to change. An increasing number of publications on sensitive skin appeared in recognized scientific journals, emphasizing the importance of the condition for research groups of the cosmetic and pharmaceutical industry and for biomedical researchers. Large epidemiological studies have been conducted on the prevalence of sensitive skin in different countries and among different ethnicities and cultures. Since especially across industrialized countries the prevalence of sensitive skin is high and seems to have a serious impact on the quality of life, the identification of the pathways underlying sensitive skin and treatments thereof became a key topic of research. Many studies used different chemical agents in order to identify subjects with sensitive skin and to discover the underlying pathways. Despite this progress, a consensus on the definition has not been reached yet and attempts to establish valid diagnostic tests to identify the profile of sensitive skin have failed.

Terms and definitions proposed in literature to describe symptoms commonly designated as sensitive skin are abundant: *susceptible skin*, *hypersensitive skin*, *reactive skin*, *hyperreactive skin*, *intolerant skin*, *hyperirritable skin*, *cosmetic intolerance syndrome*, *status cosmeticus*, *delicate skin*, and *sensory skin irritation*. Currently, the term *sensitive skin* is the one most commonly used; however, a uniform definition has not been established. Inter alia, because of the highly heterogeneous presentation of sensitive skin and the lack of an objective test, clinical studies report inconsistent results and, therefore, these pathways have not been deciphered yet.

More knowledge on the pathomechanical background and reality behind sensitive skin is of great interest for researchers and clinicians working in the area of skin irritation and skin–material interactions, who aspire to look beyond the cosmetic perspective and include objective measurements of sensitive skin. Evidence on the pathways underlying sensitive skin will enable addressing solutions for individual differences in skin reactions, which is highly desired by both patients and consumers in this new era.

Epidemiology

In order to determine the prevalence of sensitive skin and to characterize the symptom profile and its eliciting factors, several surveys have been conducted in large cohorts across different geographical areas. Studies have mainly been conducted in industrialized countries, where commercial enterprise with respect to products for personal care are highly developed and accessible to the majority of inhabitants.

Since sensitive skin is a subjective condition by its current definition, it is difficult to objectively investigate its prevalence. Many studies applied a four-point scale (13–21) in order to classify self-reported skin sensitivity, in which the classes are not universally defined but seem to be comparable: (i) the strongest classification for sensitive skin, which has roughly been described as very sensitive skin, strongly sensitive skin, or "I strongly agree with having a sensitive skin"; (ii) sensitive skin, moderately sensitive skin, rather sensitive skin, or "I somewhat agree with having a sensitive skin"; (iii) not very sensitive, slightly sensitive, somewhat sensitive skin, or "I somewhat disagree with having a sensitive skin"; and (iv) not sensitive at all, not sensitive, or "I strongly disagree with having a sensitive skin." Some studies used a two-point scale, "sensitive" or "not sensitive," or did not explain the definition of the used scale (17,22).

Surveys have been administered using different modalities as digital questionnaires, telephone interviews, or direct questions of the researcher to the subject and show that approximately 50% of people in the industrialized world report to have some degree of sensitive skin (Table 1.1). Some epidemiological studies included solely females (14,20,24,26), while other studies included a cohort comprising both genders, of which most often the majority are female. Among the European population, 60% of females (16,20,22–24) and 36% of males (16,22,23) report having sensitive skin. Three studies in the United States show that 59% of females also assess their skin as sensitive (13,14,19), and two studies show that 45% of males assess their skin as sensitive (13,19). These numbers are calculated from Table 1.1, corrected for the number of subjects included. In Brazil, Russia, and Japan, similar percentages were found for females. Among Japanese men, 52.8% report sensitive skin, while lower numbers are found among men in Brazil and Russia (22.3% and 25.4%, respectively). The overall prevalence of sensitive skin in China is lower compared to those in European countries and the United States.

The large number of people reporting to have sensitive skin might reflect that the condition of sensitive skin is commonly addressed in the media and is known among this relatively prosperous population. Cultural factors and the media might have influence on the propensity to report to self-perceived sensitive skin.

TABLE 1.1

The Prevalence of Self-Reported Sensitive Skin in Large Cohorts Identified by Surveys

	Reference	Country	N	% Females	SS (%) of Total	SS (%) of Females	SS (%) of Males
Farage (2009)	(13)	United States	1039	84	68.4	69.0	64.4
Jourdain et al. (2002)	(14)	United States	811	100	NA	52.0	NA
Misery et al. (2011)	(19)	United States	994	50.2	44.6	50.9	38.2
Misery et al. (2009)	(17)	France	1006	NA	82	59	44
Morizot et al. (2000)	(20)	France	319	100	NA	90	NA
Guinot et al. (2006)	(23)	France	8522	59.5	49	61	32
Saint-Martory et al. (2008)	(24)	France	400	100	NA	85	NA
Willis et al. (2001)	(22)	United Kingdom	2058	87.5	49.7	51.4	38.2
Sparavigna et al. (2005)	(25)	Italy	2101	88.5	NA	56.5	NA
Loffler et al. (2001)	(16)	Germany	420	38.6	75.2	63.6	82.5
Misery et al. (2009)	(17)	Europe	4506	NA	38.4	49.4	37.0
Kamide et al. (2013)	(15)	Japan	1500	51.8	54.5	56.0	52.8
Xu et al. (2013)	(21)	China	9154	57.1	13	15.9	8.6
Farage et al. (2012)	(26)	China	408	100	NA	23.0	NA
Taïeb et al. (2014)	(27)	Brazil	1022	NA	NA	45.7	22.3
Taïeb et al. (2014)	(27)	Russia	1500	NA	NA	50.1	25.4

Note: Percentages are either extracted or calculated from the result sections of the original articles. NA, not applicable; SS, subjects with sensitive skin.

Clinical Manifestation

There is no consensus on the symptom profile of sensitive skin. People assessing their skin as sensitive experience unpleasant sensations of the skin, particularly characterized by stinging, burning, or itching sensations (20,24,28). Remarkably, visible signs of skin irritation, as erythema or skin dryness, are absent in many individuals (20,22,24,29,30). Since the symptoms reported by subjects are rather nonspecific, the differentiation from or relationship with dermatological disorders such as irritant contact dermatitis, allergic contact dermatitis, rosacea, physical urticaria, and dermographism, xerosis, (atopic) dermatitis, and photodermatoses may be challenging. Deeper understanding of sensitive skin will enable placing this condition in the context of skin pathology.

Factors impeding the detection and definition of sensitive skin are the frequent absence of clinical signs and subjective character of symptoms (20,31,32) and the heterogeneity thereof (20).

Eliciting Factors

Sensitive skin perceptions are elicited by exogenous and endogenous factors that usually have a considerably low impact on individuals and frequently do not cause skin irritation (13,18,22,23,25).

In order to define the symptom profile and to address specific exogenous and endogenous factors which may elicit skin reactions, nonuniform comprehensive questionnaires were conducted in different populations (18,22,23), showing various risk factors and triggers. Among these factors, the important triggers are cosmetics and soaps (20,21,24–26), environmental climate [temperature changes (14,15,20,21), heat (14,15,20,24,25), cold (14,15,20,25), and dampness (21)], sun exposure (14,21,24), stress or emotions (20,24,25), wind (14,15,25), and friction from clothes (24).

Having a dry or greasy skin (17,21), a history of childhood atopic dermatitis (AD) (17,21,22), being female (21), and having a fair skin type (21) are important host factors increasing the risk of having sensitive skin (21).

Subject Selection in Clinical Studies

To enable conduction of clinical studies in a population with sensitive skin and with nonsensitive skin, assumptions on the definition and inclusion criteria have to be made. Erroneous selection of subjects may possibly lead to formulating wrong conclusions on pathomechanisms. Moreover, since symptoms might be subclinical in situations in which the skin is not challenged, differences in physiology may be minute and difficult to detect, and therefore careful selection of subjects with sensitive skin is of high importance.

A performed systematic literature review on objective measurements on sensitive skin identified studies including subjects by means of perception, for example, burning, stinging, itching, and general skin discomfort (33). This self-reported skin sensitivity was determined (i) by sensory skin reactions following application of specific stimuli or (ii) by questionnaire. Subsequently, the relation of the group characteristics of the selected populations and the selected study population with objective measurements were studied, both at baseline and following specific stimulations.

Subject Selection and Provocation by Stimuli

Many research groups select sensitive subjects and nonsensitive subjects as a control group by evaluation of sensory discomfort after application of a chemical agent on the skin. Lactic acid is one of the most frequently used agents (34–43), and the lactic acid stinging test (LAST) was previously even proposed as the best diagnostic test available for sensitive skin (44). LAST identifies "stingers"—subjects perceiving sensations of stinging after application of lactic acid on the nasolabial fold—which are assumed to correlate with sensitive skin. A detailed evaluation of studies including subjects by self-perceived sensitive skin and using LAST as a provocative method to enhance skin reactions shows that in subjects with sensitive skin, higher stinging scores are observed (45), time to onset and peaking of stinging response are shorter (45), and the overall stinging scores are higher (46,47). However, the test is subjective in nature and lacks sensitivity, 59.9–80% (27,45,48) of subjects with sensitive skin report a positive reaction to LAST, and specificity, 66.7% of nonsensitive subjects experience this reaction (48) for sensitive skin. Thus, lactic acid mainly elicits some, but not all key symptoms in the clinical profile of sensitive skin, predominantly skin stinging and slightly burning. This might be the reason for the insufficient sensitivity. In addition to this, studies have shown that a positive response to one substance does not predict a reaction to another substance (40,45,49–52), questioning the validity of using a single substance to test skin sensitivity. Next to using lactic acid as a challenge, studies of sensitive skin reactions and sensations have been performed using a wide range of chemical agents. They include but are not limited to sodium lauryl sulfate (SLS), capsaicin, menthol, benzoic acid, *trans*-cinnamic acid, octane, cumene, methyl nicotinate and acetyl-β-methylcholine chloride (vasodilators), ethanol, allergens, occlusion, cocamidopropyl betaine and benzalkonium chloride (surfactants), and balsam of Peru. Furthermore, material interactions (53) and electrical provocations (54) followed by noninvasive measurements of the biophysical parameters of the skin have been appraised in people reporting perceptions of sensitive skin to quantify sensory irritation and to reveal the underlying mechanisms of sensitive skin. Many provocations used in experiments resulted in sensory skin reactions, but, again, these might not be specifically addressing the sensitive skin.

Subject Selection by Questionnaire

An increasing number of studies select subjects by means of self-perceived sensitive skin inventoried by questionnaires, using different definitions of sensitive skin, as explained in the "Epidemiology" section. Some research groups included solely the question, "Do you have a sensitive skin, yes or no?" In one study, skin sensitivity was scored on a labeled magnitude scale, permitting both semantic descriptors and a continuum of intensity rankings to compare individuals (55). In contrast, other research groups conducted extensive nonuniform questionnaires addressing sensory, objective symptoms and additionally encompassing numerous potentially eliciting factors by means of inclusion of subjects with sensitive skin and with nonsensitive skin.

A ten-item questionnaire was developed by Misery et al. (56). With this questionnaire, researchers made an attempt to establish standardized patient questionnaires, which might allow scoring in a reproducible manner on a "sensitive scale" and might be suited for monitoring the evolution of the skin condition (56). However, only a selected population with sensitive skin diagnosed in a private clinic was included in this study, limiting the application of the developed scale as a diagnostic tool for selecting sensitive and nonsensitive subjects for research purposes.

Pathomechanisms and Objective Readouts

Kligman et al. (57) used a novel nomenclature for sensitive skin by proposing different subtypes of sensitive skin defined by clinical presentation or possible underlying etiology as follows: (i) *subjective irritation* refers to an irritant response without visible clinical signs; (ii) *neurosensory irritation* signifies neutrally mediated responses such as itching, stinging, burning, and tightness; (iii) *chemosensory* relates to sensory responses induced by chemicals in contrast to physical, mechanical, and environmental factors; and (iv) *psychophysical irritation* implies a psychological component. Willis et al. (22) described several clinical forms depending on the intensity of clinical symptoms: (i) *Very sensitive skin* is dry or fatty and bitterly reacting to both exogenous factors, that is, cosmetic products and environmental factors, and endogenous features. The clinical symptoms are acute and permanent, and both factors trigger determining psychological reactions. (ii) *Environmentally sensitive skin* is skin that is often clear, dry, and thin and essentially reactive to environmental factors, that is, heat and rapid temperature changes, with frequent bouts of flushing. (iii) *Cosmetically sensitive skin* is essentially reactive to cosmetics. This intolerance is lighter and often limited to some identifiable cosmetic products. Farage and Maibach also proposed a heterogeneous phenomenon with multiple etiologic aspects (58); Richters et al. (33)

critically appraised the evidence of objective measurements at baseline and following skin provocations. This research group chose an approach by including studies which had selected sensitive subjects based on perception. The translation from skin perceptions to objective measurements was made, and it was shown that the strongest evidence exists for the role of an impaired skin barrier in sensitive skin. This impaired barrier might cause sensory perceptions, and vascular reactivity might develop subsequently.

However, strong evidence and consistency on pathways underlying sensitive skin is still lacking at this moment.

Skin Barrier Impairment

Many research groups focused on the skin barrier function and measured transepidermal water loss (TEWL) as a parameter of skin barrier function. In some studies, a higher TEWL was observed in the unchallenged skin of subjects with sensitive skin compared to that in subjects with nonsensitive skin (16,29,37,59). In stingers, a higher TEWL was also measured compared to that in nonstingers (34,37,38,41,52). Additionally, a higher TEWL at baseline seems to correlate with stronger TEWL increase following provocation (34): plastic occlusion resulted in significantly longer evaporation half-life time in subjects with sensitive skin (59), and a trend to increased recovery time of TEWL following SLS stimulation was also observed. A low hydration of the stratum corneum is also associated with an impaired skin barrier. A significantly lower stratum corneum hydration in facial areas in subjects with sensitive skin (47) and in stingers (34) and a nonsignificantly lower stratum corneum hydration in facial areas in subjects with sensitive skin were found (37). Challenging the skin chemically resulted in a significantly lower stratum corneum hydration in stingers compared to that in nonstingers (41). Clinically, a dryer skin is also observed (25). In contrast to these findings, other studies found no difference in stratum corneum hydration between subjects with sensitive skin and subjects with nonsensitive skin (16,29) or between stingers and nonstingers (34,37,41) either challenged or unchallenged. The skin of stingers with self-reported sensitive skin appears to be rougher since Fast Fourier transform evaluation of tapes after tape-stripping the stratum corneum in 243 stingers reveals lower contents of cells (42). This implies a more irregular, rougher, and possibly less hydrated skin as well as impaired intercorneocyte adhesion. Objectively measured skin elasticity and distensibility show no correlation with hypersensitivity (43).

The literature is insufficient and inconclusive with regard to the role of sebum secretion in sensitive skin perceptions. No differences were observed with respect to sebum and surface pH between sensitive and nonsensitive subjects (43,47) and between stingers and nonstingers (34). However, in one study, significantly lower sebum and higher surface pH were measured in subjects with sensitive skin compared to those in subjects with nonsensitive skin (9).

Hypersensitivity: Neurologic Aspects

Sensitive skin has a predominantly subjective character, as stinging, burning, itching, and sensations of tightness are reported, implying that the neurons of subjects with a sensitive skin dysfunction easily respond to mild stimuli. Stander et al. also addressed the role of the neural system and neuromediators in skin sensitivity (60). Differences in pain perceptions were observed in subjects with sensitive skin by functional magnetic resonance imaging (46). Skin discomfort induced by lactic acid leads to the activation of different parts of the cerebral cortex. Quatresooz et al. also measured the electrical current perception threshold (CPT) in subjects with reactive and nonreactive skin and concluded that some subjects with reactive skin and a lower CPT showed a higher density of mast cells in the dermis (54). This is in line with the findings of Kim et al., who detected a lower CPT to 5 Hz electric current on the forearm in subjects with sensitive skin compared to CPT in subjects with nonsensitive skin (38). Five hertz is a selective stimulator of the C fibers of sensory nerves (38). C fibers are unmyelinated fibers playing a role in the perception of pain, itch, and warmth. Additionally, an inverse correlation was shown between the clinical detection thresholds of capsaicin and sensitive skin indexed by questionnaire (61). When the skin comes in contact with capsaicin, noxious heat, or low pH, transient receptor potential vanilloid 1 is activated (62,63) and results in nociceptor-mediated burning pain. An overexpression of this receptor could play a key role in the pathomechanism of sensitive skin, as inhibition results in reduced burning sensation following capsaicin application (64).

Vascular Responses

Next to neurosensory signs, objective signs such as skin redness are also frequently reported by individuals with sensitive skin, implying a key role for vascular or even inflammatory responses in the pathomechanism of sensitive skin. As a readout for erythema visual assessment (35,37,40,47), colorimetry and spectrophotometry (29,35,38,41,48,65) and laser Doppler flowmetry are used (16,29,37–39,41,65). At baseline, in one study, significant differences in skin redness were found; a lower a^* value was found in self-reported sensitive skin compared to that in nonsensitive skin (29). The literature is inconclusive on differences in skin redness between sensitive and nonsensitive subjects following stimulation of the skin. With respect to endothelium markers (CD31), no different quantity is found between subjects with reactive skin and low CPT and subjects with less reactive skin and high CPT (54). Lactic acid, SLS, capsaicin, and cumene application did not result in higher erythema responses in subjects with sensitive skin compared to subjects with nonsensitive skin (29,38,41). In contrast, octane, acetyl-β-methylcholine chloride, methyl nicotinate, and allergen patch testing did result in relatively stronger erythema responses in sensitive subjects (1,41,47). A proposed explanation for vascular reactivity is that when the skin barrier function is impaired in subjects with sensitive skin, subsequently higher concentrations of chemical agents can be reached, eliciting vascular responses more strongly (66).

Allergic Predisposition

AD is considered to be a predisposing factor for the development of sensitive skin, since more individuals with sensitive skin report to have atopy compared to nonsensitive subjects (17,22,67). Stinging is also frequently reported in AD (67). Subjects with AD are more prone to develop skin irritation following application of a patch with SLS (68–72).

However, sensitive subjects selected by LAST seem not to develop stronger objective skin irritation responses following the application of SLS (40,49). A correlation was only demonstrated by Lammintausta et al. showing stronger increase in laser Doppler blood flow (51). Histologically, increased numbers of mast cells are found in subjects with reactive skin and a low CPT (54). This, in combination with an impaired skin barrier function, implies the potential of sensitive skin pathophysiology with that of AD, which should be explored in future studies.

Limitations

Many clinical studies are observational studies, mainly or solely comprising the female gender. Relatively young populations are often included, with a mean age younger than 40 years (14,29,34,37–40,42,47,48, 54,65,73). Many studies unfortunately lack statistical power, since only small populations are included and potential selection bias, confounders, and information bias are frequently not addressed. Many authors do not specify age, ethnicity, skin type, or concomitant skin diseases. Skin diseases are extraneous variables affecting skin sensitivity, especially variables such as skin barrier function and clinical inflammatory parameters. Abnormal physiological pathways such as, impaired skin barrier function and increased inflammatory responses in AD or psoriasis should be excluded from explorative studies on the pathomechanism of sensitive skin. The existing heterogeneity of study designs reported so far complicates the comparison of results; various selection methods have been used which are different natures, and many provocations have been performed. In addition, different body sites are stimulated (40), which are not comparable with respect to skin sensitivity; different time points and devices have been applied; and studies have been performed under various conditions with respect to environmental climate.

Future Perspectives

Since sensitive skin is highly prevalent in the Western world and has an impact on the quality of life, understanding of the physiological reality and managing sensitive skin is of high importance. Approaches focused on identifying pathomechanisms causing perceptions of skin discomfort designated as sensitive skin could enable an evidence-based diagnosis and rational interventions for patients with sensitive skin, implementing personalized medicine, highly aspired in these modern times. New approaches in this research field might encompass highly reproducible in vivo skin models in order to enable studying skin reactions in subjects with sensitive skin. By eliciting skin responses, the mechanisms underlying sensitive skin might be enhanced and become measurable; moreover, when elicited in a standardized way, skin reactions in subjects with different conditions will be comparable.

Processes set off may be studied in a dynamic fashion by exploring parameters at several moments in time following the stimulus. In addition, a better understanding of the morphology and physiology of reactions might be established by exploration of different potential mechanisms applying different perspectives: clinical, biophysical, and immunohistochemical. These methodologies could be complementary and could enable decisively answering questions on the contribution of physiological impairments, and a suitable definition can be established. The hypothesis of multiple etiologies underlying sensitive skin would not be farfetched as also proposed by Farage and Maibach (58). An impaired skin barrier function is strongly hypothesized in literature to be a key player in the pathomechanism of sensitive skin. However, consistent evidence is lacking. Immunohistochemistry could function as a reference in order to validate or investigate in detail the stratum corneum. This enables further research by noninvasive analysis of the skin barrier, for example. Focus should be given to the quantification of components of the stratum corneum, encompassing ceramides, lipid composition, and natural moisturizing factor. Advanced biophysical techniques, such as confocal Raman spectroscopy, can accurately quantify these components in a noninvasive way. However, of note, differences in biophysical measurements do not ensure differences in skin sensitivity since these parameters have high interindividual variability in the general population. Additional parameters measuring the same process could strengthen specific pathways and might explain previously described inconsistencies in study outcomes.

Next to a different perspective on measurements, clinical studies require new methods on the selection of subjects. By including "extreme subjects" with subjectively severe sensitive skin and subjects with subjectively no complaints of sensitive skin, potential differences might become highlighted. It would be interesting when the selection of subjects would become more uniform and comparable. Quantification of perceptions of the sensitive subject could enable the comparison. Translation of these perceptions to biophysical properties and detailed histological data might be the best approach to measuring this dominantly subjective skin condition. One of the criteria which should be included in the selection tool is skin reaction to multiple stimuli, to prevent measuring irritant or allergic contact dermatitis or heat intolerance, for example. Perception-based selection of subjects through a questionnaire spanning a range of provocations, including those of chemical, mechanical, and thermal origin and including multiple signs and symptoms, might be a more valid and applicable selection tool than selection by reaction to one chemical agent skin provocation.

Currently, scientists are still being challenged by this relatively unexplored phenomenon. An integral approach is recommended to unravel the sensitive skin phenomenon, taking into the picture the clinical, biophysical, and histological hallmarks of this condition. A new step in diagnosis and treatment of the condition could be taken only by conducting cross-disciplinary, collaborative research, including experts' contribution in dermatology, cosmetic sciences, psychology, and biophysics.

REFERENCES

1. Berardesca E, Cespa M, Farinelli N, Rabbiosi G, Maibach H. In vivo transcutaneous penetration of nicotinates and sensitive skin. *Contact Dermatitis*. 1991;25(1):35–8.
2. Berardesca E, Maibach HI. Sensitive and ethnic skin: A need for special skin-care agents? *Dermatologic Clinics*. 1991;9(1):89–92.
3. Draelos ZD. Sensitive skin: Perceptions, evaluation, and treatment. *American Journal of Contact Dermatitis*. 1997;8(2):67–78.
4. Issachar N, Gall Y, Borell MT, Poelman MC. pH measurements during lactic acid stinging test in normal and sensitive skin. *Contact Dermatitis*. 1997;36(3):152–5.
5. Issachar N, Gall Y, Borrel MT, Poelman MC. Correlation between percutaneous penetration of methyl nicotinate and sensitive skin, using laser Doppler imaging. *Contact Dermatitis*. 1998;39(4):182–6.

6. Mills Jr OH, Berger RS. Defining the susceptibility of acne-prone and sensitive skin populations to extrinsic factors. *Dermatologic Clinics.* 1991;9(1):93–8.

7. Muizzuddin N, Marenus KD, Maes DH. Factors defining sensitive skin and its treatment. *American Journal of Contact Dermatitis.* 1998;9(3):170–5.

8. Paquet F, Pierard-Franchimont C, Fumal I, Goffin V, Paye M, Pierard GE. Sensitive skin at menopause: Dew point and electrometric properties of the stratum corneum. *Maturitas.* 1998;28(3):221–7.

9. Seidenari S, Francomano M, Mantovani L. Baseline biophysical parameters in subjects with sensitive skin. *Contact Dermatitis.* 1998;38(6):311–5.

10. Simion AF, Rau AH. Sensitive skin: What is it and how to formulate for it. *Cosmetics & Toiletries.* 1994;109:43s.

11. Bernstein ET. Cleansing of sensitive skin; with determination of the pH of the skin following use of soap and a soap substitute. *The Journal of Investigative Dermatology.* 1947;9(1):5–9.

12. Maibach HI, Lammintausta K, Berardesca E, Freeman S. Tendency to irritation: Sensitive skin. *Journal of the American Academy of Dermatology.* 1989;21(4 Pt 2):833–5.

13. Farage MA. How do perceptions of sensitive skin differ at different anatomical sites? An epidemiological study. *Clinical and Experimental Dermatology.* 2009;34(8):e521–30.

14. Jourdain R, de Lacharriere O, Bastien P, Maibach HI. Ethnic variations in self-perceived sensitive skin: Epidemiological survey. *Contact Dermatitis.* 2002;46(3):162–9.

15. Kamide R, Misery L, Perez-Cullell N, Sibaud V, Taïeb C. Sensitive skin evaluation in the Japanese population. *The Journal of Dermatology.* 2013;40(3):177–81.

16. Loffler H, Dickel H, Kuss O, Diepgen TL, Effendy I. Characteristics of self-estimated enhanced skin susceptibility. *Acta Dermato-Venereologica.* 2001;81(5):343–6.

17. Misery L, Boussetta S, Nocera T, Perez-Cullell N, Taïeb C. Sensitive skin in Europe. *Journal of the European Academy of Dermatology and Venereology.* 2009;23(4):376–81.

18. Misery L, Myon E, Martin N, Verriere F, Nocera T, Taïeb C. Sensitive skins in France: An epidemiological approach. [French]. *Annales de Dermatologie et de Vénéréologie* 2005;132(5):425–9.

19. Misery L, Sibaud V, Merial-Kieny C, Taïeb C. Sensitive skin in the American population: Prevalence, clinical data, and role of the dermatologist. *International Journal of Dermatology.* 2011;50(8):961–7.

20. Morizot F, Guinot C, Lopez J, LaFus I, Tschachler E. Sensitive skin: Analysis of symptoms, perceived causes and possible mechanisms. *Cosmetics & Toiletries.* 2000;115:83–9.

21. Xu F, Yan S, Wu M, Li F, Sun Q, Lai W et al. Self-declared sensitive skin in China: A community-based study in three top metropolises. *Journal of the European Academy of Dermatology and Venereology.* 2013;27(3):370–5.

22. Willis CM, Shaw S, De Lacharriere O, Baverel M, Reiche L, Jourdain R et al. Sensitive skin: An epidemiological study. *The British Journal of Dermatology.* 2001;145(2):258–63.

23. Guinot C, Malvy D, Mauger E, Ezzedine K, Latreille J, Ambroisine L et al. Self-reported skin sensitivity in a general adult population in France: Data of the SU.VI.MAX cohort. *Journal of the European Academy of Dermatology and Venereology.* 2006;20(4):380–90.

24. Saint-Martory C, Roguedas-Contios AM, Sibaud V, Degouy A, Schmitt AM, Misery L. Sensitive skin is not limited to the face. *British Journal of Dermatology.* 2008;158(1):130–3.

25. Sparavigna A, Di Pietro A, Setaro M. "Healthy skin": Significance and results of an Italian study on healthy population with particular regard to "sensitive" skin. *International Journal of Cosmetic Science.* 2005;27(6):327–31.

26. Farage M, Mandl C, Berardesca E, Maibach H. Sensitive skin in China. *Journal of Cosmetics, Dermatological Sciences and Applications.* 2012;2(3):184–95.

27. Taïeb C, Auges M, Georgescu V, Perez Cullell N, Misery L. Sensitive skin in Brazil and Russia: An epidemiological and comparative approach. *European Journal of Dermatology.* 2014;24(3):372–6.

28. Misery L, Myon E, Martin N, Consoli S, Boussetta S, Nocera T et al. Sensitive skin: Psychological effects and seasonal changes. *Journal of the European Academy of Dermatology and Venereology.* 2007;21(5):620–8.

29. Diogo L, Papoila AL. Is it possible to characterize objectively sensitive skin? *Skin Research and Rechnology.* 2010;16(1):30–7.

30. Primavera G, Berardesca E. Sensitive skin: Mechanisms and diagnosis. *International Journal of Cosmetic Science.* 2005;27(1):1–10.

31. Farage MA, Katsarou A, Maibach HI. Sensory, clinical and physiological factors in sensitive skin: A review. *Contact Dermatitis.* 2006;55(1):1–14.

32. Green BG. Measurement of sensory irritation of the skin. *American Journal of Contact Dermatitis.* 2000;11(3):170–80.

33. Richters R, Falcone D, Uzunbajakava N, Verkruysse W, van Erp P, van de Kerkhof P. What is sensitive skin? A systematic literature review of objective measurements. *Skin Pharmacology and Physiology.* 2015;28(2):75–83.

34. An S, Lee E, Kim S, Nam G, Lee H, Moon S et al. Comparison and correlation between stinging responses to lactic acid and bioengineering parameters. *Contact Dermatitis.* 2007;57(3):158–62.

35. Berardesca E, Abril E, Serio M, Cameli N. Effects of topical gluco-oligosaccharide and collagen tripeptide F in the treatment of sensitive atopic skin. *International Journal of Cosmetic Science.* 2009;31(4):271–7.

36. de Campos Dieamant G, Velazquez Pereda MDL, Eberlin S, Nogueira C, Werka RM, Queiroz MLS. Neuroimmunomodulatory compound for sensitive skin care: In vitro and clinical assessment. *Journal of Cosmetic Dermatology.* 2008;7(2):112–9.

37. Distante F, Rigano L, D'Agostino R, Bonfigli A. Intra- and inter-individual differences in sensitive skin. *Cosmetics & Toiletries.* 2002;117(7):39–46.

38. Kim SJ, Lim SU, Won YH, An SS, Lee EY, Moon SJ et al. The perception threshold measurement can be a useful tool for evaluation of sensitive skin. *International Journal of Cosmetic Science.* 2008;30(5):333–7.

39. Lee E, An S, Lee TR, Kim HK. Development of a novel method for quantitative evaluation of sensory skin irritation inhibitors. *Skin Research and Technology.* 2009;15(4):464–9.

40. Marriott M, Holmes J, Peters L, Cooper K, Rowson M, Basketter DA. The complex problem of sensitive skin. *Contact Dermatitis.* 2005;53(2):93–9.

41. Schliemann S, Antonov D, Manegold N, Elsner P. Sensory irritation caused by two organic solvents—Short-time single application and repeated occlusive test in stingers and non-stingers. *Contact Dermatitis.* 2011;65(2):107–14.

42. Sparavigna A, Pietro A, Setaro M. Sensitive skin: Correlation with skin surface microrelief appearance. *Skin Research and Technology.* 2006;12(1):7–10.

43. Vijver van de LPL, Boelsma E, Rausch-Goldbohm RA, Roza L. Subjective skin condition and its association with objective skin measurements. *Cosmetics & Toiletries.* 2003;118(7):45–54.

44. Frosch PJ, Kligman AM. A method for appraising the stinging capacity of topically applied substances. *Journal of the Society of Cosmetic Chemists.* 1977;28:197–209.

45. Bowman JP, Floyd AK, Znaniecki A, Kligman AM, Stoudemayer T, Mills OH. The use of chemical probes to assess the facial reactivity of women, comparing their self-perception of sensitive skin. *Journal of Cosmetic Science.* 2000;51:67–273.

46. Querleux B, Dauchot K, Jourdain R, Bastien P, Bittoun J, Anton JL et al. Neural basis of sensitive skin: An fMRI study. *Skin Research and Technology.* 2008;14(4):454–61.

47. Roussaki-Schulze AV, Zafiriou E, Nikoulis D, Klimi E, Rallis E, Zintzaras E. Objective biophysical findings in patients with sensitive skin. *Drugs under Experimental and Clinical Research.* 2005;31 Suppl:17–24.

48. Cho HJ, Chung BY, Lee HB, Kim HO, Park CW, Lee CH. Quantitative study of stratum corneum ceramides contents in patients with sensitive skin. *Journal of Dermatology.* 2012;39(3):295–300.

49. Basketter DA, Griffiths HA. A study of the relationship between susceptibility to skin stinging and skin irritation. *Contact Dermatitis.* 1993;29(4):185–8.

50. Coverly J, Peters L, Whittle E, Basketter DA. Susceptibility to skin stinging, nonimmunologic contact urticaria and acute skin irritation: Is there a relationship? *Contact Dermatitis.* 1998;38(2):90–5.

51. Lammintausta K, Maibach HI, Wilson D. Mechanisms of subjective (sensory) irritation: Propensity to non-immunologic contact urticaria and objective irritation in stingers. *Dermatosen in Beruf und Umwelt: Occupation and Environment.* 1988;36(2):45–9.

52. Wu Y, Wang X, Zhou Y, Tan Y, Chen D, Chen Y et al. Correlation between stinging, TEWL and capacitance. *Skin Research and Technology.* 2003;9(2):90–3.

53. Farage MA, Maibach H. Cumulative skin irritation test of sanitary pads in sensitive skin and normal skin population. *Cutaneous and Ocular Toxicology.* 2007;26(1):37–43.

54. Quatresooz P, Pierard-Franchimont C, Pierard GE. Vulnerability of reactive skin to electric current perception—A pilot study implicating mast cells and the lymphatic microvasculature. *Journal of Cosmetic Dermatology.* 2009;8(3):186–9.

55. Robinson MK, Perkins MA. Evaluation of a quantitative clinical method for assessment of sensory skin irritation. *Contact Dermatitis*. 2001;45(4):205–13.
56. Misery L, Jean-Decoster C, Mery S, Georgescu V, Sibaud V. A new ten-item questionnaire for assessing sensitive skin: The Sensitive Scale-10. *Acta Dermato-Venereologica*. 2014;94(6):635–9.
57. Kligman AM, Sadiq I, Zhen Y, Crosby M. Experimental studies on the nature of sensitive skin. *Skin Research and Technology*. 2006;12(4):217–22.
58. Farage MA, Maibach HI. Sensitive skin: Closing in on a physiological cause. *Contact Dermatitis*. 2010;62(3):137–49.
59. Pinto P, Rosado C, Parreirao C, Rodrigues LM. Is there any barrier impairment in sensitive skin? A quantitative analysis of sensitive skin by mathematical modeling of transepidermal water loss desorption curves. *Skin Research and Technology*. 2011;17(2):181–5.
60. Stander S, Schneider SW, Weishaupt C, Luger TA, Misery L. Putative neuronal mechanisms of sensitive skin. *Experimental Dermatology*. 2009;18(5):417–23.
61. Jourdain R, Bastien P, de Lacharriere O, Rubinstenn G. Detection thresholds of capsaicin: A new test to assess facial skin neurosensitivity. *Journal of Cosmetic Science*. 2005;56(3):153–66.
62. Clapham DE. TRP channels as cellular sensors. *Nature*. 2003;426(6966):517–24.
63. Dhaka A, Viswanath V, Patapoutian A. Trp ion channels and temperature sensation. *Annual Review of Neuroscience*. 2006;29:135–61.
64. Kueper T, Krohn M, Haustedt LO, Hatt H, Schmaus G, Vielhaber G. Inhibition of TRPV1 for the treatment of sensitive skin. *Experimental Dermatology*. 2010;19(11):980–6.
65. Aramaki J, Kawana S, Effendy I, Happle R, Loffler H. Differences of skin irritation between Japanese and European women. *British Journal of Dermatology*. 2002;146(6):1052–6.
66. Lee BH, Park CK, Kim HO, Jo HJ, Park CW, Lee CH. The skin irritations of corrosive and non-corrosive irritants in patients with sensitive skin. *Korean Journal of Dermatology*. 2007;45(6):551–9.
67. Pons-Guiraud A. Sensitive skin: A complex and multifactorial syndrome. *Journal of Cosmetic Dermatology*. 2004;3(3):145–8.
68. Agner T, Serup J. Sodium lauryl sulphate for irritant patch testing—A dose–response study using bioengineering methods for determination of skin irritation. *The Journal of Investigative Dermatology*. 1990;95(5):543–7.
69. Cowley NC, Farr PM. A dose–response study of irritant reactions to sodium lauryl sulphate in patients with seborrhoeic dermatitis and atopic eczema. *Acta Dermato-Venereologica*. 1992;72(6):432–5.
70. Nassif A, Chan SC, Storrs FJ, Hanifin JM. Abnormal skin irritancy in atopic-dermatitis and in atopy without dermatitis. *Archives of Dermatology*. 1994;130(11):1402–7.
71. Basketter DA, Miettinen J, Lahti A. Acute irritant reactivity to sodium lauryl sulfate in atopics and nonatopics. *Contact Dermatitis*. 1998;38(5):253–7.
72. Loffler H, Effendy I. Skin susceptibility of atopic individuals. *Contact Dermatitis*. 1999;40(5):239–42.
73. Sahlin A, Edlund F, Loden M. A double-blind and controlled study on the influence of the vehicle on the skin susceptibility to stinging from lactic acid. *International Journal of Cosmetic Science*. 2007;29(5):385–90.

2

Sensitive Skin: A Review of Prevalence Worldwide

Charles Taïeb and Laurent Misery

Sensitive skin is very common. Several epidemiological studies have been conducted and published during the past decade, and some previously. To fulfill the objective of consistency, we chose to compare only publications that cover 14 countries throughout the world (Belgium, France, Germany, Greece, Italy, Portugal, Spain, Switzerland, United States, Brazil, India, Korea, Japan, and Russia) (1–8) and that were carried out with the same methodology. These 14 countries have a population that exceeds 2.4 billion individuals, including 1.8 billion people of 15 years and more.

We have also added the results of an evaluation of sensitive skin in China (9) that was performed with the same methodology but with a different recruitment of samples. Including China, we go beyond three billion individuals!

In all studies (1–9), Consumer Science & Analytics (CSA) Santé (CSA Health Institute) performed surveys on samples of the population aged 15 years and older that were representative according to the quota method (gender, age, occupation of household head, type of geographical area, and region) (10).

This approach guaranteed the representativeness of the population of each country and allowed the inclusion of all people, without ignoring those who rarely meet dermatologists (such as elderly people, men, and poor people). Except in China, where a community-based study was undertaken in three major cities in China, Beijing, Shanghai, and Guangzhou, the participants in the study were screened by cluster sampling, and were investigated by interview at their own homes.

A systematic check of the interviews was performed by calling back 20% of the interviewees. If this procedure had revealed an abnormal finding in a single questionnaire, all the interviews conducted by the interviewer concerned would be checked. No such abnormal finding was observed.

The first part of the questionnaire was related to demographics (geographical area, age, gender, and social status) and to skin type. The second part addressed facial skin sensitivity. The subjects were requested to rate their skin as "very sensitive," "sensitive," "slightly sensitive," or "not sensitive." The interviewees responded to an open question regarding their perception of the onset of tingling, burning, or irritation in the presence of different factors, such as emotional stimuli, cold, heat, sun exposure, cosmetics, dry air, air-conditioning, water, air pollution, and variations in temperature. The participants were also asked if they had ever suffered from rashes without an apparent cause, if their facial skin was easily irritated, if they had visited a dermatologist during the previous year, and whether they had any skin diseases.

The relatively low rate of nonresponse to the question, "Do you have sensitive skin?" in all countries (less than 1.5% except in Russia and Brazil, which have a nonresponse rate of nearly 10%) suggests that the term *sensitive skin* makes sense for a very large number of individuals whatever their country of residence is.

To characterize sensitive skin in the population, the characteristics of the subjects with sensitive or very sensitive skin (the "sensitive skin" group) were compared with those of the subjects with "not very sensitive" or "not sensitive at all" skin ("nonsensitive skin" group).

The worldwide prevalence of sensitive skin is close to 40% (36.9%).

A global approach might be defined according to four continents: Europe, North America, South America, and Asia; the prevalences were respectively 41%, 33.7%, 44.6%, and 34.2% for Europe, Asia, North America, and South America.

The sensitive skin group might be divided into the "very sensitive skin" and "relatively or rather sensitive skin" groups. People reporting slightly sensitive skin were considered the same as people without sensitive skin.

Table 2.1 details the distributions for each continent between these four categories.

If we focus more precisely on countries, very sensitive skins were declared by 8.6% of people worldwide, from 6.3% in India to 17.7% in Italy. In six countries (India, Japan, Greece, United States, Russia, and Brazil), less than 10% of individuals declared that they suffered from very sensitive skin. A prevalence of very sensitive skin expressed by more than 15% of the population was found in two countries (Germany and Italy).

No sensitive skin was declared by 26.8% of the interviewed people, from 9.4% in Italy to 41% in Germany. In five countries (Japan, Italy, Korea, Switzerland, and Germany), less than 10% of individuals reported that they did not have sensitive skin. In three countries (India, Brazil, and Belgium), more than 30% of individuals 15 years and older said that they do not have sensitive skin.

Table 2.2 describes these results in detail.

Sensitive skin is thought to be a feminine problem. All studies show that it is more frequent in women, but many men also have sensitive skins (Tables 2.3 through 2.5).

Concerning China, a community-based study was undertaken in three major cities in China—Beijing, Shanghai, and Guangzhou—from November 2009 to January 2010. A total of 9154 questionnaires were completed (3931 men and 5223 women). The mean prevalence of very sensitive and sensitive skins in the three cities was 13% (17.12% in Beijing, 9.10% in Shanghai, and 22.39% in Guangzhou). The mean prevalence was 8.62% in men and 15.93% in women, with significant difference between men and women in three selected cities ($P < .001$). The total prevalence of very sensitive and sensitive skins was 16.44%

TABLE 2.1

Prevalence of Sensitive Skin by Continent

	Europe (%)	North America (%)	South America (%)	Asia (%)
Very sensitive	13.1	9.3	9.9	6.8
Rather sensitive	27.9	35.3	24.3	26.8
Slightly sensitive	35.6	34.7	32.6	37.2
Not sensitive	23.4	20.7	33.2	28.9

TABLE 2.2

Prevalence of Sensitive Skin by Country

	Very Sensitive (%)	Sensitive (%)	Slightly Sensitive (%)	Not Sensitive (%)
Belgium	10.46	16.53	33.26	39.75
Brazil	9.93	24.30	32.55	33.24
France	12.00	40.10	28.70	19.20
Germany	16.23	19.44	23.25	41.08
Greece	8.83	21.77	39.43	29.98
India	6.30	23.70	37.10	32.80
Italy	17.65	36.92	35.90	9.53
Japan	8.47	46.00	40.13	5.40
Korea	14.20	42.60	32.60	9.60
Portugal	14.03	13.43	56.51	16.03
Russia	10.35	29.37	38.18	22.10
Spain	12.65	19.08	54.82	13.45
Switzerland	12.75	18.42	28.74	40.08
United States	9.26	35.31	34.71	20.72

TABLE 2.3

Prevalence of Sensitive Skin by Continent in Men

	Europe (%)	North America (%)	South America (%)	Asia (%)
Sensitive	32.4	38.0	22.5	30.0
Not sensitive	67.6	62.0	77.5	70.0

TABLE 2.4

Prevalence of Sensitive Skin by Continent in Women

	Europe (%)	North America (%)	South America (%)	Asia (%)
Sensitive	48.2	50.9	45.9	37.3
Not sensitive	51.8	49.1	54.1	62.7

TABLE 2.5

Prevalence of Sensitive Skin according to Sex

	Men (%)	Women (%)	Global (%)
Belgium	22.2	31.2	26.9
Brazil	22.5	45.9	34.5
France	44.1	59.4	52.0
Germany	27.5	43.5	35.7
Greece	23.0	37.7	30.5
India	26.2	33.7	29.9
Italy	51.5	57.5	54.6
Japan	52.9	56.0	54.5
Korea	54.4	59.2	56.8
Portugal	28.5	26.5	27.5
Russia	25.4	50.1	38.9
Spain	27.9	35.4	31.7
Switzerland	22.5	38.8	30.8
United States	38.0	50.9	44.6

in the <25 years group, 14.14% in the 25–49 years group, and 9.73% in the ≥50 years group. Moreover, 18.54% of participants claimed to have dry skin, 16.70% claimed to have greasy skin, and 8.04% with normal skin claimed to have the symptoms of sensitive skin.

We can see that the prevalence data of sensitive skin in the three cities of China are much lower than those in Europe and the United States. There was significant difference in the prevalence of sensitive skin among the three cities, which are located in different climatic and latitude regions, and between men and women. The prevalence gradually decreased with increasing age.

From these studies, we can conclude that there are differences between countries. However, there is consistency among the data:

- Sensitive skin is very common.
- The prevalence of sensitive skin is higher in women than in men.
- Skin sensitivity occurs in people with or without any skin disease, but it is more common in individuals with a history of atopic dermatitis or other skin diseases.

Some other studies performed by other methodologies confirm these data. To our knowledge, the first one was conducted in England (11). Because several studies were performed in the United States, this allows some comparisons. Hence, the comparison of four studies (with different methodologies) suggests that the frequency of sensitive skin might increase (12).

REFERENCES

1. Misery L, Myon E, Martin N, Verrière F, Nocera T, Taïeb C. Sensitive skin in France: An epidemiological approach. *Ann Dermatol Venereol.* 2005; 132: 425–9.
2. Misery L, Boussetta S, Nocera T, Perez-Cullell N, Taïeb C. Sensitive skin in Europe. *J Eur Acad Dermatol Venereol.* 2009; 23: 376–81.
3. Misery L, Myon E, Martin N et al. Sensitive skin: Psychological effects and seasonal changes. *J Eur Acad Dermatol Venereol.* 2007; 21: 620–6.
4. Misery L, Sibaud V, Taïeb C. Sensitive skin in the American population: Prevalence, clinical data and role of the dermatologist. *Int J Dermatol* 2011; 50: 961–7.
5. Kamide R, Misery L, Perez-Cullell N, Sibaud V, Taïeb C. Sensitive skin evaluation in the Japanese population. *J Dermatol* 2013; 40: 177–81.
6. Taïeb C, Auges M, Georgescu V, Perez-Cullell N, Misery L. Sensitive skin in Brazil and Russia: An epidemiological and comparative approach. *Eur J Dermatol* 2014; 24: 372–6.
7. Brenaut E, Misery L, Taïeb C, Sheth R. Sensitive skin in India: An epidemiological and comparative approach. In press.
8. Misery L, Taïeb C. *Sensitive Skin in Korea: An Epidemiological and Comparative Approach.* San Francisco: American Academy of Dermatology. 2015.
9. Xu F, Yan S, Wu M, Li F, Sun Q, Lai W, Shen X, Rahhali N, Taïeb C, Xu J. Self-declared sensitive skin in China: A community-based study in three top metropolises. *J Eur Acad Dermatol Venereol.* 2013; 27: 370–5.
10. Hansen MH, Hurwitz WN, Madow WG. *Sample Survey Methods and Theory, Volume 1: Methods and Applications.* New York: Wiley. 1993.
11. Willis CM, Shaw S, de Lacharrière O, Baverel M, Reiche L, Jourdain R, Bastien P, Wilkinson JD. Sensitive skin: An epidemiological approach. *Br J Dermatol.* 2001; 145: 258–63.
12. Farage MA, Miller KW, Wippel AM, Berardesca E, Misery L, Maibach H. Sensitive skin in the United States: Surveys of regional differences. *Family Med Medical Sci Res* 2013; 2: 112.

3

Skin Structure and Function

Golara Honari

Introduction

Skin as one of the largest organs in the body has multiple key features required for interacting dynamically with the environment. Its primary functions include a barrier function against environmental hazards such as ultraviolet (UV) radiation, chemical and physical insults, and microorganisms. Skin also prevents dehydration, regulates temperature, and has self-healing properties. Dynamic and complex arrangement of a variety of cells; element of the extracellular matrix; and vascular, appendageal, and nervous structures each play a role. Knowledge of skin penetration pathways is essential in the assessment of chemical safety, drug delivery systems, and formulation of cosmetic products. At the same time, understanding of the somatosensory system and its interactions with environmental and endogenous factors is essential in the evaluation of individuals with sensitive skin, who experience unpleasant sensations of stinging, burning, and prickling with subtle environmental assaults.

This chapter overviews the essential structural elements of the skin and their key functions relevant to skin absorption pathways and sensations and somatosensory systems, which are discussed in detail in the following sections.

Structure and Function

Normal skin consists of three main layers: epidermis, dermis, and hypodermis.

- Epidermis: The epidermis provides barrier function, innate immunity, and UV protection.
- Dermis: The dermis, the largest component of the skin, is an integrated system of fibrous cellular and acellular matrix. Many cell types reside in the dermis including fibroblasts, macrophages, and mast cells. Vascular, lymphatic, and nervous networks are present in the dermis.
- Hypodermis (subcutis): The hypodermis (subcutis) provides mechanical and physiologic support and contains a larger source of vessels and nerves.

There are regional variations in the skin thickness and presence of different appendages such as hair, sebaceous glands, and sweat glands, which can affect the functional properties of the skin. For example, hair-bearing skin is typically thinner and more permeable than non-hair-bearing skin of the palms and soles.

Epidermis

The epidermis is the outermost layer of the skin and is about 0.05–1 mm in thickness depending on body part. Three main populations of cells reside in the epidermis: keratinocytes, melanocytes, and Langerhans cells. Keratinocytes are the predominant cells in the epidermis, which are constantly

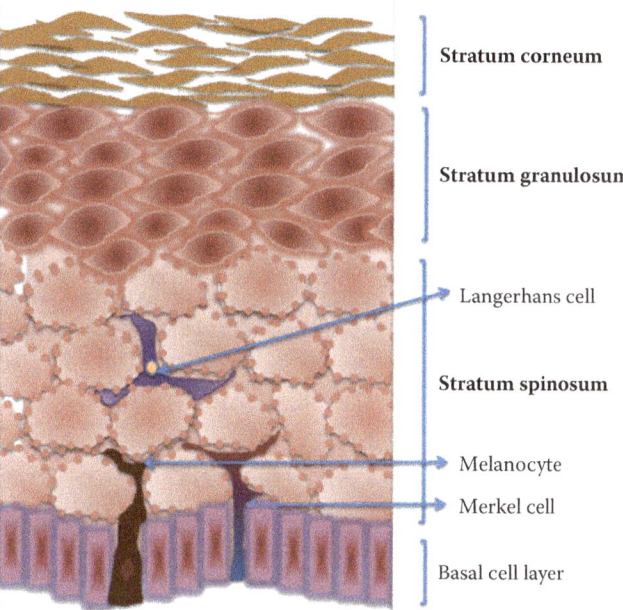

Stratum corneum

Stratum granulosum

Langerhans cell

Stratum spinosum

Melanocyte

Merkel cell

Basal cell layer

FIGURE 3.1 Schematic of epidermis. The basal cell layer is the deepest layer of the epidermis differentiating to spinous cells then to granular cells and eventually terminally differentiating to stratum corneum.

generated in the basal lamina and go through maturation, differentiation, and migration to the surface. As keratinocytes differentiate, they form three layers above the basal layer known as stratum spinosum, stratum granulosum, and stratum corneum (SC) (Figure 3.1). The keratinocyte transit time from the basal layer up to the SC is about 14 days (1), and the turnover time within the SC is also around 14 days (2); certain inflammatory conditions can affect these turnover times.

The SC is the outer layer of the epidermis and serves as the main functional barrier. A theoretical model is a *brick-and-mortar*-like structure where bricks represent terminally differentiated nonviable keratinocytes, also known as *corneocytes*, embedded in intercellular lipid membranes (3). As corneodesmosomes (protein bridges between corneocytes) degrade, lacunar spaces are created within the SC referred to as an aqueous *pore* pathway. These spaces can extend and form continuous networks, creating a pathway for penetration across the SC (4).

The major components of the SC lipid membranes are free fatty acids, ceramides, and esterols (5). Melanocytes are neural crest-derived, pigment-synthesizing dendritic cells that reside primarily in the basal layer. Merkel cells are mechanosensory receptors also present in the basal layer. Langerhans cells are dendritic antigen-processing and antigen-presenting cells in the epidermis (6). They form 2–8% of the total epidermal cell population, mostly found in a suprabasal position. The dermal–epidermal junction (DEJ) is a basement membrane zone that forms the interface between the epidermis and the dermis. The major functions of the DEJ are to attach the epidermis and dermis to each other and to provide resistance against external shearing forces.

Dermis

The dermis is an integrated system of fibrous cellular and acellular matrices that accommodates nervous and vascular structures as well as epidermally derived appendages. Many cell types reside in the dermis including fibroblasts, macrophages, mast cells, and circulating immune cells. The dermis is responsible for skin elasticity, pliability, and tensile strength. It provides protection against mechanical injury, retains water, and aids in thermal regulation. It also contains and supports receptors of sensory stimuli and is a key element in wound healing (7).

Hypodermis

The hypodermis is primarily composed of adipose tissue, which insulates the body and serves as a reserve energy supply. It cushions and protects the skin and supports nerves, vessels, and lymphatics located within the septa, supplying the overlying region.

Skin Appendages

Skin appendages include nails, hair, sebaceous glands, eccrine (sweat) glands, and apocrine glands. They have two distinct components: superficial and deeper components in the dermis, which are downgrowths of the epidermis. The dermal component regulates differentiation of the appendage. During embryonic development, dermal–epidermal interactions are critical for the induction and differentiation of these structures.

Skin as a Route of Entry

The SC is 3–20 μm in thickness, composed of 15–25 layers of corneocytes. It provides an effective barrier against transcutaneous water loss and entry of exogenous materials.

Extracellular lipids contribute to the barrier function and the route taken through the SC by all molecules. Arrangement of extracellular lipids, their hydrophobicity, their composition, and distribution of key components (ceramides, cholesterol, and free fatty acids) provide more barrier function (8). Skin absorption varies between different body parts and between individuals; these regional intra- and interindividual variations are partly related to variations in lipid composition and SC thickness (8). A range of biological factors can influence the rate and extent of percutaneous penetration including the anatomical site, age, appendageal density, SC morphology, and composition. Routes through which chemicals can cross the SC (Figure 3.2) include the following (9):

- Intercellular (or extracellular), in which chemicals pass exclusively through the lipid matrix
- Intracellular or transcellular, in which chemicals pass both through the lipid matrix and through the corneocytes themselves

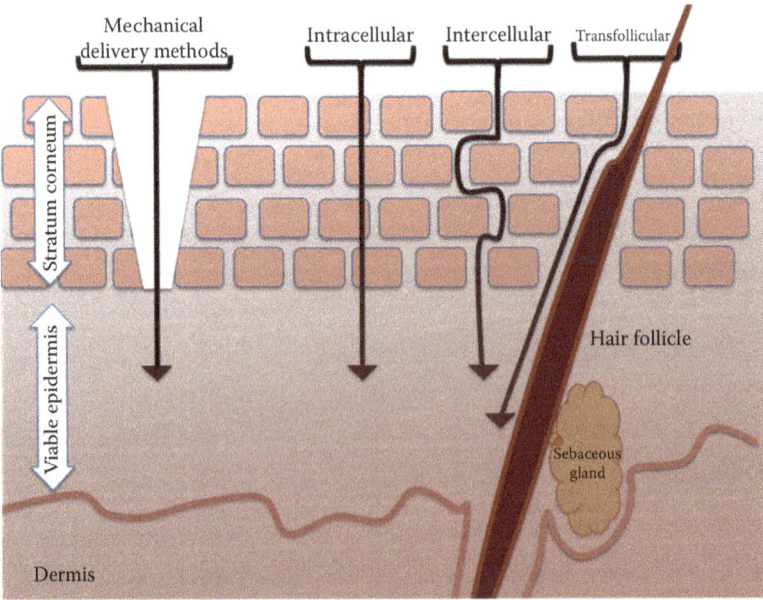

FIGURE 3.2   Schematic pathways of penetration into the skin with arrangement of corneocytes in a brick-and-mortar model.

- Through skin appendages
- Mechanical methods to remove SC such as stripping, ablation, and microneedles

In vivo measurement of skin absorption to quantify and rate the extent of absorption is of fundamental importance in the risk assessment of compounds that are active via the dermal route of entry, although the details are beyond the scope of this chapter. The skin as part of the somatosensory system is reviewed in the following chapter.

Measuring the Skin

Measuring the physical characteristics of the skin using biophysical instruments provides key information about various skin parameters. Many noninvasive techniques and equipment are available with increasing applications within dermatotoxicology, allowing the study of the skin in real time and providing objective, quantitative data, which can also be used in the evaluation of individuals affected by sensitive skin.

Parameters measured with these techniques provide information about a particular aspect of the skin. Using multiple parameters measured simultaneously, along with clinical assessment, provides more of a comprehensive analysis. Histological studies may be used to complement these analyses. Few parameters and techniques are briefly introduced in this chapter, and additional texts are available for comprehensive study (10,11). Raman spectroscopy is discussed in detail later in the book.

Skin Surface pH

Skin pH is normally acidic, ranging in pH values of 4–6, while the pH in the internal environment of the body is near neutral, ranging from 7 to 9 (12). The term *acid mantle* refers to the inherent acidic nature of the SC. Skin pH affects barrier function and SC cohesion. The elevation of pH in the normal skin creates a disturbed barrier (13). Measurement of skin surface pH is used to assess the acidity of the surface of the skin, which can vary according to the time of the day, the skin site, and between individuals. There are several instruments available for the measurement of skin pH; basically, any standard, portable pH meter with a planar electrode should suffice.

Sebum

Sebum is a light yellow viscous fluid, composed of triglycerides, free fatty acids, squalene, wax and sterol esters, and free sterols. Sebum is produced by sebaceous glands and contributes to moisture balance in the SC. Sebum production is mainly influenced by androgens and varies among individuals and races, but its average rate in adults is approximately $1 \text{ mg}/10 \text{ cm}^2$ every 3 hours (14). Sebum production less than $0.5 \text{ mg}/10 \text{ cm}^2$ every 3 hours is associated with dry skin, and values of $1.5–4.0 \text{ mg}/10 \text{ cm}^2$ every 3 hours are associated with seborrhea (15). Sebum can be measured using a gravimetric or a variety of photometric techniques.

Methods used in the past for the measurement of skin lipids included skin swabbing by absorbing pads followed by soaking them in solvents or by weighing the absorptive tapes (gravimetric analysis) (16). Also, photometric analyses such as *grease-spot* photometry and UV-visible spectrophotometry are used. Photometric techniques can provide additional information, such as droplet size and distribution (8). Multiple commercially available devices can provide quantitative measures of sebum secretion.

Desquamation

Loss of superficial SC is a natural process called *desquamation*, which can be affected in certain diseases. Desquamation is used to assess the structure and biological dynamics of SC and to investigate the effect of drugs and topical products on the skin. Techniques for desquamation measurement usually involve stripping the surface layers for analysis or visual assessment through skin imaging.

Squamometry involves stripping of corneocytes from the surface of the SC using adhesive disks followed by staining with toluidine blue-basic fuchsin ethanol-based solution and reading the colorimetric variable (17). Image analysis systems are also used to assess desquamation (18–20). These techniques are rapid, reliable, and sensitive.

Thickness

Epidermal and SC thickness can be measured in vivo using noninvasive methods such as ultrasound-based devices, confocal microscopy, and spectroscopic techniques (21–25). These measurements have investigative and clinical applications.

The Measurement of Transepidermal Water Loss

Transepidermal water loss (TEWL) is the amount of water that passively evaporates through the skin to the external environment due to water vapor pressure gradient on both sides of the skin barrier and is used to characterize skin barrier function. The average TEWL in humans is about 300–400 mL/day; however, it can be affected by environmental and intrinsic factors. In high humidity, the amount of water loss will decrease due to the drop in the water vapor pressure gradient. TEWL varies in different anatomic sites and is inversely related to the corneocyte size. Skin sites with smaller corneocytes have higher TEWL values (26–28). Multiple instruments are commercially available to measure TEWL, providing valuable data with applications in clinical settings, toxicology, and product development. TEWL is a sensitive indicator of skin irritation and is widely used in objective analysis of irritancy potential or protective properties of topical products. The accuracy of TEWL measurements can be influenced by environmental factors such as humidity, temperature, and ventilation and intrinsic factors. It is essential that these measurements be conducted under standard conditions (29).

Hydration Measurement

The water content of SC in normal conditions is estimated to be around 5–10% in the outer layer and about 30% near the viable epidermis (30). The water contents of the skin influence its physical properties, viscoelastic characteristics, and functional properties such as drug penetration and barrier function. In disease states such as atopic dermatitis, SC cannot properly stay hydrated. Hydration status of SC is considered a measure of toxicity. Hydration measurements are extensively used in the assessment of topical product safety and efficacy.

Various methods have been introduced to indirectly measure hydration. One method uses electrical properties of the skin such as capacitance, impedance, resistance, and conductance to calculate hydration levels (31). Another method measures transient thermal transfer by using a probe to transfer a constant generated thermal pulse to the epidermis, while it simultaneously obtains high-precision measurements of skin temperature. The water content of SC is calculated based on the changes detected in the temperature (32). The third technique, nuclear magnetic resonance (NMR) spectroscopy, directly measures the total water content of the epidermis and the outer dermis, using magnetic fields (33). NMR provides direct measurements and is considered a reference technique for skin hydration studies. However, all the available techniques can complement each other (34).

Measurement of Vascular Perfusion

Skin microcirculation and perfusion can be affected by a number of exogenous and endogenous factors. Changes in cutaneous vascular perfusion may reflect a physiologic response such as thermoregulation or a pathologic response such as inflammation caused by exposure to chemical irritants and concomitant release of inflammatory mediators. Also, exposure to topical vasoactive drugs can affect skin circulation. Laser Doppler instruments measure the Doppler shift induced by the laser light that is being scattered by moving red blood cells. A signal is quantified based on the average red blood cell concentration and velocity. Since this measure is not an exact measure, it is referred to as *flux*, which has a linear relationship with the actual flow (35–37). Two distinct laser Doppler tools are used: the first is the laser Doppler flowmetry (LDF), which has a small probe touching the skin, measuring blood flow over a small volume (1 mm^3 or smaller), and the second method is laser Doppler imaging (LDI), in which the laser beam is emitted at a certain distance above the skin surface and reflected by a computer-driven mirror to scan an area of the skin. LDI provides two-dimensional images mapping the perfusion but is a slow method. Quantifying fast changes in blood flow is easier with LDF compared to LDI (35).

Laser speckle contrast imaging (LSCI) is a noncontact imaging technique that provides information on skin perfusion over large areas (up to 100 cm^2) with a high frequency (up to 100 images per second). These images are obtained based on the generation of a high-contrast grainy pattern when a laser hits a matte surface. This pattern is called the *speckled pattern*, which fluctuates when objects move. The images created by LSCI reflect fast changes in skin blood flux over wide skin areas (35,38).

These techniques along with the other methods briefly mentioned in this chapter are among the many tools used to assess skin parameters and to provide objective measures for investigators and clinicians. Many bioengineering methods are subject to operational guidelines and have limitations. Data obtained from various methods can complement each other.

REFERENCES

1. Weinstein G, Van Scott E. Autoradiographic analysis of turnover times of normal and psoriatic epidermis. *J Invest Dermatol*. 1965;45(4):257–262.
2. Bergstresser P, Taylor J. Epidermal "turnover time"—A new examination. *Br J Dermatol*. 1977;96(5): 503–509.
3. Michaels AS, Chandrasekaran SK, Shaw JE. Drug permeation through human skin: Theory and in vitro experimental measurements. *AICHE J*. 1975;21(5):985–996.
4. Menon GK, Elias PM. Morphologic basis for a pore-pathway in mammalian stratum corneum. *Skin Pharmacol*. 1997;10(5–6):235–246.
5. Lee D, Ashcraft JN, Verploegen E, Pashkovski E, Weitz DA. Permeability of model stratum corneum lipid membrane measured using quartz crystal microbalance. *Langmuir*. 2009;25(10):5762–5766.
6. Mutyambizi K, Berger CL, Edelson RL. The balance between immunity and tolerance: The role of Langerhans cells. *Cell Mol Life Sci*. 2009;66(5):831–840.
7. Chu DH. Chapter 7. Development and structure of skin. In: Goldsmith LA, Katz SI, Gilchrest BA, Paller AS, Leffell DJ, Wolff K., eds. *Fitzpatrick's Dermatology in General Medicine*. 8th ed. New York: McGraw-Hill; 2012.
8. Elias PM. The epidermal permeability barrier: From the early days at Harvard to emerging concepts. *J Invest Dermatol*. 2004;122(2):xxxvi–xxxix.
9. Prausnitz MR, Mitragotri S, Langer R. Current status and future potential of transdermal drug delivery. *Nat Rev Drug Discov*. 2004;3(2):115–124.
10. Fluhr WJ, Elsner P, Berardesca E, Maibach HI. *Bioengineering of the Skin: Water and the Stratum Corneum, 2nd Edition (Dermatology: Clinical & Basic Science)*. 2nd ed. Boca Raton, FL: CRC Press; 2004.
11. Agache P, Humbert P. *Measuring the Skin*. Heidelberg: Springer; 2004.
12. Ali SM, Yosipovitch G. Skin pH: From basic science to basic skin care. *Acta Derm Venereol*. 2013; 93(3):261–267.
13. Hachem JP, Crumrine D, Fluhr J, Brown BE, Feingold KR, Elias PM. pH directly regulates epidermal permeability barrier homeostasis, and stratum corneum integrity/cohesion. *J Invest Dermatol*. 2003;121(2):345–353.
14. Plewig G, Kligman A. *Acne and Rosacea*. Berlin: Springer; 2000.
15. Bolognia JL, Jorizzo JL, Schaffer JV. *Dermatology*. 3rd ed. China: Elsevier; 2012.
16. Pande SY, Misri R. Sebumeter. *Indian J Dermatol Venereol Leprol*. 2005;71(6):444–446.
17. Pierard-Franchimont C, Henry F, Pierard GE. The SACD method and the XLRS squamometry tests revisited. *Int J Cosmet Sci*. 2000;22(6):437–446.
18. Black D, Boyer J, Lagarde JM. Image analysis of skin scaling using D-Squame samplers: Comparison with clinical scoring and use for assessing moisturizer efficacy. *Int J Cosmet Sci*. 2006;28(1):35–44.

19. Wilhelm KP, Kaspar K, Schumann F, Articus K. Development and validation of a semiautomatic image analysis system for measuring skin desquamation with D-Squames. *Skin Res Technol.* 2002;8(2):98–105.

20. Xhauflaire-Uhoda E, Loussouarn G, Haubrechts C, Leger DS, Pierard GE. Skin capacitance imaging and corneosurfametry: A comparative assessment of the impact of surfactants on stratum corneum. *Contact Dermatitis.* 2006;54(5):249–253.

21. El Gammal S, El Gammal C, Kaspar K, Pieck C, Altmeyer P, Vogt M, Ermert H. Sonography of the skin at 100 MHz enables in vivo visualization of stratum corneum and viable epidermis in palmar skin and psoriatic plaques. *J Invest Dermatol.* 1999;113(5):821–829.

22. Kaspar K, Vogt M, Ermert H, Altmeyer P, El Gammal S. 100 MHz sonography in the visualization of the palmar stratum corneum after application of various creams and ointments. *Ultraschall Med.* 1999;20(3):110–114.

23. Corcuff P, Bertrand C, Leveque JL. Morphometry of human epidermis in vivo by real-time confocal microscopy. *Arch Dermatol Res.* 1993;285(8):475–481.

24. Caspers PJ, Lucassen GW, Carter EA, Bruining HA, Puppels GJ. In vivo confocal Raman microspectroscopy of the skin: Noninvasive determination of molecular concentration profiles. *J Invest Dermatol.* 2001;116(3):434–442.

25. Egawa M, Hirao T, Takahashi M. In vivo estimation of stratum corneum thickness from water concentration profiles obtained with Raman spectroscopy. *Acta Derm Venereol.* 2007;87(1):4–8.

26. Rougier A, Lotte C, Corcuff P, Maibach HI. Relationship between skin permeability and corneocyte size according to anatomic site, age and sex in man. *J Soc Cosmet Chem.* 1988;39(1):15–26.

27. Machado M, Salgado TM, Hadgraft J, Lane ME. The relationship between transepidermal water loss and skin permeability. *Int J Pharm.* 2010;384(1–2):73–77.

28. Hadgraft J, Lane ME. Transepidermal water loss and skin site: A hypothesis. *Int J Pharm.* 2009; 373(1–2):1–3.

29. Sotoodian B, Maibach HI. Noninvasive test methods for epidermal barrier function. *Clin Dermatol.* 2012;30(3):301–310.

30. Blank IH, Moloney J 3rd, Emslie AG, Simon I, Apt C. The diffusion of water across the stratum corneum as a function of its water content. *J Invest Dermatol.* 1984;82(2):188–194.

31. Berardesca E, Borroni G. Instrumental evaluation of cutaneous hydration. *Clin Dermatol.* 1995;13(4): 323–327.

32. Berardesca E, Fideli D, Borroni G, Rabbiosi G, Maibach H. In vivo hydration and water-retention capacity of stratum corneum in clinically uninvolved skin in atopic and psoriatic patients. *Acta Derm Venereol.* 1990;70(5):400–404.

33. Foreman MI. A proton magnetic resonance study of water in human stratum corneum. *Biochim Biophys Acta.* 1976;437(2):599–603.

34. Girard P, Beraud A, Sirvent A. Study of three complementary techniques for measuring cutaneous hydration in vivo in human subjects: NMR spectroscopy, transient thermal transfer and corneometry—Application to xerotic skin and cosmetics. *Skin Res Technol.* 2000;6(4):205–213.

35. Roustit M, Cracowski JL. Assessment of endothelial and neurovascular function in human skin microcirculation. *Trends Pharmacol Sci.* 2013;34(7):373–384.

36. Stern MD. In vivo evaluation of microcirculation by coherent light scattering. *Nature.* 1975; 254(5495):56–58.

37. Ahn H, Johansson K, Lundgren O, Nilsson GE. In vivo evaluation of signal processors for laser Doppler tissue flowmeters. *Med Biol Eng Comput.* 1987;25(2):207–211.

38. Briers JD. Laser Doppler, speckle and related techniques for blood perfusion mapping and imaging. *Physiol Meas.* 2001;22(4):R35–R66.

4

The Somatosensory System

Francis McGlone and David Reilly

Somatosensation

The primary sensory modality subserving the body senses is collectively described as the somatosensory system and comprises all the peripheral afferent nerve fibers and specialized receptors subserving proprioceptive (joint, muscle) and cutaneous sensitivity. The former processes information about limb position and muscle forces, which the central nervous system (CNS) uses to monitor and control limb movements and, via elegant feedback and feedforward mechanisms, ensures that a planned action or movement is executed fluently. This chapter will focus on sensory inputs arising from the skin surface—cutaneous sensibility—and describe the neurobiological processes that enable the skin to be *sensitive*. Skin sensations are multimodal and are classically described as subserving the three submodalities of touch, temperature, and pain. We will also consider the growing evidence for a fourth submodality, present only in hairy skin, that is preferentially activated by slowly moving, low-force, mechanical stimuli.

This brief introduction to somatosensation will start with the discriminative touch system. The component that is relayed via the spinal cord includes the entire body from the neck down; information from the face is relayed by cranial nerves, but both parts of this system share a common central organization. Sensation enters the periphery via sensory axons that have their cell bodies sitting just outside the spinal cord in the dorsal root ganglia, with one ganglion for each spinal nerve root. Neurons are the building blocks of the nervous system, and somatosensory neurons are unique in that, unlike most neurons, the electrical signal does not pass through the cell body, but the cell body sits off to one side, without dendrites, the signal passing directly from the distal axon process to the proximal process which enters the dorsal half of the spinal cord and immediately turns up the spinal cord forming a white matter column, the dorsal columns, which relay information to the first brain relay nucleus in the medulla. These axons are called the *primary afferents* because they are the same axons that carry the signal into the spinal cord. Sensory input from the face does not enter the spinal cord but instead enters the brainstem via the trigeminal nerve (one of the cranial nerves). Just as with inputs from the body, there are three modalities of touch, temperature, and pain, with each modality having different receptors traveling along different tracts projecting to different targets in the brainstem. Once the pathways synapse in the brainstem, they join the pathways from the body on their way up to the thalamus and higher cortical structures. Sensory information arising from the skin is represented in the brain in the primary and secondary somatosensory cortices, where the contralateral body surfaces are mapped in each hemisphere. In line with other sensory modalities, information is then fed forward to higher-order neural systems controlling perception, recognition, attention, and emotion, as well as systems that integrate this information with other sensory modalities, such as vision, to enable the brain to maximize the information that it receives from the senses about conditions in the external world.

The Peripheral Nervous System

The skin is the most extensive and versatile organ of the body, and in a fully grown adult, it covers a surface area approaching 2 m². This surface (despite the comment made by the UK comedian, Spike

Milligan: "Oh wonderful stuff is skin. It's the stuff that keeps you in!") is far more than just a passive barrier. Apart from its role in the etiology of *sensitive skin*, the topic of this book, the skin contains in excess of two million sweat glands and five million hairs that may be either fine vellus types covering all surfaces, apart from the soles of the feet and the palms of the hands (glabrous skin), or over 100,000 of the coarser type found on the scalp. Evidence is also emerging that nonglabrous skin contains a system of nerves that specifically code for the pleasant properties of touch. It consists of an outer, waterproof, stratified squamous epithelium of ectodermal origin—the epidermis—plus an inner, thicker, supporting layer of connective tissue of mesodermal origin—the dermis. The thickness of this layer, and thereby its susceptibility to irritation, varies from 0.5 mm over the eyelid to 5.0 mm over the palm and sole of the foot.

Touch

Most primate research into skin sensory processing has focused on the glabrous surface of the hand, in particular, the digits, and a description of this somatic site will provide a good general understanding of somatosensation (1–6). Of the three *classical* submodalities of the somatosensory system, discriminative touch subserves the perception of pressure, vibration, and texture and relies upon four different receptors in the digit skin—(1) Meissner's corpuscles, (2) Pacinian corpuscles, (3) Merkel's disks, and (4) Ruffini endings—collectively known as *low-threshold mechanoreceptors* (LTMs), a class of cutaneous receptors that are specialized to transduce mechanical forces impinging the skin into nerve impulses. The first two are classified as fast adapting (FA), as they only respond to the initial and final contacts of a mechanical stimulus on the skin, and the second two are classified as slowly adapting (SA), as they continue firing during a constant mechanical stimulus. A further classification relates to the receptive field (RF) of the LTMs, that is, the surface area of the skin to which they are sensitive. The RF is determined by the anatomical location of the LTMs within the skin with those near the surface at the dermal/epidermal boundary, Meissner's corpuscles, and Merkel's disks, having small RFs, and those lying deeper within the dermis, Pacinian corpuscles, and Ruffini endings, having large RFs.

Psychophysical procedures have been traditionally employed to study the sense of touch, and as in hearing research where the sensory receptor is another type of specialized mechanoreceptor, different frequencies of vibration are used to quantify the response properties of this sensory system. Von Bekesy (7) was the first to use vibratory stimuli as an extension of his research interests in audition. In a typical experiment, participants are asked to respond with a simple button press when they can just detect the presence of a vibration presented to a digit within one of the two time periods. This two-alternative forced choice paradigm provides a threshold-tuning curve, the slopes of which provide information about a particular class of the response properties of LTMs. As can be seen from Figure 4.1, a U-shaped function is generated, with

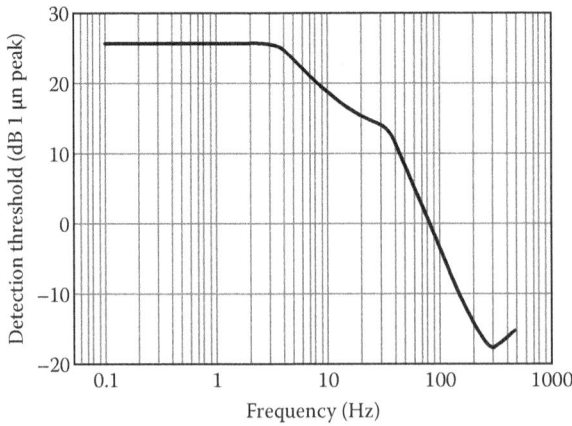

FIGURE 4.1   Absolute detection thresholds for sinusoidal stimuli, where it can be seen that as the vibration frequency increases, the detection thresholds decrease. (Reproduced from Bolanowski, S. J., Gescheider, G. A., Verrillo, R. T., and Checkosky, C. M., *J Acoustic Soc Am*, 84, 1680–1694, 1988, with the permission of the Acoustical Society of America.)

increasingly lower detection thresholds being measured as vibrotactile frequency increases to a *peak* at around 300 Hz, at which point the curve begins to increase again as sensitivity decreases.

By carefully controlling the spatial configuration of the vibrating probe (i.e., its diameter and the gap between it and a static surround), the vibratory frequency, the amplitude, the stimulus duration, the skin surface temperature, and the use of various masking techniques, Verrillo et al. (8,9–12) proposed that there are four distinct psychophysical channels mediating tactile perception in the glabrous skin of the hand. This model proposes that each psychophysically determined channel is represented by one of the four anatomical end organs and nerve fiber subtypes with frequencies in the 40–500 Hz range providing a sense of vibration, transmitted by Pacinian corpuscles (Pacinian corpuscle channel or fast-adapting I [FAI]), Meissner's corpuscles being responsible for the sense of *flutter* in the 2–40 Hz range (non-Pacinian I [NPI] channel or fast-adapting II [FAII]), the sense of *pressure* being mediated by Merkel's discs in the 0.4–2.0 Hz range (non-Pacinian III [NPIII] or slowly adapting I [SAI]), and Ruffini end organs producing a *buzzing* sensation in the 100–500 Hz range (non-Pacinian III [NPII] or slowly adapting II [SAII]). Neurophysiological studies have by and large supported this model, but there is still some way to go to link the anatomy with perception (see Table 4.1 for a summary of the properties of these LTMs).

There have been relatively few studies of tactile sensitivity on hairy skin, the cat being the animal of choice for most of these studies. Mechanoreceptive afferents (Aβ fibers) have been described that are analogous to those found in human glabrous skin (FAI, FAII, SAI, and SAII), and Essick and Edin (13) have described sensory fibers with these properties in human facial skin. The relationship between these sensory fibers and tactile perception is still uncertain, and this is exemplified by the response properties of SAI afferents. Harrington and Merzenich (14) found that these afferents are responsive to levels of stimulation that are below perceptual thresholds, and Jarvilehto et al. (15) describe high levels of activity in human hairy skin SAIs that are not perceivable, in contrast to the responses of this class of afferent in glabrous skin where SAI nerve activity is directly correlated with a sense of pressure.

Sensory axons are classified according to their degree of myelination, the fatty sheath that surrounds the nerve fiber. The degree of myelination determines the speed with which the axon can conduct nerve impulses and, hence, the conduction velocity (CV) of the nerves. The largest and fastest axons are called A-α and include some of the proprioceptive neurons, such as the muscle stretch receptors. The second largest group, called A-β, includes all the discriminative touch receptors being described here. Pain and temperature include the third and fourth groups, A-δ and C fibers, and will be dealt with in the section "Temperature" (Table 4.1).

Electrophysiological studies by Vallbo and Johansson (16), on single peripheral nerve fibers innervating the human hand, have provided a generally accepted model of touch that relates the four anatomically defined types of cutaneous or subcutaneous sense organs to their neural response patterns.

The technique that they employed and developed is called *microneurography* and involves inserting a fine tungsten microelectrode, with tip diameter of <5 μm, through the skin of the wrist and into the underlying median nerve which innervates the thumb and the first two digits. A sensitive biological

TABLE 4.1

Main Characteristics of Primary Sensory Afferents Innervating Human Skin

Class	Modality	Axonal Diameter (μm)	CV (m/s)
Myelinated			
A-α	Proprioceptors from muscles and tendons	20	120
A-β	LTMs	10	80
A-δ	Cold, noxious, thermal	2.5	12
Unmyelinated			
C-pain	Noxious, heat, thermal	1	<1
C-tactile	Light stroking, gentle touch	1	<1
C-autonomic	Autonomic, sweat glands, vasculature	1	<1

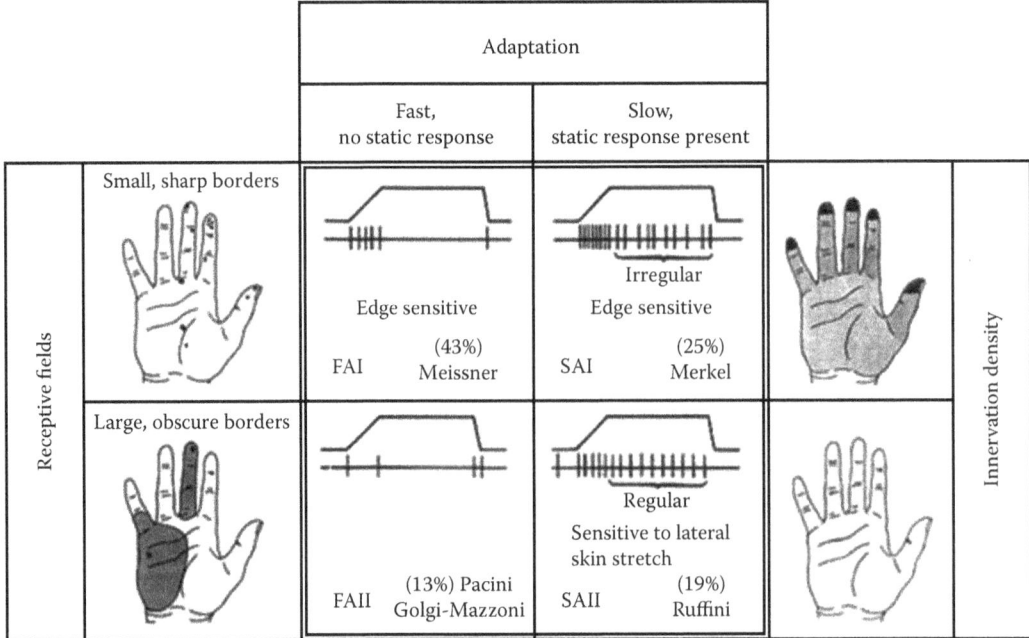

FIGURE 4.2   The four types of LTMs in human glabrous skin are depicted. The four panels in the center show the nerve-firing responses to a ramp-and-hold indentation, and in percentage, the frequency of occurrence and putative morphological correlate. The black dots in the left panel show the RFs of type 1 (*top*) and type 2 (*bottom*) afferents. The right panel shows the average density of type 1 (*top*) and type 2 (*bottom*) afferents with darker area depicting higher densities. Abbreviations: LTM: low-threshold mechanoreceptor; RF: receptive field. (After Westling, G. K., Sensori-Motor Mechanisms during Precision Grip in Man, Medical dissertation, Umea University, Sweden, 1986.)

amplifier records and amplifies the spike discharges conveyed by the axons and feeds these to a loud-speaker to enable the experimenter to hear the spike activity and *home-in* on a single unit. The skilled manual micromanipulation of the electrode, coupled with stroking across the hand to stimulate LTMs, first results in a population response being recorded, that is, neural activity in a nerve fascicle containing hundreds of peripheral axons until finally, sometimes after many hours, a single axon is isolated. At this stage, the RF of the single unit is mapped with a Von Frey hair and the unit subtype (i.e., FA or SA) identified. Once this stage is completed, a small pulsed current of a few microamperes (typically <10 μA) is delivered to the nerve that provides a final, perceptual confirmation of the unit subtype.

If, for example, an RA unit has been isolated, microstimulation is perceived as a *flutter* or *vibration*, depending on the frequency of the electrical pulses, and is perceptually localized to the previously mapped RF. Figure 4.2 depicts the relationships between RF, adaptation rate, and unit type from studies carried out on the human hand (17).

Temperature

The cutaneous somatosensory system detects changes in ambient temperature over an impressive range, initiated when thermal stimuli that differ from a homeostatic set point excite temperature-specific sensory nerves in the skin, and relays this information to the spinal cord and brain. It is important to recognize that these nerves code for temperature change, not absolute temperature, as a thermometer does. The system does not have specialized receptor end organs, such as those found in LTMs, but uses free nerve endings throughout the skin to sense changes in temperature. Within the innocuous thermal-sensing range, there are two populations of thermosensory fibers, one that responds to warmth (warm receptors) and one that responds to cold (cold receptors), and include fibers from the A-δ and C ranges. Specific cutaneous cold and warm receptors have been defined as slowly conducting units that exhibit a steady-state discharge at constant skin temperature and a dynamic response to temperature changes (18,19). Cold- and warm-specific receptors can be distinguished from nociptors that respond to noxious low and high temperatures (<20°C and >45°C) (20,21) and also from thermosensitive mechanoreceptors (18,22). Konietzny (22) recorded from 13 cold-specific units in humans employing the microneurography technique and measured CVs which were in the C fiber range (0.43–2.04 m/s).

Serra et al. (23) reported a number of spontaneously active fibers employing microneurography, which were sensitive to small temperature changes and that were described as cold-specific units, but all had CVs in the C fiber range (0.43–1.27 m/s). Standard medical textbooks describe the cutaneous cold sense in humans as being mediated by myelinated A fibers with CVs in the range of 12–30 m/s (24), but a work from Campero et al. (25) concludes that either human cold-specific afferent fibers are incompletely myelinated *BC* fibers, described by Duclaux et al. (26) as having electrophysiological and morphological properties of C fibers in their distal part and B fibers in their proximal part, or there are C as well as A cold fibers, with the C fiber group contributing little to sensation. For example, the resting discharge at room temperature (21°C) is characterized by a low-frequency discharge (~1 Hz), and this steady-state activity is suppressed by sudden warming of the RF and increased by cooling the RF.

The free nerve endings for cold- or warm-sensitive nerve fibers are located just beneath the skin surface. The terminals of an individual temperature-sensitive fiber do not branch profusely or widely. Rather, the endings of each fiber form a small, discretely sensitive point, which is separate from the sensitive points of neighboring fibers. The total area of the skin occupied by the receptor endings of a single temperature-sensitive nerve fiber is relatively small (1 mm in diameter) with the density of these thermosensitive points varying in different body regions. For example, there are up to 15–25 cold points per square centimeter in the lips, 3–5 cold points per square centimeter in the finger, and less than 1 cold point per square centimeter in some broad areas of the trunk. There are 3–10 times as many cold-sensitive points as warm-sensitive points in most areas of the body.

It is well established from physiological and psychological testing that warm- and cold-sensitive nerve fibers are distinctively different from one another in both structure and function.

Pain

Here, we consider a system of peripheral sensory nerves that innervate all cutaneous structures and whose sole purpose is to protect the skin against potential or actual damage. These primary afferents include A-δ and C fibers which respond selectively and linearly to the levels of thermal, mechanical, and chemical intensities/strengths that are tissue threatening, that is, having the potential to damage the skin. This initial encoding mechanism is termed *nociception* and describes the sensory process detecting any overt, or impending, tissue damage. The term *pain*, on the other hand, describes the perception of irritation, stinging, burning, soreness, or painful sensations arising from the skin.

It is important to recognize, especially when we are investigating an area such as sensitive skin, that the perception of pain depends not only on nociceptor inputs, but also on other processes and pathways giving information about, for example, emotional or contextual components. Pain is, therefore, described in terms of an *experience* rather than just a simple sensation. There are again submodalities within the nociceptive system which, at the peripheral anatomical level, are evident with respect to the degree of myelination of the nerve fibers (A-δ and C) subserving nociception (Table 4.2). A-δ fibers are thin (1–5 μm), poorly myelinated axons of mechanical nociceptors, thermal receptors, and mechanoreceptors with axon potential CVs averaging 12 m/s, and C fibers are very thin (<1 mm) slowly conducting axons (<1 m/s). Mechanical nociceptors are in the A-δ range and possess RFs distributed as 5–20 small sensitive spots over an area approximately 2–3 mm in diameter. In many cases, the activation of these spots depends upon stimuli intense enough to produce tissue damage, such as a pinprick. A-δ units with a short latency response to intense thermal stimulation in the range of 40–50°C have been described as well as other units excited by heat after a long latency—usually with thresholds in excess of 50°C. Over 50% of the unmyelinated axons (C fibers) of a peripheral nerve respond not only to intense mechanical stimulation, but also to heat and noxious chemicals, and are therefore classified as polymodal nociceptors (27) or C-mechanoheat (CMH) nociceptors (28). A subgroup of polymodal nociceptors has been reported to respond to extreme cold; however, many of these units develop an excitatory response to

TABLE 4.2

Major Findings by Bolanowski et al. (8) and Previous Work Done by These Researchers at the Institute
for Sensory Research at Syracuse University

Channel	Pacinian	NPI	NPII	NPIII
Frequency response (Hz)	40–80	3–100	15–400	<0.3 to >100
Threshold (at 1 μm)	<−20 dB at 300 Hz	28 dB at 3 Hz	10 dB at 300 Hz	28 dB at 3 Hz
Sensation	Vibration	Flutter	Not known	Pressure
Temporal summation	Yes	No	Yes	No
Spatial summation	Yes	No	Not known	No
Receptor type	FAI Pacinian corpuscle	FAII Meissner's corpuscle	SAII Ruffini end organ	SAI Merkel's disk

Source: Bolanowski, S. J., Gescheider, G. A., Verrillo, R. T., and Checkosky, C. M., *J Acoustic Soc Am*, 84, 1680–
1694, 1988; Gescheider, G. A., O'Malley, M. J., and Verrillo, R. T., *J Acoustic Soc Am*, 74, 474–485, 1983;
Gescheider, G. A., Sklar, B. F., Van Doren, C. L., and Verrillo, R. T., *J Acoust Soc Am*, 78, 534–543, 1985;
Gescheider, G. A., Verrillo, R. T., and Van Doren, C. L., *J Acoustic Soc Am*, 72, 1421–1426, 1982; Verrillo,
R. T., *J Acoustic Soc Am*, 35, 1962–1966, 1963.

cooling after prior exposure to noxious heat. A small number of C fibers have mechanical thresholds
in the nociceptor range with no response to heat, whereas others have been found to respond preferentially to noxious heating. RFs consist of single zones with distinct borders, and in this respect, they
differ from A-δ nociceptors that have multipoint fields. Innervation densities are high, and responses
have been reported to a number of irritant chemicals such as dilute acids, histamine, bradykinin, and
capsaicin. By employing microneurography, Schmidt et al. (29) described not only CMH-responsive
units, but also a novel class of C nociceptors responding only to mechanical stimuli (CM), units
responding only to heating (CH), and units that were insensitive to mechanical and heating stimuli and
also to sympathetic provocation tests (CMiCHi). Of relevance here is that some CM, CH, and CMiCHi
units were sensitized to thermal and/or mechanical stimuli after topical application of skin irritants
such as mustard oil or capsaicin; these units then acquired responsiveness to stimuli to which they
were previously unresponsive. The recruitment of these *silent nociceptors* implies spatial summation
to the nociceptive afferent barrage at central levels and may, therefore, contribute to primary hyperalgesia after chemical irritation and to secondary hyperalgesia as a consequence of central sensitization
(detailed subsequently).

Nociceptors do not show the kinds of adaptation response found with rapidly adapting LTMs (i.e.,
they fire continuously to tissue damage), but pain sensation may come and go, and pain may be felt in the
absence of any nociceptor discharge. They rely on chemical mediators around the nerve ending, which
are released from nerve terminals and skin cells in response to tissue damage. Koltenzenburg et al. (30)
showed that nerve growth factor (NGF) is an important mediator in painful inflammatory skin states,
with levels increasing in inflamed tissue. Following carrageenan inflammation of rodent skin, a marked
increase in the proportion of nociceptors which displayed an ongoing activity was observed, and this
was reflected in a significant increase in the average ongoing discharge activity. Spontaneously active C
fibers were sensitized to heat and displayed a more than twofold increase in their discharge to a standard
noxious heat stimulus. Furthermore, the number of nociceptors responding to the algesic mediator bradykinin increased significantly from 28% to 58%.

In contrast, the mechanical threshold of nociceptive afferents did not change during inflammation.
When the NGF-neutralizing molecule tropomyosin receptor kinase A (TrkA) immunoglobulin G (IgG)
was coadministered with carrageenan at the onset of the inflammation, primary afferent nociceptors
did not sensitize and displayed essentially normal response properties, although the inflammation as
evidenced by tissue edema developed normally, demonstrating that NGF is a crucial component for the
sensitization of primary afferent nociceptors associated with tissue inflammation.

The axon terminals of nociceptive axons possess no specialized end organ structure and, for that
reason, are referred to as *free nerve endings*. This absence of any encapsulation renders them sensitive
to chemical agents, both intrinsic and extrinsic, and inflammatory mediators released at a site of injury

can initiate or modulate activity in surrounding nociceptors over an area of several millimeters leading to two kinds of sensory responses termed *hyperalgesia*—the phenomenon of increased sensitivity of damaged areas to painful stimuli; primary hyperalgesia occurs within the damaged area, and secondary hyperalgesia occurs in undamaged tissues surrounding this area.

One further sensation mediated by afferent C fibers is that of itch, and this is dealt with in detail in Chapter 7.

Pleasure

It is generally accepted that human tactile sensibility is solely mediated by LTMs with fast-conducting large myelinated afferents (as described earlier). However, a growing body of evidence has been accumulating, from anatomical, psychophysical, electrophysiological, and neuroimaging studies, that a further submodality of afferent slowly conducting unmyelinated C fibers exists in human hairy skin that are neither nociceptive nor pruritic but that respond preferentially to low-force, slowly moving mechanical stimuli traversing across their RFs. These nerve fibers have been classified as C-tactile afferents (CT afferents) and were first described by Nordin in 1990 (31) in the face and previously by Johansson et al. (32) in the same region, employing the technique of microneurography.

Evidence of a more general distribution of CT afferents has subsequently been found in the arm and the leg, but never in glabrous skin sites such as the palms of the hands or the soles of the feet (33–35). It is well known that the mechanoreceptive innervation of the skin of many mammals is subserved by A- and C-afferents (27,36,37), but until the observations of Nordin and Vallbo, C-mechanoreceptive afferents in human skin appeared to be lacking entirely. The functional role of CT afferents is not fully known (38), but their neurophysiological response properties, fiber class, and slow CVs preclude their role in any rapid mechanical discriminative or cognitive tasks and point to a more limbic function, particularly the emotional aspects of tactile perception (39,40). However, the central neural identification of low-threshold C-mechanoreceptors, responding specifically to light touch, and the assignment of a functional role in human skin have been achieved. In a study on a unique patient lacking large myelinated A-β fibers, it was discovered that the activation of CT afferents produced a faint sensation of pleasant touch, and functional neuroimaging showed activation in the insular cortex but no activation in the primary sensory cortex identifying CT afferents as a system for limbic touch that might underlie emotional, hormonal, and affiliative responses to skin-to-skin contacts between individuals engaged in grooming and bonding behaviors—pleasant touch (41,42). If pain is elicited via sensory C- and A-δ fibers, then it is reasonable to speculate that the same system may be alternatively modulated to deliver a sensation of pleasure. One hypothesis is that pleasant touch stimulates opioid and cannabinoid receptors on these peripheral nerve fibers (both opioids and cannabinoids also have antinociceptive and anti-inflammatory activities) and that this signal is decoded in areas of the brain such as the insular cortex, which is associated with pleasure. Further evidence of the representation of pleasant touch in the brain has been provided by Francis et al. (43), where it was shown that discriminative and affective aspects of touch are processed in different brain areas. The activation of the primary somatosensory cortex was found in the physical aspects of stimulation, whereas the orbitofrontal cortex (an area of the frontal lobes involved in emotion) was activated by pleasant aspects. This area has also been shown to represent painful as well as pleasant touch, demonstrating the relevance of this brain region for representing the emotional dimensions of skin sensitivity—the positive and the negative (44).

Work is in progress to identify this class of C fibers anatomically and histologically, and a study employing the pan-neuronal marker PGP9.5 and confocal laser microscopy has identified a population of free nerve endings located solely within the epidermis that may represent the putative anatomical substrate for this submodality (45).

Sympathetic Nerves

Although this chapter deals with the sensory aspects of skin innervation, it is important to briefly review the role of a class of efferent (motor) nerves that innervate various skin structures: (a) blood vessels, (b) cutaneous glands, and (c) unstriated muscle in the skin, for example, the erectors of the hairs. In sensitive skin conditions and some painful neuropathic states, sympathetic nerves play a role in exacerbating inflammation and irritation. The efferent sympathetic fibers that leave the CNS in connection with certain cranial and spinal nerves and end in sympathetic ganglia are known as *preganglionic fibers*. From these ganglia, postganglionic fibers arise and conduct nerve impulses to the different organs in the skin such as the vasoconstrictor fibers to the blood vessels, the pilomotor fibers to the hairs, and the motor fibers to the sweat glands. Most of the postganglionic neurons utilize the organic chemical noradrenalin as their neurotransmitter, which is released at the effector synapse where the neuron ends. Noradrenaline and adrenaline stimulate two types of adrenergic receptors, namely α and β receptors. Adrenaline stimulates both α and β receptors almost equally, whereas noradrenaline acts more pronouncedly on the α receptors. The stimulation of the two different types can produce different results; for example, the stimulation of the α receptors on capillaries causes vasoconstriction, whereas the stimulation of the β receptors causes vasodilation. Most of the postganglionic neurons are adrenergic; however, those which serve the sweat glands are cholinergic in their action except those on the palms of the hands, which are adrenergic.

In some cases, the sympathetic nervous system has been purported to play an important role in sustaining pain in some theories, suggesting that pain receptors in the affected part of the body become responsive to a family of nervous system messengers known as *catecholamines*. Animal studies indicate that noradrenaline, released from sympathetic nerves, acquires the capacity to activate pain pathways after tissue or nerve injury. Complex regional pain syndrome is a chronic pain condition that is believed to be the result of dysfunction in the CNS or the peripheral nervous systems. Typical features include dramatic changes in the color and temperature of the skin over the affected limb or body part, accompanied by intense burning pain, skin sensitivity, sweating, and swelling.

Receptors and Channels

Signaling of stimuli such as heat, pain, or chemical challenge acting on nociceptors is peripherally controlled via a complex regulation of activity in a series of ion channels. A candidate receptor for chemosensory agents such as capsaicin and menthol eluded scientific characterization until 1997 and 2002, respectively (46,47). Developments in molecular cloning of receptor types (e.g., the vanilloid receptor and associated thermo-transient receptor potential [TRP] channels—a subset of TRP ion channels) combined with electrophysiological and receptor–ligand characterization have shed new light on the understanding of how noxious stimuli are encoded at the cellular level (48). The vanilloid receptor subtype 1 (VR1, also referred to as TRPV1) is a classical cation channel and is expressed in cutaneous sensory nerve fibers, mast cells, and epithelial cells of appendage structures (49). Interestingly, the activity for temperature (heat and cold) and pain and chemesthetic activity can all be explained in terms of the plasticity of a family of thermo-TRP cation channels (50). The development of transgenic mouse models lacking expression of the VR1 gene shows that phenotypic characteristics in VR1 null (−/−) mice support a functional role for VR1 in sensory transduction of nociceptive stimuli, although it was apparent that another unidentified receptor could partially compensate for the loss of VR1 function (51,52).

As an understanding of the process involved in sensing temperature and chemical stimulation of nociceptors has evolved, it has become apparent that there are additional non-TRP proteins and receptors which also play a role in nociception, for example, the acid-sensing ion channels and the P2X3 adenosine triphosphate receptor (53,54).

Opioids

The pain relief produced by opiates, such as morphine, derived from the opium poppy (*Papaver somniferum*), has been used and studied extensively for more than 5000 years. In addition to narcotic effects caused by activities within the CNS, opioids are also known for their antinociceptive and anti-inflammatory effects in the periphery. Coggeshall et al. (55) used light microscopic techniques to demonstrate the presence of μ- and δ-opioid receptors on ummyelinated afferents in human skin. In 2002, Stander et al. (56) showed a colocalization of μ-opioid receptor isoform 1A (MOR 1A) and calcitonin gene-related peptide in sensory fibers, suggesting a functional relationship for opiate agonists in terms of anti-inflammatory and antinociceptive activities. Opiates also cause vasodilatation of the skin, although this does not appear to account for a reduction in pain via a local warming mechanism; that is, the analgesic effect is clearly μ opioid receptor (MOR) mediated (57). The activity of opiates in the periphery does appear to be dependent on the extent of inflammation and local tissue damage, and this may account for many of the discrepancies reported by various authors (58–60).

A range of cell types, including neurons, keratinocytes, and immune cells, produces endogenous opioids. There are three families of peptides identified to date, each arising from alternate processing of the gene products for proopiomelanocortin (POMC), proencephalin, and prodynorphin. In the skin, the opioid, β-endorphin, is produced by posttranslational cleavage of the POMC gene and acts both on MORs on nerves and keratinocytes (61). The expression of MOR on keratinocytes and the involvement in the pathogenesis of clinical skin disease such as psoriasis suggest an additional role for opiates as immunoregulatory molecules in the skin (62).

Cannabinoids

Cannabis (*Cannabis sativa* L.), such as the opiates, has long been used for its narcotic effects. The discovery of specific cannabinoid receptors and endogenous ligands, produced in the periphery, has led to a new therapeutic potential as an analgesic and an anti-inflammatory molecule (63,64). To date, two G protein-coupled cannabinoid receptors, referred to as cannabinoid (CB) 1 and CB2, have been identified in both the CNS and the peripheral nervous systems (65,66). Differential localization using in situ hybridization and immunohistochemistry has shown the presence of CB receptors on both nociceptive and nonnociceptive afferents, in addition to staining on nonneuronal tissues, for example, keratinocytes and leukocytes (67,68).

Several studies have shown that both classical agonists, such as HU210, and endogenous cannabinoid (endocannabinoids) agonists, such as anandamide, have anti-inflammatory and antinociceptive benefits (69,70). The lipid metabolic pathways leading to production of endocannabinoids, their interactions with receptors, deactivation, and clearance pathways have been reviewed by Piomelli (71).

An interesting development in the understanding of the role of endocannabinoids in the skin has been the observation that they can also activate VR1. Anandamide has been shown to activate VR1 (72,73), and this may explain the ability of anandamide to act as a vasodilator, although there is still some controversy over the levels required to activate VR1 and its physiological relevance.

The Central Projections

The submodalities of skin sensory receptors and nerves that convey information to the brain about mechanical, thermal, and painful stimulations of the skin are grouped into three different pathways in the spinal cord and project to different target areas in the brain. They differ in their receptors, pathways, and targets and also in the level of decussation (crossing over) within the CNS. Most sensory systems en route to the cerebral cortex decussate at some point, as projections are mapped contralaterally. The discriminative touch system crosses in the medulla, where the spinal cord joins the brain; the pain system crosses at the point of entry into the spinal cord.

Spinal Cord

All the primary sensory neurons described earlier have their cell bodies situated outside the spinal cord in the dorsal root ganglion, there being one ganglion for every spinal nerve. Sensory neurons have a unique property in that, unlike most neurons, the nerve signal does not pass through the cell body but, as the cell body sits off to one side, the signal passes directly from the distal axon process to the proximal process, which enters the dorsal half of the spinal cord.

Tactile primary afferents, or first-order neurons, immediately turn up the spinal cord toward the brain, ascending in the dorsal white matter and forming the dorsal columns. In a cross section of the spinal cord at cervical levels, two separate tracts can be seen—the midline tracts comprise the gracile fasciculus conveying information from the lower half of the body (legs and trunk) and the outer tracts comprise the cuneate fasciculus conveying information from the upper half of the body (arms and trunk). At the medulla, situated at the top of the spinal cord, the primary tactile afferents make their first synapse with second-order neurons, where fibers from each tract synapse in a nucleus of the same name—the gracile fasciculus axons synapse in the gracile nucleus and the cuneate axons synapse in the cuneate nucleus. The neurons receiving the synapse provide the secondary afferents and immediately cross to form a new tract on the contralateral side of the brainstem—the medial lemniscus—which ascends through the brainstem to the next relay station in the midbrain, the thalamus.

As with the tactile system, pain, and thermal afferents, primary afferents synapse ipsilaterally and then the secondary afferents cross, but the crossings occur at different levels. Pain and temperature afferents enter the dorsal horn of the spinal cord and synapse within one or two segments, forming Lissauer's tract as they do so. The dorsal horn is a radially laminar structure; the thin outermost layer is called the *posterior marginalis layer*, the second layer is the substantia gelatinosa, and the layer deeper to that is the nucleus proprius. The two types of pain fibers, C and A-δ, enter different layers of the dorsal horn. A-δ fibers enter the posterior marginalis and the nucleus proprius and synapse on a second set of neurons. These are the secondary afferents which will relay the signal to the thalamus. The secondary afferents from both layers cross to the opposite side of the spinal cord and ascend in the spinothalamic tract. The C fibers enter the substantia gelatinosa and synapse, but they do not synapse on secondary afferents. Instead, they synapse on interneurons—neurons which do not project out of the immediate area but relay the signal to the secondary afferents in either the posterior marginalis or the nucleus proprius. The spinothalamic tract ascends the entire length of the cord and the entire brainstem and, by the time that it reaches the midbrain, appears to be continuous with the medial lemniscus. These tracts enter the thalamus together.

It is important to note that although the bulk of afferent input adheres to the plan outlined earlier, there is degree mixing that goes on between the tracts. Some light touch information, for example, travels in the spinothalamic tract with the result that the damage to the dorsal columns does not completely remove touch and pressure sensation. Some proprioception also travels in the dorsal columns and follows the medial lemniscus all the way to the cortex, so there is conscious awareness of body position and movement. The pain and temperature system also has multiple targets in the brainstem and other areas.

We have concentrated on somatosensory inputs from the body thus far, but as facial skin is often the source of sensitive reactions to topical applications, its peripheral and central anatomy/neurophysiology will be briefly summarized here. The trigeminal nerve innervates all facial skin structures (including the oral mucosa), and just as with the spinal afferents, these neurons have their cell bodies outside of the CNS in the trigeminal ganglion with their proximal processes entering the brainstem. Just as in the spinal cord, the three modalities of touch, temperature, and pain have different receptors in the facial skin, travel along different tracts, and have different targets in the brainstem—the trigeminal nucleus, a relatively large structure that extends from the midbrain to the medulla.

The large-diameter (A-β) fibers enter directly into the main sensory nucleus of the trigeminal and, as with the somatosensory neurons of the body, synapse and then decussate, the secondary afferents joining the medial lemniscus as it projects to the thalamus. The small-diameter fibers conveying pain and temperature enter the midbrain with the main fifth cranial nerve but then descend down the brainstem to the caudal medulla where they synapse and cross. These descending axons form a tract, the spinal tract of V, and synapse in the spinal nucleus of V, so called because it reaches as far down as the upper cervical spinal cord. The spinal nucleus of V comprises three regions along its length: the subnucleus oralis, the subnucleus interpolaris, and the subnucleus caudalis. The secondary afferents from the subnucleus caudalis cross to the opposite side and join the spinothalamic tract where the somatosensory information from the face joins that from the body, entering the thalamus in a separate nucleus, the ventroposterior medial (VPM) nucleus.

Brain

The third-order thalamocortical afferents (from thalamus to cortex) travel up through the internal capsule to reach the primary somatosensory cortex, located in the postcentral gyrus, a fold of cortex just posterior to the central sulcus. The thalamocortical afferents convey all the signals, whether from ventro-postero lateral or VPM to primary somatosensory cortex where the sensory information from all body surfaces is mapped in a somatotopic (body-mapped) manner (74,75), with the legs represented medially, at the top of the head, and the face represented laterally. Within the cortex, there are thought to be nine separate areas primarily subserving somatosensation: primary somatosensory cortex, SI, comprised four subregions (2, 1, 3a, and 3b); secondary somatosensory cortex, SII, located along the superior bank of the lateral sulcus (76–80); insular cortex (81); and the posterior parietal cortex, areas 5 and 7b.

As with studies of the peripheral nervous system, the technique of microneurography has also been employed to study the relationship between skin sensory nerves and their central projections, as evidenced by the use of concurrent functional magnetic resonance imaging (fMRI). The microstimulation of individual LTM afferents, projecting to RFs on the digit, produces robust, focal, and orderly (somatotopic) hemodynamic blood oxygen level-dependent responses in both primary and secondary somatosensory cortices (82), in accordance with the findings of Penfield and Boldrey (83). It is expected that this technique will permit the study of many different topics in somatosensory neurophysiology, such as sampling from FA and SA mechanoreceptors and C fibers with neighboring or overlapping RFs on the skin and quantifying their spatial and temporal profiles in response to electrical chemical and/or mechanical stimulation of the skin areas that they innervate, as well as perceptual responses to microstimulation.

Finally, the forward projections from these primary somatosensory areas to limbic and prefrontal structures have been studied with fMRI to understand the effective representations of skin stimulation for both pain and pleasure (43,84) and it is hoped that studies of this nature will help us to better understand the emotional aspects of both negative (sensitive skin) and positive (pleasant touch) skin sensations.

REFERENCES

1. Johansson RS. Receptive field sensitivity profile of mechanosensitive units innervating the glabrous skin of the human hand. *Brain Res* 1976; 219:13–27.
2. Darian-Smith I. The sense of touch: Performance and peripheral neural processes. In: Brookhart JM, Mountcastle VB, eds. *Handbook of Physiology: Section 1: The Nervous System.* Vol. 3. Oxford: Oxford University Press, 1984:739–878.
3. Gescheider GA, Bolanowski SJ, Verrillo RT. Sensory, cognitive and response factors in the judgement of sensory magnitude. In: Algom D, ed. *Psychophysical Approaches to Cognition.* Amsterdam: Elsevier, 1992:575–621.
4. Greenspan JD, Lamotte RH. Cutaneous mechanoreceptors of the hand: Experimental studies and their implications for clinical testing of tactile sensation. *J Hand Ther* 1993; 6:75–82.
5. Vallbo AB, Hagbarth K, Torebjork E, Wallin BG. Somatosensory, proprioceptive and sympathetic activity in human peripheral nerves. *Physiol Rev* 1979; 59:919–957.
6. Willis WD, Coggeshall RE. *Sensory Mechanisms of the Spinal Cord.* 2nd ed. New York: Plenum Press, 1991.
7. von Bekesy G. Uber die Vibrationsempfindung [On the vibration sense]. *Akustische Zeitschrift* 1939; 4:315–334.
8. Bolanowski SJ, Gescheider GA, Verrillo RT, Checkosky CM. Four channels mediate the mechanical aspects of touch. *J Acoustic Soc Am* 1988; 84:1680–1694.
9. Gescheider GA, O'Malley MJ, Verrillo RT. Vibrotactile forward masking: Evidence for channel independence. *J Acoustic Soc Am* 1983; 74:474–485.
10. Gescheider GA, Sklar BF, Van Doren CL, Verrillo RT. Vibrotactile forward masking: Psychophysical evidence for a triplex theory of cutaneous mechanoreception. *J Acoust Soc Am* 1985; 78:534–543.
11. Gescheider GA, Verrillo RT, Van Doren CL. Prediction of vibrotactile masking functions. *J Acoustic Soc Am* 1982; 72:1421–1426.
12. Verrillo RT. Effect of contactor area on the vibrotactile threshold. *J Acoustic Soc Am* 1963; 35:1962–1966.
13. Essick GK, Edin BB. Receptor encoding of moving tactile stimuli in humans. II: The mean response of individual low-threshold mechanoreceptors to motion across the receptive field. *J Neurosci* 1995; 15:848–864.
14. Harrington T. Merzenich M. Neural coding in the sense of touch; Human sensations of skin indentation compared with responses of slowly adapting mechanoreceptive afferents innervating the hairy skin of monkeys. *Exp Brain Res* 1970; 10:251–264.

15. Jarvilehto T, Hamalainen H, Laurinen P. Characteristics of single mechanoreceptive fibres innervating hairy skin of the human hand. *Exp Brain Res* 1976; 25:45–61.
16. Vallbo AB, Johansson RS. The tactile sensory innervation of the glabrous skin of the human hand. In: Gordon G. ed. *Active Touch*. New York: Pergamon, 1978:29–54.
17. Westling GK. Sensori-motor mechanisms during precision grip in man. Umea University Medical dissertation. New Series 171, Umea, Sweden, 1986.
18. Hensel H. Boman KKA. Afferent impulses in cutaneous sensory nerves in human subjects. J Neurophysical 1960; 23:564–578.
19. Hensel H. Cutaneous thermoreceptors. In: Iggo, A. ed. Somatosensory System. Berlin: Spring, 1973:79–110.
20. Torebjörk, Hallin. A new method for classification of C-unit activity in intact human skin nerves. In: Bonica JJ, Albe-Fessard D, eds. Advances in Pain Research and Therapy. New York: Raven Press, 1976:29–34.
21. Campero M, Serra J, Ochoa JL. C-polymodal nociceptors activated by noxious low temperature in human skin. *J Physiol* 1966; 497:565–572.
22. Konietzny F. Peripheral neural correlates of temperature sensations in man. *Hum Neurobiol* 1984; 3:21–32.
23. Serra J. Campero M, Ochoa JL, Bostock H. Activity-dependent slowing of conduction differentiates functional subtypes of C fibres innervating human skin. *J Physiol* 1999; 515:799–811.
24. Darian-Smith I, ed. Thermal sensibility. In: Handbook of Physiology, Section 1, The Nervous System, Vol. 3, Sensory Processes, Part 2. Bethesda, MD: American Physiological Society, 1984:879–913.
25. Campero M, Serra J, Bostock H, Ochoa JL. Slowly conducting afferents activated by innocuous low temperature in human skin. *J Physiol* 2001; 535:855–865.
26 Duclaux R, Mei N, Ranieri F. Conduction velocity along afferent vagal dendrites: A new type of fibre. *J Physiol* 1976; 260:487–495.
27. Bessou M, Perl ER. Response of cutaneous sensory units with unmyelinated fibres to noxious stimuli. *J Neurophysiol* 1969; 32:1025–1043.
28. Campbell JN, Raja SN, Cohen RH, Manning DC, Khan AA, Meyer RA. Peripheral neural mechanisms of nociception. In: Wall PD, Melzack R, eds. *Textbook of Pain*. New York: Churchill Livingstone, 1989:22–45.
29. Schmidt R, Schmelz M, Forster C, Ringkamp M, Torebjork E, Handwerker H. Novel classes of responsive and unresponsive C nociceptors in humans skin. *J Neurosci* 1995; 15:333–341.
30. Koltenzenburg M, Bennett DL, Shelton DL, McMahon SB. Neutralization of endogenous NGF prevents the sensitization of nociceptors supplying inflamed skin. *Eur J Neurosci* 1999; 11:1698–1704.
31. Nordin M. Low threshold mechanoreceptive and nociceptive units with unmyelinated (C) fibres in the human supraorbital nerve. *J Physiol* 1990; 426:229–240.
32. Johansson RS, Trulsson M, Olsson KA, Westberg KG. Mechanoreceptor activity from the human face and oral mucosa. *Exp Brain Res* 1988; 72:204–208.
33. Vallbo AB, Hagbarth K-E, Torebjork HE, Wallin BG. Somatosensory, proprioceptive, and sympathetic activity in human peripheral nerves. *Physiol Rev* 1979; 59:919–957.
34. Löken L, Wessberg J, Morrison I, McGlone F, Olausson, H. Coding of pleasant touch by unmyelinated afferents in humans. *Nat Neurosci* 2009; 5:547–548.
35. McGlone F, Wessberg J, Olausson H. Discriminative and Affective touch: Sensing and feeling. *Neuron* 2014; 82:737–755.
36. Zotermann Y. Touch, pain and tickling: An electrophysiological investigation on cutaneous sensory nerves. *J Physiol* 1939; 95:1–28.
37. Iggo A, Korhuber HHA. A quantitative study of C-mechanoreceptors in the hairy skin of the cat. *J Physiol* 1977; 271:549–565.
38. MacKenzie RA, Burke D, Skuse NF, Lethlean AK. Fibre function and perception during cutaneous nerve block. *J Neurol Neurosurg Psychiatry* 1975; 38:865–873.
39. Vallbo AB, Olausson H, Wessberg J, Norsell U. A system of unmyelinated afferents for innocuous mechanoreception in the human skin. *Brain Res* 1993; 628:301–304.
40. Essick G, James A, McGlone FP. Psychophysical assessment of the affective components of non-painful touch. *Neuroreport* 1999; 10:2083–2087.

41. Olausson H, Lamarre Y, Backlund H, Morin C, Wallin BG, Starck S, Strigo K, Worsley K, Vallbo AB, Bushnell MC. Unmyelinated tactile afferents signal touch and project to the insular cortex. *Nat Neurosci* 2002; 5:900–904.

42. Wessberg J, Olausson H, Fernstormm KW, Vallbo AB. Receptive field properties of unmyelinated tactile afferents in the human skin. *J Neurophysiol* 2003; 89:1567–1575.

43. Francis ST, Rolls ET, Bowtell R, McGlone F, O'Doherty JO, Browning A, Clare S, Smith E. The representation of pleasant touch in the brain and its relationship with taste and olfactory areas. *Neuroreport* 1999; 10:453–459.

44. Rolls ET, O'Doherty JO, Kringelbach ML, Francis S, Bowtell R, McGlone F. Representations of pleasant and painful touch in the human orbitofrontal cortices. *Cereb Cortex* 2003; 13:308–317.

45. Reilly DM, Ferdinando D, Johnston C, Shaw C, Buchanan KD, Green M. The epidermal nerve fibre network: Characterization of nerve fibres in human skin by confocal microscopy and assessment of racial variations. *Br J Dermatol* 1997; 137:163–170.

46. Caterina MJ, Schumaker MJ, Tominaga M, Rosen TA, Levin JD, Julius D. The capsaicin receptor: A heat-activated ion channel in the pain pathway. *Nature* 1997; 389:816–824.

47. McKemy DD, Neuhausser WM, Julius D. Identification of a cold receptor reveals a general role for TRP channels in thermosensation. *Nature* 2002; 416:52–58.

48. Patapoutian A, Peier AM, Story GM, Viswanath V. ThermoTRP channels and beyond: Mechanisms of temperature sensation. *Nat Rev Neurosci* 2003; 4:529–538.

49. Stander S, Moormann C, Schumacher M, Buddenkotte J, Artuc M, Shpacovitch V, Brzoska T et al. Expression of vanilloid receptor subtype 1 in cutaneous sensory nerve fibres, mast cells, and epithelial cells of appendage structures. *Exp Dermatol* 2004; 13:129–139.

50. Montell C, Birnaumer L, Flockerzi V. The TRP channels, a remarkably functional family. *Cell* 2002; 108:595–598.

51. Caterina MJ, Leffer A, Malmberg AB, Martin WJ, Trafton J, Petersen-Zeitz M, Koltzenburg M, Basbaum Ai, Julius D. Impaired nociception and pain sensation in mice lacking the capsaicin receptor. *Science* 2000; 288:306–313.

52. Davis JB, Gray J, Gunthorpe MJ, Hatcher JP, Davey PT, Overend P, Harries MH et al. Vanilloid receptor-1 is essential for inflammatory thermal hyperalgesia. *Nature* 2000; 405:183–187.

53. Askwith CC, Benson CJ, Welsh MJ, Snyder PM. DEG/EnaC ion channels involved in sensory transduction are modulated by cold temperature. *PNAS* 2001; 98:6459–6463.

54. Souslova V, Cesare P, Ding Y, Akopian AN, Stanfa L, Suzuki R, Carpenter K et al. Warm-coding deficits and aberrant inflammatory pain in mice lacking P2X3 receptors. *Nature* 2000; 407:1015–1017.

55. Coggeshall RE, Zhou S, Carlton SM. Opioid receptors on peripheral sensory axons. *Brain Res* 1997; 764:126–132.

56. Stander S, Gunzer M, Metze D, Luger T, Steinhoff M. Localization of m-opioid receptor 1A on sensory nerve fibres in human skin. *Regul Pept* 2002; 110:75–83.

57. Holland RL, Harkin NE, Coleshaw RK, Jones DA, Peck AW, Telekes A. Dipipanone and nifedipine in cold induced pain: Analgesia not due to skin warming. *Br J Clin Pharmacol* 1987; 24:823–826.

58. Yuge O, Matsumoto M, Kitahata LM, Collins JG, Senami M. Direct opioid application to peripheral nerves does not alter compound action potentials. *Anesth Analg* 1985; 64:667–671.

59. Frank GB, Sudha TS. Effects of encephalin, applied intracellularly, on action potentials in vertebrate A and C nerve fibre axons. *Neuropharmacology* 1987; 26:61–66.

60. Antoijevic I, Mousa SA, Schafer M, Stein C. Perineural defect and peripheral opioid analgesia during inflammation. *J Neurosci* 1995; 15:165–172.

61. Bigliardi PL, Bigliardi-Qi M, Buechner S, Ruffi T. Expression of m-opiate receptor in human epidermis and keratinocytes. *J Invest Dermatol* 1998; 111:297–301.

62. Bigliardi-Qi M, Bigliardi PL, Eberle AN, Buechner S, Ruffi T. b-Endorphin stimulates cytokeratin 16 expression and downregulates m-opiate receptor expression in human epidermis. *J Invest Dermatol* 1998; 114:527–532.

63. Dvorak M, Watkinson A, McGlone F, Rukweid R. Histamine-induced responses are attenuated by a cannabinoid receptor agonist in human skin. *Inflamm Res* 2003; 52:238–245.

64. Johanek LM, Simone DA. Activation of peripheral cannabinoid receptors attenuates cutaneous hyperalgesia produced by a heat injury. *Pain* 2004; 109:432–442.

65. Matsuda LA. Molecular aspects of cannabinoid receptors. *Crit Rev Neurobiol* 1997; 11:143–166.

66. Munro S, Thomas KL, Abu-Shaar M. Molecular characterization of a peripheral receptor for cannabinoids. *Nature* 1993; 365:61–65.
67. Price TJ, Helesic G, Parghi D, Hargreaves KM, Flores CM. The neuronal distribution of cannabinoid receptor type 1 in the trigeminal ganglion of the rat. *Neuroscience* 2003; 120:155–162.
68. Galiegue S, Mary S, Marchand J, Dussossoy D, Carriere D, Carayon P, Bouaboula M, Shire D, Le Fur G, Casellas P. Expression of central and peripheral cannabinoid receptors in human immune tissues and leukocytes subpopulations. *Eur J Biochem* 1995; 232:54–61.
69. Rukweid R, Watkinson A, McGlone F, Dvorak M. Cannabinoid agonists attenuate capsaicin-induced responses in human skin. *Pain* 2003; 102:283–288.
70. Walker JM, Huang SM, Strangman NM, Tsou K, Sanudo-Pena MN. Pain modulation by release of the endogenous cannabinoid anandamide. *PNAS* 1999; 96:12198–12203.
71. Piomelli D. The molecular logic of endocannabinoid signalling. *Nat Rev Neurosci* 2003; 4:873–884.
72. DiMarzo V, Bisogno T, Melck D, Ross R, Brochic H, Stevenson L, Pertwee R, DePetrocellis L. Interactions between synthetic vanilloids and the endogenous cannabinoid system. *FEBS Lett* 1998; 436:449–454.
73. DiMarzo V, Bisogno T, Petrocellis L. Anandamide: Some like it hot. *Trends Pharmacol Sci* 2001; 22:346–349.
74. Penfield R, Rasmussen T. *The Cerebral Cortex of Man*. New York: Macmillan, 1952.
75. Maldjian JA, Gotschalk A, Patel RS, Detre JA, Alsop DC. The sensory somatotopic map of the human hand demonstrated at 4 T. *Neuroimage* 1999; 10:55–62.
76. Woolsey C. Second somatic receiving areas in the cerebral cortex of the cat, dog and monkey. *Fed Proc* 1946; 55–56.
77. Maeda K, Kakigi R, Hoshiyama M, Koyama S. Topography of the secondary somatosensory cortex in humans: A magentoencephalographic study. *Neuroreport* 1999; 10:301–306.
78. Coghill RC, Talbot JD, Evans AC, Meyer E, Gjedde A, Bushnell MC, Duncan GH. Distributed processing of pain and vibration by the human brain. *J Neurosci* 1994; 14:4095–4108.
79. Francis ST, Kelly EF, Bowtell R, Dunseath WJ, Folger SE, McGlone FP. FMRI of the responses to vibratory stimulation of digit tips. *Neuroimage* 2000; 11:188–202.
80. McGlone FP, Kelly EF, Trulsson M, Francis ST, Westling G, Bowtel R. Functional neuroimaging studies of human somatosensory cortex. *Behav Brain Res* 2002; 135:147–158.
81. Schneider RJ, Friedman DP, Mishkin M. A modality-specific somatosensory area within the insula of the rhesus monkey. *Brain Res* 1993; 621:116–120.
82. Trulsson M, Francis ST, Kelly EF, Westling G, Bowtell R, McGlone FP. Cortical responses to single mechanoreceptive afferent microstimulation revealed with fMRI. *Neuroimage* 2001; 13:613–622.
83. Penfield R, Boldrey E. Somatic motor and sensory representation in the cerebral cortex of man as studied by electrical stimulation. *Brain* 1937; 60:389–443.
84. Rolls E, O'Doherty J, Kringelbach M, Francis S, Bowtell R, McGlone F. Representation of pleasant and painful touch in the human orbitofrontal cortex. *Cereb Cortex* 2003; 10:284–294.

Section II

Pathophysiology of Sensitive Skin

5

Stratum Corneum and Sensitive Skin

Enzo Berardesca

Stratum Corneum and Sensitive Skin

Subjects with sensitive skin report exaggerated reactions when their skin is in contact with cosmetics, soaps, and sunscreens, and they often report worsening after exposure to dry and cold climates. Epidemiologic studies have been carried out to assess whether there is a correlation with sex, age, skin type, or race and are described elsewhere in this book.

Subjects with sensitive skin may have a thinner SC with a reduced corneocyte area causing a higher transcutaneous penetration of water-soluble chemicals (1). Frosch and Kligman (2), by testing different irritants, showed a 14% incidence of sensitive skin in the normal population, likely correlated to a thin permeable SC, which makes these subjects more susceptible to chemical irritation.

Moreover, the declined barrier function in sensitive skin has already been reported as the result of an imbalance of intercellular lipid of SC (3). Although impaired barrier function is easily understood as a mechanism of sensitive skin, other factors are also possible implications such as changes in the nerve system and/or the structure of the epidermis. In a study (4), detailed characteristics of sensitive skin have been investigated using noninvasive methods. Sensitive skin has been classified into three different types based on their physiological parameters. Type 1 has been defined as the low barrier function group. Type 2 has been defined as the inflammation group with normal barrier function and inflammatory changes. Type 3 has been specified as the pseudohealthy group in terms of normal barrier function and no inflammatory changes. In all types, a high content of nerve growth factor has been observed in the SC, relative to that of nonsensitive skin. In both types 2 and 3, the sensitivity to electrical stimuli was high (4). Since these data suggest that the hypersensitive reaction of sensitive skin is closely related to nerve fibers innervating the epidermis, Yamasaki and Gallo (5) proposed that the innate immune system triggers an abnormal inflammatory reaction that mediates the symptoms of rosacea and sensitive skin. If so, flushing and blushing erythema may be due to chronic inflammation. In particular, cathelicidin may play a role in inducing the cytokine cascade. Indeed, some forms of cathelicidin peptides were known to have a unique capacity to be both vasoactive and proinflammatory (5).

Direct connections were observed between unmyelinated nerve fibers and mast cells; stress in animal models induces substance P (SP) in unmyelinated nerve fibers, which triggers mast cell degranulation with subsequent histamine release (6). Stress is commonly reported as a trigger for sensitive skin, and mast cell degranulation is supported by the finding that sensitive skin sufferers had higher density of mast cells and size of lymphatic microvasculature (7). Neurogenic inflammation probably results from the release of neurotransmitters such as SP, calcitonin gene-related peptide (CGRP), and vasoactive intestinal peptide, which induce vasodilatation and mast cell degranulation. Nonspecific inflammation may also be associated with the release of interleukins. Indeed, sensitive skin could be the result of an inflammatory process resulting from the abnormal penetration in the skin of potentially irritating substances because of skin barrier dysfunction (8). In addition, the presence of a nonspecific reaction has been related to cutaneous sensory innervation in the establishment of skin sensitivity (9,10). Neuropeptides released from cutaneous nerves and skin resident cells such as SP, CGRP, and POMC peptides (such as β-endorphin and encephalin) are mandatory for a fine-tuned regulation of cutaneous immune responses and tissue maintenance and repair (11,12). In response to noxious stimuli, SP and CGRP lead to vasodilatation and mast cell degranulation, originating in a process called *neurogenic inflammation*. Classical pathways are then activated causing a nonspecific inflammation in consequence of released cytokines and eicosanoids such as interleukin-1 α (IL-1α), tumor necrosis factor alpha, prostaglandin E2, and prostaglandin F2 (13). On the other hand, POMC activities include antagonism and downregulation of adhesion molecules and reduced inflammation by the modulation of IL-10 production, which contributes to the amelioration of the subjective neurosensory forms of discomfort.

Several research studies, however, are investigating the molecular basis for sensory hyperreactivity. Transient receptor potential, vanilloid family 1 (TRPV1) is a nonreceptive, thermosensitive ion channel which reacts to noxious stimuli, most notably noxious heat and low pH. TRPV1 is expressed on fibroblasts, mast cells, and endothelial cells; activation results in pain or pruritus with a burning component. TRPV1 is also dramatically upregulated by inflammatory mediators (14) as well as heat and capsaicin. It has been hypothesized that the development of sensitive skin may be related to the dysregulation of muscle contraction and relaxation process (15); actin-bound myosin cross bridges in sensitive skin had more compacted shape than those in nonsensitive skin, indicating more contracted cross-bridge state in sensitive skin tissues. This could also be linked to altered adenosine triphosphate metabolism and response of skin pH. These data demonstrated that subjects with sensitive skin showed impaired pH homeostasis after lactic acid stimulation and increase of detection ability for pH upon internal or external stimuli such as lactic acid (15). Enhanced acidity might induce pain via the stimulation of TRPV1, acid-sensing ion channel subunit 3, and CGRP in the human sensitive skin. SC microbiome has also been investigated in subjects affected by sensitive skin, and no differences versus normal controls have been reported (16).

The existing overlap between atopic population and subjects affected by sensitive skin is well documented. Using TEWL modeling, statistically significant differences have been detected in the parameters obtained in the sensitive skin group, which supports the thesis that individuals with increased skin susceptibility have impaired barrier function (17). However, few studies have investigated the SC lipid composition in subjects affected by sensitive skin. Cho et al. (18) compared the average amounts of ceramides in the SC on various parts of the body (right cheek, forearm, thigh, leg, back, palm) between the sensitive group and the nonsensitive group. The results indicated that the mean values of the amounts of ceramides in other parts of the body surface except the face were lower in the sensitive group than in the nonsensitive group, but the difference was not statistically significant. However, on the face, the sensitive group showed a statistically significant decrease in the mean value of the amounts of ceramides compared to the nonsensitive, indicating that the amount of ceramides in the SC on the facial skin has a correlation with skin sensitivity.

Changes in SC thickness and therefore of transcutaneous penetration may explain regional differences or specialized areas of sensitive skin. The face has demonstrated to be the most common site of skin sensitivity, physiologically predictable due to the larger and multiple number of products used on the face (particularly in women), a thinner barrier in facial skin, and a greater density of nerve endings (19). The nasolabial fold was reported to be the most sensitive region of the facial area, followed by the malar eminence, chin, forehead, and upper lip (20,21). Saint-Martory et al. (22) found that hand, scalp, feet, neck, torso, and back sensitivity followed facial sensitivity in descending order of prevalence. Significant numbers of individuals experience sensitivity of the scalp (23,24). One-third of the population interviewed reported sensitive scalp with higher levels in women than in men. Interestingly, the prevalence declared that sensitivity of the scalp increases with age. The authors explain that this could be due to alterations of nerve endings due to the aging process or increased proclivity to irritation as a consequence of chronic exposure to surfactants contained in shampoos. The genital area is another site frequently affected by sensitive skin.

In a study of 1039 men and women, 56.2% reported sensitivity of genital skin (25), an area of particular interest since it is formed partially from embryonic endoderm and therefore differs from the skin at other body sites (26). A surprising 56.2% of responders claimed sensitive genital skin, with significantly more African Americans than Caucasians (66.4%; $P < .0001$) claiming sensitivity of this area. Rough fabrics were found to be the most common offender for sensitive skin in the genital area (27).

In conclusion, SC plays a central role in the determination of sensitive skin. This could be due to differences not only in structure and intercellular lipids, but also in proclivity to release neuromodulators and proinflammatory agents causing hyperreactions and sensations. Further studies are needed to fully elucidate these mechanisms.

REFERENCES

1. Berardesca E, Cespa M, Farinelli N et al. In vivo transcutaneous penetration of nicotinates and sensitive skin. *Contact Dermatitis* (1991) 25, 35–38.
2. Frosch PJ, Kligman AM. A method for appraising the stinging capacity of topically applied substances. *J Soc Cosmet Chem* (1977) 28, 197–209.
3. Ohta M, Hikima R, Ogawa T. Physiological characteristics of sensitive skin classified by stinging test. *J Cosmet Sci Soc Jpn* (2000) 23, 163–167.
4. Yokota T, Matsumoto M, Sakamaki T et al. Classification of sensitive skin and development of a treatment system appropriate for each group. *IFSCC Magazine* (2003) 6, 303–307.
5. Yamasaki K, Gallo RL. The molecular pathology of rosacea. *J Dermatol Sci* (2009) 55, 77–81.
6. Kumagai M, Nagano M, Suzuki H et al. Effects of stress memory by fear conditioning on nerve-mast cell circuit in skin. *J Dermatol* (2011) 38, 553–561.
7. Quatresooz P, Piérard-Franchimont C, Piérard GE. Vulnerability of reactive skin to electric current perception—A pilot study implicating mast cells and the lymphatic microvasculature. *J Cosmet Dermatol* (2009) 8, 186–189.
8. Yosipovitch G, Yarnitzky D. Quantitative sensory testing. In: Maibach HI, Marzulli FN, eds. *Dermatotoxicology Methods: The Laboratory Worker's Vade Mecum*. New York: Taylor & Francis (1997) 120–135.
9. Primavera G, Berardesca E. Sensitive skin: Mechanisms and diagnosis. *Int J Cosmet Sci* (2005) 27, 1–10.
10. Misery L, Myon E, Martin N et al. Sensitive skin: Psychological effects and seasonal changes. *J Eur Acad Dermatol Venereol* (2007) 21, 620–628.
11. Peters EMJ, Ericson ME, Hosoi J et al. Neuropeptide control mechanisms in cutaneous biology: Physiological and clinical significance. *J Invest Dermatol* (2006) 126, 1937–1947.
12. Luger TA, Lotti T. Neuropeptides: Role in inflammatory skin diseases. *J Eur Acad Dermatol Venereol* (1998) 10, 207–211.
13. Luger TA. Neuromediators—A crucial component of the skin immune system. *J Dermatol Sci* (2002) 30, 87–93.
14. Kueper T, Krohn M, Haustedt LO et al. Inhibition of TRPV1 for the treatment of sensitive skin. *Exp Dermatol* (2010) 19, 980–986.
15. Kim EJ, Lee DH, Kim YK et al. Decreased ATP synthesis and lower pH may lead to abnormal muscle contraction and skin sensitivity in human skin. *J Dermatol Sci* (2014) 76, 214–221.
16. Hillion M, Mijouin L, Jaouen T et al. Comparative study of normal and sensitive skin aerobic bacterial populations. *Microbiologyopen* (2013) 2, 953–961.
17. Pinto P, Rosado C, Parreirão C et al. Is there any barrier impairment in sensitive skin?: A quantitative analysis of sensitive skin by mathematical modeling of transepidermal water loss desorption curves. *Skin Res Technol* (2011) 17, 181–185.
18. Cho HJ, Chung BY, Lee HB et al. Quantitative study of stratum corneum ceramides contents in patients with sensitive skin. *J Dermatol* (2012) 39, 295–300.
19. Chew A, Maibach H. Sensitive skin. In: Loden M, Maibach H, eds. *Dry Skin and Moisturizers: Chemistry and Function*. Boca Raton, FL: CRC Press (2000) 429–440.
20. Marriott M, Holmes J, Peters L et al. The complex problem of sensitive skin. *Contact Dermatitis* (2005) 53, 93–99.
21. Distante F, Bonfigli A, Rigano L et al. Intra- and inter-individual differences in facial skin biophysical properties. *Cosmet Toiletries* (2002) 7, 149–158.
22. Saint-Martory C, Roguedas-Contios AM, Sibaud V et al. Sensitive skin is not limited to the face. *Brit J Dermatol* (2008) 158, 130–133.
23. Misery L, Sibaud V, Ambronati M et al. Sensitive scalp: Does this condition exist? An epidemiological study. *Contact Dermatitis* (2008) 58, 234–238.
24. Misery L, Rahhali N, Ambonati M et al. Evaluation of sensitive scalp severity and symptomatology by using a new score. *J Eur Acad Dermatol Venereol* (2011) 25, 1295–1298.
25. Frosch PJ, Kligman AM. A method for appraising the stinging capacity of topically applied substances. *J Soc Cosmet Chem* (1977) 28, 197–209.
26. Farage M, Maibach HI. The vulvar epithelium differs from the skin: Implications for cutaneous testing to address topical vulvar exposures. *Contact Dermatitis* (2004) 51, 201–209.
27. Farage MA. Perceptions of sensitive skin of the genital area. *Curr Probl Dermatol* (2011) 40, 142–154.

6

Altered Somatosensory Pathways

Eun Ju Kim, Dong Hun Lee, and Jin Ho Chung*

Sensorineural Basis of Sensitive Skin

Sensitive skin is a hyperreactive skin condition to various exogenous or endogenous factors, character-ized by sensory symptoms such as tightness, stinging, prickling, burning, tingling, pain, and itching. The nature of sensitive skin is primarily sensory, without visible signs of irritation and inflammation. Increasing evidence suggests that sensitive skin is closely related to the altered sensorineural pathways in the skin, particularly in the aspects of dysfunctional neural responses and neurogenic inflammation (1–3). When sensory nerve fibers were stimulated with three different currents (2 kHz, 250 Hz, 5 Hz), only subjects with sensitive skin showed lowered sensory perception thresholds for unmyelinated C fiber at 5 Hz electric current (a current known to selectively stimulate C fibers), indicating that the neurologi-cal instability of C fiber nociception may play a role in abnormal sensory perception of sensitive skin (4). Moreover, subjects with self-perceived sensitive skin showed a greater and specific cerebral activation in fMRI, compared with those with nonsensitive skin, when stimulated by a lactic acid sting test (5). In this chapter, we first introduce the modern concept of neurogenic inflammation as one of the possible neuronal mechanisms responsible for causing sensitive skin. Then, recognized roles of the vanilloid receptors, particularly TRPV1, in sensitive skin will be reviewed. Finally, we will summarize our find-ings that dysfunction of muscle contraction, carbohydrate and lipid metabolism, acidic homeostasis, and ion balance are important in the pathogenesis of sensitive skin.

Concept of Neurogenic Inflammation and Hyper/Dysesthesia

The skin is densely innervated by peripheral nerve fibers, forming an integrative neuroimmunologic network. Derived from dorsal root ganglion (DRG), there are three types of sensory nerve fibers (A-β, A-δ, C fibers) in the skin (6–9).

1. A-β fibers (largest; moderately myelinated): Touch, vibration, pressure, and pain (mechanono-ciceptor) sensation
2. A-δ fibers (smaller; thinly myelinated): Cold and pain (mechanonociceptor) sensation
3. C fibers (slowest; smaller, nonmyelinated): Heat, cold, pruritus, pain (polymodal nociceptor), and autonomic peripheral functions

Primary sensory nerves from DRG consist of mostly A-δ fibers (~80%) and C fibers (~20%). In human skin, mechanoheat responsive, mechanosensitive, and heat-sensitive C fibers constitute 45%, 13%, and 6% of cutaneous afferent nerves, respectively (8). These C and A-δ fibers convey afferent signals to the CNS in response to a variety of physical (heat, cold, nociception, mechanical distension, UV light) and chemical (toxic agents, allergens, microbes, proteases) stimuli from the external environment. Moreover, internal stimuli such as pH changes, hormones, and inflammatory mediators can induce the activation of

---

* Dong Hun Lee and Jin Ho Chung share senior authorship.

primary afferent neurons (8,10). On the other hand, relatively sparse autonomic nerve fibers in the skin (limited in the dermis) produce neurotransmitters such as acetylcholine and catecholamines, which may play a role in inflammation, blood and lymphatic hemodynamics, and regulation of skin appendages (10,11). There is some evidence that inflammatory skin disorders such as chronic atopic dermatitis and psoriasis are associated with increased skin innervation (8,12), although it is unknown that sensitive skin tissues have an altered density in nerve fibers.

In contrast to the traditional view that the peripheral nervous system and the immune system serve separate functions, it is now evident that the peripheral nervous system directly communicates with the immune system (11). Pioneering experiments by Bayliss in 1901 revealed cutaneous vasodilation after the stimulation of cut dorsal nerve roots (13), which led to the concept of *neurogenic inflammation*. Neurogenic inflammation is the inflammation caused by the activation of primary sensory nerve terminals, which is characterized by four hallmarks of inflammation, that is, redness (*rubor*) and warmth (*calor*) (secondary to vasodilation), swelling (*tumor*, secondary to plasma extravasation), and pain/hypersensitivity (*dolor*, secondary to altered excitability of sensory neurons) in addition to granulocyte infiltration in postcapillary venules.

To be more specific, polymodal C fibers and, to a lesser extent, A-δ fibers, not only conduct afferent signals to the spinal DRG and brain orthodromically upon stimulation, but also transmit efferent action potentials antidromically to the periphery (*axon reflex*). These action potentials, along with local depolarization, trigger a rapid and local release of neural mediators from both peripheral axons and terminals (8,10,11,14–17). Mast cells rapidly degranulate and release a variety of bioactive substances such as cytokines, prostaglandins (PGs), serotonin, and histamine (18,19). It is reported that a subgroup of subjects with sensitive skin has a higher density of skin mast cells than those with nonsensitive skin (20). In response to bioactive mediators from nerves and target cells, sensory nerve fibers can become sensitized and lower their activation thresholds, leading to sustained release of neuropeptides. Consequently, this process may be self-sustaining and self-amplifying via positive feedback loops, which involve regulation of calcium influx mainly through G protein-coupled receptors and TRP channels (14,15) (Figure 6.1). Nonspecific inflammation is associated with the production of interleukins (IL-1, IL-8, PG E_2, PG F_2, and tumor necrosis factor [TNF]-α) (1,21).

Hyperesthesia is a condition that involves an abnormal increase in cutaneous sensitivity including pain, touch, and thermal sensation. Hyperesthesia is observed in many neurologic disorders such as herpes zoster, peripheral neuropathy, and radiculopathies. One of the possible mechanisms underlying hyperesthesia is that pain thresholds are lowered in areas with tissue inflammation or injury. Another explanation is that inflammation activates silent nociceptors and/or elicits perpetuating nerve signals, leading to long-lasting changes and nociceptor sensitization. These phenomena contribute to the amplification and persistence of pain. On the other hand, *allodynia* is pain caused by excitation of low-threshold sensory nerve fibers in response to nonnociceptive stimuli, whereas *hyperalgesia* is exaggerated pain to noxious stimuli (22–24).

When activated by noxious stimuli, skin cells as well as nociceptors release a multitude of neural mediators which act on target cells via a paracrine, juxtacrine, or endocrine pathway to initiate neurogenic inflammation as well as sensory symptoms such as pruritus. Neurogenic inflammation is mediated mainly by the action of neuropeptides SP and CGRP from nociceptors, on vascular endothelial and smooth muscle cells (11,25). Specifically, SP induces enhanced capillary permeability and resultant plasma extravasation and edema, while CGRP causes potent vasodilation (26–28). As neurogenic inflammation is implicated in the pathogenesis of sensitive skin, it is likely that SP and CGRP are upregulated in sensitive skin. Indeed, sensitive skin tissues showed an increased expression of CGRP (29), and we herein focus on the functions of SP and CGRP associated with skin inflammation.

The expression of SP is regulated by proinflammatory mediators and neurotrophins. Keratinocytes, mast cells, endothelial cells, fibroblasts, lymphocytes, leukocytes, macrophages, Langerhans cells, and Merkel cells express functional neurokinin (NK) receptors. SP induces vascular responses and pruritus by the production of TNF-α, histamine, and PG D_2 from mast cells, which may participate in a positive feedback mechanism. SP also enhances leukocyte–endothelial interactions by the upregulation of cell adhesion molecules (intercellular adhesion molecule 1, vascular cell adhesion molecule 1) and chemotaxis of neutrophils and eosinophils. SP stimulates the production of the proinflammatory cytokines such

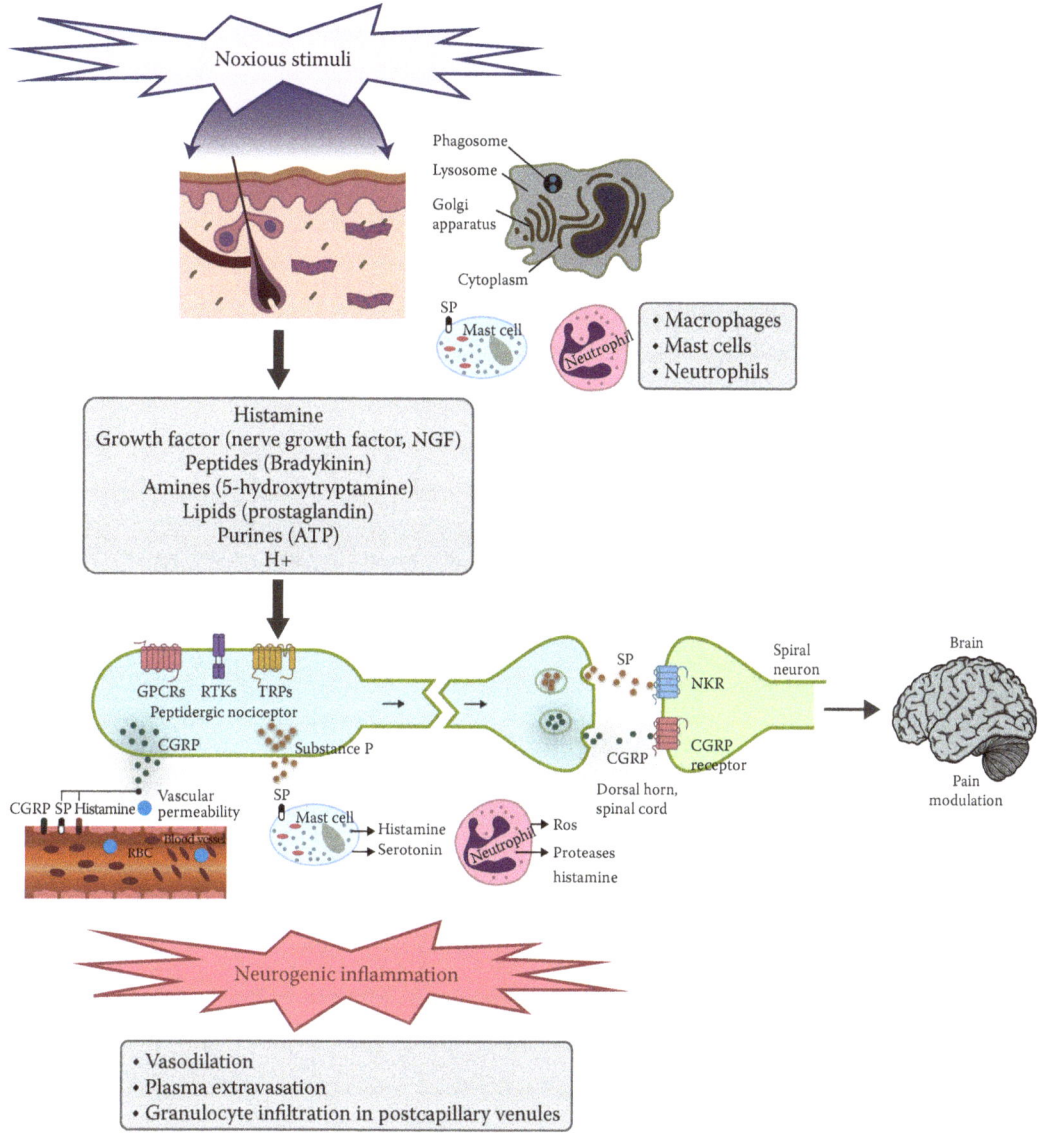

FIGURE 6.1 Overview of neurogenic inflammation.

as IL-1α, IL-1β, and IL-8 and regulates the important transcription factors such as nuclear transcription factor κB, nuclear factor of activated T cells, and activator protein 1 (8,10,16).

CGRP predominantly induces arteriole vasodilation and stimulates the proliferation of keratinocytes and vascular endothelial cells via interaction with a CGRP receptor. It is one of the most potent vasodilators and generally mediates anti-inflammatory and neurotrophic action. However, under certain circumstances, CGRP increases the adhesion of neutrophils and monocytes, enhances neutrophil accumulation and edema formation, and promotes the release of TNF-α from mast cells, indicating its proinflammatory role. It inhibits the degradation of SP by neutral endopeptidase (NEP) and triggers SP release (8,10,16).

Moreover, there are about 30 other neurotransmitters identified in the skin, for example, NK A, neurotensin, vasoactive intestinal peptide, pituitary adenylate cyclase-activating polypeptide, neuropeptide Y, somatostatin, gastrin-releasing hormone, β-endorphin, enkephalin, and galanin. There are excellent review papers on other neuropeptides in the skin elsewhere (8,10,30–34). Collectively, neural mediators from nociceptors promote (a) chemotaxis and activation of neutrophils, macrophages, and lymphocytes and degranulation of mast cells; (b) increased blood flow, vascular leakage, and edema; and (c) priming of dendritic cells for T cell differentiation (11).

Moreover, many cells with neuropeptide receptors also produce neuropeptide-degrading enzymes such as NEP or angiotensin-converting enzyme to limit the extent or duration of neurogenic inflammation (8,10).

The coordinated interaction between the peripheral nervous system and the immune system is mediated by different types of peripheral nerves and target cells in the skin such as keratinocytes, mast cells, endothelial cells, fibroblasts, and other immune cells (10,14). These interactions are implicated in cutaneous disease states such as urticaria, psoriasis, atopic dermatitis, hypersensitivity reactions, rosacea, UV-induced inflammation, and sensitive skin as well as normal homeostasis (8,10,16,19,29,33,35–41).

Taken together, neurogenic inflammation is a multidirectional and interactive cross talk between the peripheral nervous system, the immune system, and skin cells such as keratinocytes. Targeting neurogenic inflammation is a promising target of novel therapeutic approaches for sensitive skin.

The Role of Vanilloid Receptors in Sensitive Skin

Many subjects with sensitive skin report untoward sensory feelings such as pruritus, burning, and pain to changes in temperature (1). This phenomenon led to the notion that receptors and pathways that mediate both temperature sensation and sensory symptoms are implicated in the pathogenesis of sensitive skin. Moreover, the stinging test using capsaicin or lactic acid has been employed as a robust method to diagnose sensitive skin objectively (2,6,42).

Capsaicin, the main pungent ingredient of hot chili pepper, is a natural agonist of TRPV1. Since the successful cloning of TRPV1 in 1997 (43), significant progress has been made in the field of TRPV1 biology (8,22,44–46). Six related subfamilies (TRPV [vanilloid], TRP canonical, TRP melastatin, TRP polycystin, TRP mucolipin, and the TRP ankyrin groups) based on the amino acid sequence homology comprise mammalian TRP channels. TRP channels are composed of six putative transmembrane domains, a pore-forming loop between the fifth and sixth domains, and intracellular NH_2 and COOH termini that assemble as homo- or heterotetramers to form cation-permeable channels (22,47). TRPV1 forms cation channels with varying selectivity to diverse cations. For example, capsaicin-activated TRPV1 channels have roughly a 10:1 selectivity (permeability ratio) of Ca^{2+} over Na^+, whereas heat-activated TRPV1 channels have a 4:1 selectivity (22,48). In addition to Ca^{2+} influx, Ca^{2+} release from internal stores, such as the Golgi apparatus, the endoplasmic reticulum, or the sarcoplasmic reticulum in muscle cells, contributes to changes in intracellular Ca^{2+} (22).

TRPV1 is a key molecular sensor and signaling integrator of thermal, chemical, and other sensory stimuli (49). TRPV1 is expressed on keratinocytes, fibroblasts, mast cells, endothelial cells, and sensory C and A-δ fibers (50–53). TRPV1 is a crucial contributor to pain, itch, and neurogenic inflammation (54–56). TRPV1 can be activated by low pH (<5.9), noxious heat (>43°C), and various chemicals such as adenosine triphosphate (ATP), anandamide, leukotriene B4, and resiniferatoxin (22) (Table 6.1; Figure 6.2). Long-term application of capsaicin causes TRPV1-mediated depletion of neuropeptides, leading to the *desensitization* of nerves (long-lasting refractory state unresponsive to further seemingly innocuous stimuli), and the amelioration of inflammatory responses (8,44).

The channel activity of TRPV1 can be markedly enhanced by low pH or inflammatory mediators via the activation of protein kinase A (PKA), PKC, PLC, and Ca^{2+}/CaMKII pathways, leading to *receptor sensitization*, which lowers sensory perception thresholds (22,57–59). Pain sensation is augmented by acidic milieu during ischemia or inflammation. A-δ and C fiber neurons transduce extracellular protons via at least two different classes of cation-selective channels, TRPV1 and acid-sensing ion channels (ASICs) (60). On the contrary, TRPV1 can be inhibited by phosphorylation by cyclic adenosine monophosphate-dependent protein kinase (61).

The transmembrane influx of cations into the cytoplasm depolarizes the cells and elicits neuronal action potential propagation and muscle contraction. In nonexcitable cells such as keratinocytes and fibroblasts, membrane depolarization by TRPV1 leads to the stimulation of voltage-dependent channels and is associated with various physiological and pathological functions such as proliferation, differentiation,

TABLE 6.1

Properties of TRPV1 Proteins

Expression in the skin	Keratinocytes, fibroblasts, mast cells, dermal blood vessels, hair follicles, sebocytes, sweat glands, smooth muscle, skeletal muscle, Langerhans cells, C, A-δ fibers
Direct activation	Noxious heat (>43°C)
	Vanilloid compounds
	Capsaicin, resiniferatoxin, olvanil
	Endocannabinoid lipids
	Anandamide, arachidonylethanolamide, 2-arachidonoyl glycerol
	Eicosanoids
	5-(*S*)-HETE, 12-(*S*)-HETE, 5-(*S*)-HPETE, 2-(*S*)-HPETE
	Leukotriene B4
	Extracellular proton (pH <5.9)
	Allicin
	ATP (via protein kinase C [PKC])
	Bradykinin (via PKC)
	Camphor
	Eugenol
	NGF (via PKC)
	Oleoylethanolamide
	PGE_2/PGI_2 (via PKA)
	Piperine (black pepper)
	Serotonin (via PKC)
	Zingerone (ginger)
Sensitizing pathways	PKA
	PKC
	Phospholipase C (PLC)
	Ca^{2+}/calmodulin-dependent kinase II (CaMKII)
Inhibitors	Capsazepine, ruthenium red, iodoresiniferatoxin, (*N*-(4-tertiarybutylphenyl)-4-(3-cholorphyridin-2-yl)tetrahydropryazine-1(2*H*)-carbox-amide), phosphatidylinositol-4,5-bisphosphate
Functions	Pain, noxious temperature sensation, bladder distension sensing, neurogenic inflammation

Source: Nilius, B., Owsianik, G., Voets, T., and Peters, J. A., *Physiol Rev*, 87, 165–217, 2007; Ramsey, I. S., Delling, M., and Clapham, D. E., *Annu Rev Physiol*, 68, 619–647, 2006; Veldhuis, N. A., Poole, D. P., Grace, M., McIntyre, P., and Bunnett, N. W., *Pharmacol Rev*, 67, 36–73, 2015.

Note: HETE: hydroxyeicosatetraenoic acid; HPETE: hydroperoxyeicosatetraenoic acid.

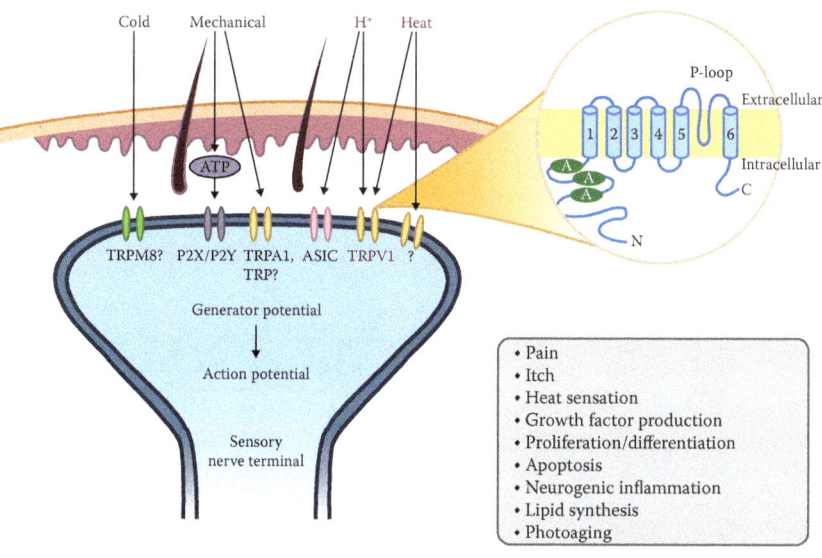

FIGURE 6.2 Overview of TRPV1.

apoptosis, and inflammation (22,44,47,48). Previously, our group has identified the role of TRPV1 in intrinsic and extrinsic skin aging (induced by UV irradiation and heat) as well as UV-induced inflammation (62–66).

Kueper et al. (2) showed that selective TRPV1 antagonist *trans*-4-*tert*-butylcyclohexanol could inhibit capsaicin-induced human TRPV1 (hTRPV1) activation in vitro in hTRPV1-overexpressing HEK293 cells and oocytes. Moreover, in a clinical study involving 30 women, the compound was effective in reducing capsaicin-induced burning in vivo (2). These findings strongly suggest that TRPV1 activation is important in the pathogenesis of sensitive skin and that TRPV1 antagonists can be used for the treatment of sensitive skin.

Novel Pathomechanism of Sensitive Skin

As previously summarized, sensitive skin is related to altered somatosensory systems, especially lowered pain threshold and enhanced pain induction elicited by neurogenic inflammation and TRPV1 activation. In addition, sensitive skin is associated with impaired skin barrier function and altered immune responsiveness (3,67). More recently, we employed an unbiased microarray analysis of skin samples obtained from subjects with sensitive or nonsensitive skin and identified the unexpected gene signature in sensitive skin, which is closely associated with the dysfunction of muscle contraction, metabolic homeostasis, and ion balance. These alterations may result in decreased synthesis of ATP and enhanced proton, leading to skin sensitivity (29,68).

Sensitive Skin Showed Decreased Expression of Muscle Contraction-Related Genes

Healthy volunteers with sensitive or nonsensitive skin were classified based on self-assessment questionnaires and a 10% lactic acid stinging test. Those with underlying skin diseases such as rosacea were excluded. Microarray analyses using the skin from volunteers revealed an unexpected and distinct gene expression signature that while 17 upregulated genes in sensitive skin are associated with the inflammatory and immune responses, 29 downregulated genes in sensitive skin represent muscle composition/ contraction, carbohydrate/lipid metabolism, and ion transport/ionic balance (Tables 6.2 and 6.3).

Many downregulated genes are associated with muscle contraction and relaxation process as well as muscle structure. In human facial skin, striated muscle fibers are found in the reticular dermis and subcutis (69), along with smooth muscles accompanying the hair follicles (arrector pili). The sarcomere, a functional unit of muscle, is composed mainly of thick filaments (myosin, slow-type myosin-binding protein C), thin filaments (actin, troponin, alpha tropomyosin 1, nebulin), and elastic components (titin). In the presence of Ca^{2+} from sarcoplasmic reticulum and ATP, the myosin head binds to the actin that enables the thin filament to slide along the thick filament, allowing for the shortening of the sarcomere (*cross-bridge cycling*) (70). Actin-bound myosin cross bridges in sensitive skin had more compacted shape than those in nonsensitive skin, indicating more contracted cross-bridge state in sensitive skin tissues (Figure 6.3). Further supporting experiments demonstrated that the decreased expressions of muscle-related genes in sensitive skin were not due to either a sampling bias or differences in anatomical sites. Our results suggest that sensitive skin may be associated with abnormal muscle contraction/relaxation process (29).

Sensitive Skin Showed Dysfunction of Metabolic Homeostasis, Impaired Aerobic ATP Synthesis, and Abnormal Muscle Contraction/Relaxation

Muscle contraction and relaxation require ATP regeneration through metabolic pathways such as phosphocreatine, anaerobic glycolysis, or oxidative metabolism. Carbohydrate and fat are the principal substrates for oxidative metabolism (71). The genes related to carbohydrate (genes for enolase 3; glycogenin 2; phosphorylase, glycogen, muscle; phosphoenolpyruvate carboxykinase 1) and fat metabolism (genes for lipase E, hormone-sensitive type, perilipin 1, glycerol-3-phosphate acyltransferase, mitochondrial, fatty acid-binding protein 4, lipoprotein lipase) were downregulated in sensitive skin. Myoglobin and carbonic anhydrase III (muscle-specific), which are involved in aerobic ATP synthesis, were also

TABLE 6.2

Downregulated Genes in Human Sensitive Skin

Gene Title	Gene Symbol	Entrez Gene	S/NS(−)	S/NS(+)
Structural Constituent of Muscle and Muscle Contraction				
Titin	*TTN*	7273	0.08	0.08
Actin, alpha 1, skeletal muscle	*ACTA1*	58	0.18	0.09
Myosin binding protein C, slow type	*MYBPC1*	4604	0.22	0.10
Myozenin 1	*MYOZ1*	58529	0.26	0.14
Tropomyosin 1 (alpha)	*TPM1*	7168	0.28	0.16
Nebulin	*NEB*	4703	0.33	0.29
Kelch like family member 41	*KLHL41*	10324	0.10	0.08
Carbohydrate Metabolism				
Enolase 3	*ENO3*	2027	0.29	0.25
Glycogenin 2	*GYG2*	8908	0.31	0.27
Protein phosphatase 1, regulatory inhibitor subunit 1A	*PPP1R1A*	5502	0.42	0.28
Glycogen phosphorylase, muscle associated	PYGM	5837	0.24	0.28
Phosphoenolpyruvate carboxykinase 1	*PCK1*	5105	0.58	0.35
Lipid Metabolism				
Lipase E, hormone sensitive type	*LIPE*	3991	0.41	0.31
Perilipin 1	*PLIN1*	5346	0.34	0.32
Glycerol-3-phosphate acyltransferase, mitochondrial	*GPAM*	57678	0.52	0.34
Fatty acid binding protein 4	*FABP4*	2167	0.43	0.34
Lipoprotein lipase	*LPL*	4023	0.43	0.35
Ion Transport and Ionic Balance				
Calsequestrin 1	*CASQ1*	844	0.45	0.23
Myoglobin	*MB*	4151	0.16	0.14
Carbonic anhydrase III, muscle specific	*CA3*	761	0.42	0.18
ATPase H+ transporting V1 subunit B1	*ATP6V1B1*	525	0.58	0.51
Signaling Pathway				
Adiponectin, C1Q and collagen domain containing	*ADIPOQ*	9370	0.42	0.39
Phosphodiesterase 3B	*PDE3B*	5140	0.48	0.40
Activin A receptor, type IC	*ACVR1C*	130399	0.43	0.42
Others				
G0/G1 switch 2	*G0S2*	50486	0.36	0.28
Cell death inducing DFFA like effector c	*CIDEC*	63924	0.45	0.35
Tenomodulin	*TNMD*	64102	0.59	0.46
Retinol binding protein 4	*RBP4*	5950	0.35	0.26
Cysteine rich secretory protein 3	*CRISP3*	10321	0.33	0.58

Source: *J Dermatol Sci*, 76, Kim, E. J., Lee, D. H., Kim, Y. K., Kim, M. K., Kim, J. Y., Lee, M. J. et al., Decreased ATP synthesis and lower pH may lead to abnormal muscle contraction and skin sensitivity in human skin, 214–221, Copyright (2014), with permission from Elsevier.

Note: S: sensitive skin; NS: nonsensitive skin; (−): − lactic acid; (+): + lactic acid.

TABLE 6.3

Upregulated Genes in Human Sensitive Skin

Gene Title	Gene Symbol	Entrez Gene	S/NS(−)	S/NS(+)
Immune Response				
Immunoglobulin light chain variable region complementarity determining region (CDR3) mRNA	−	−	2.11	6.60
Major histocompatibility complex, class I, C	*HLA*-C	3107	1.65	3.86
Immunoglobulin heavy constant alpha 1 /// immunoglobulin heavy constant alpha 2	*IGHA1* /// *IGHA2*	3493 /// 3494	1.89	2.79
Inflammation Response				
S100 calcium binding protein A8	*S100A8*	6279	1.49	2.63
Others				
Transferrin receptor	*TFRC*	7037	1.32	2.65
Cadherin 1	*CDH1*	999	1.90	2.23
Serpin family B member 13	*SERPINB13*	5275	1.28	2.38
Actin related protein 2 homolog	*ACTR2*	10097	1.55	2.19
TNF receptor superfamily member 19	*TNFRSF19*	55504	1.40	2.07
GM2 ganglioside activator	*GM2A*	2760	1.68	2.06
Tyrosine 3-monooxygenase/tryptophan 5-monooxygenase activation protein zeta	*YWHAZ*	7534	1.31	2.01
FK506 binding protein 5	*FKBP5*	2289	1.37	2.01
Peptidase inhibitor 3	*PI3*	5266	2.11	1.97
Phosphoserine phosphatase	*PSPH*	5723	1.56	1.96
HORMA domain containing 1	*HORMAD1*	84072	2.25	1.88
ETS homologous factor	*EHF*	26298	1.21	2.37
Transcription elongation factor A (SII), 1	*TCEA1*	6917	1.88	2.84
Tumor protein p63	*TP63*	8626	1.63	2.29
Small proline-rich protein 2G	*SPRR2G*	6706	1.83	1.76

Source: *J Dermatol Sci*, 76, Kim, E. J., Lee, D. H., Kim, Y. K., Kim, M. K., Kim, J. Y., Lee, M. J. et al., Decreased ATP synthesis and lower pH may lead to abnormal muscle contraction and skin sensitivity in human skin, 214–221, Copyright (2014), with permission from Elsevier.

Note: S: sensitive skin; NS: nonsensitive skin; (−): − lactic acid; (+): + lactic acid.

downregulated in sensitive skin. Consequently, sensitive skin stored significantly less ATP than nonsensitive skin. Lack of ATP in muscles leads to abnormal muscle contraction/relaxation, fatigue, and pain (72). Thus, the lower expression of genes involved in metabolic pathways could result in a lower level of ATP, which may result in abnormal muscle contraction and pain in sensitive skin.

Enhanced Acidity May Cause Skin Sensitivity and Abnormal Muscle Contraction in Human Sensitive Skin

Muscle exposed to anaerobic state triggers the overproduction of carbon dioxide and H^+, leading to enhanced acidity (73), which is known to elicit pain via TRPV1 and ASIC3 (43,74,75). Subjects with sensitive skin showed impaired pH homeostasis after lactic acid stimulation. The expressions of TRPV1, ASIC3, and CGRP were significantly induced in human sensitive skin. Moreover, rhabdomyosarcoma (RD) (skeletal muscle) cells treated with low pH showed significantly increased expressions of TRPV1, ASIC3, and CGRP. Finally, by using a well-established muscle contraction model in vitro, we confirmed that low pH could induce a state of abnormal muscle contraction, which was similar to that of sensitive skin. Collectively, our results suggest that sensitive skin may be associated with pain provocation through TRPV1, ASIC3, and CGRP due to impaired acidic homeostasis.

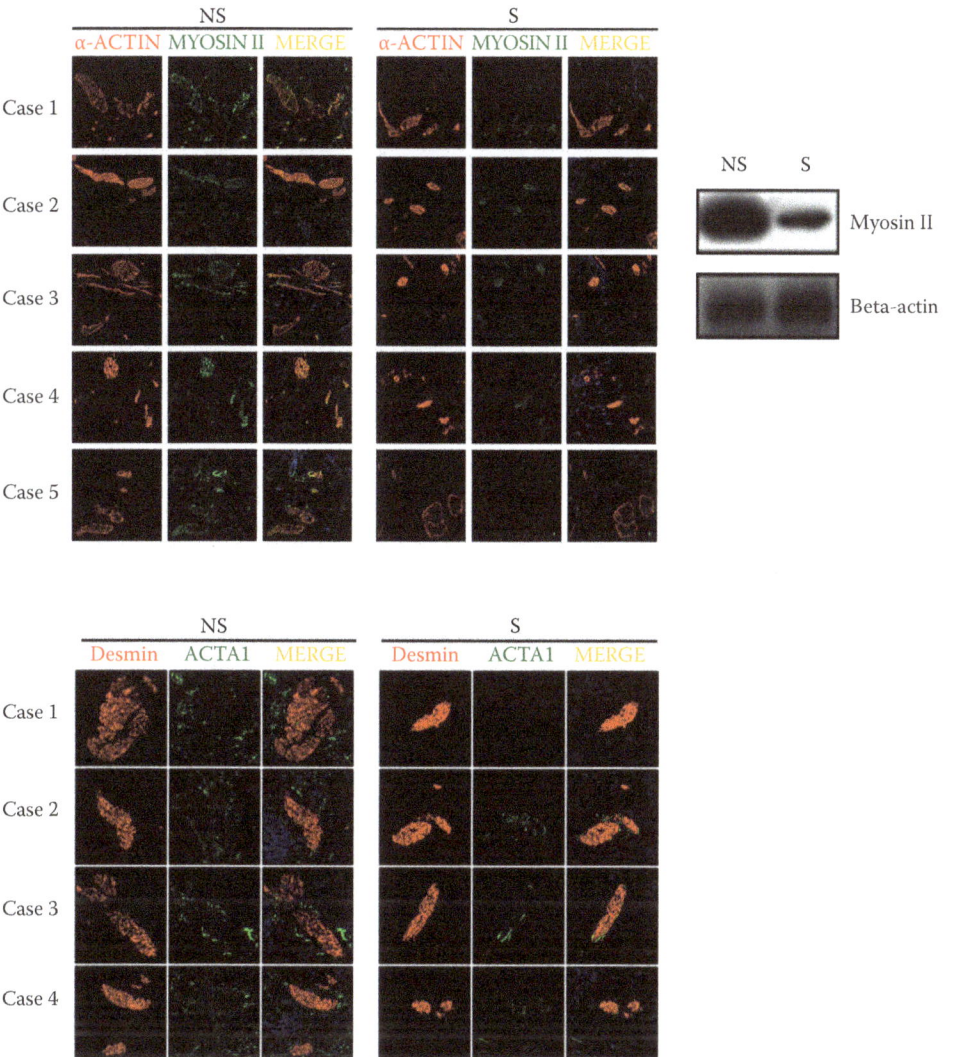

FIGURE 6.3 Actin-bound myosin cross bridges in sensitive skin. (Reprinted from *J Dermatol Sci*, 76, Kim, E. J., Lee, D. H., Kim, Y. K., Kim, M. K., Kim, J. Y., Lee, M. J. et al., Decreased ATP synthesis and lower pH may lead to abnormal muscle contraction and skin sensitivity in human skin, 214–221, Copyright (2014), with permission from Elsevier.)

ADIPOQ Mediates Sensitivity in Human Skin

Adiponectin, C1Q and collagen domain containing (ADIPOQ) is an adipocyte-derived adipokine with multiple salutary effects, such as antiapoptotic and anti-inflammatory activities (76). The expression of ADIPOQ and adiponectin receptor was markedly downregulated in sensitive skin. Adenosine monophosphate-activated protein kinase, a downstream regulator of glucose and lipid metabolism, was also downregulated in sensitive skin (77). Intriguingly, the transient knockdown of ADIPOQ in vitro recapitulated the distinct gene expression signature in human sensitive skin in vivo (29) and showed abnormal muscle contraction, and lower ATP concentration, lower pH, but greater expression of pain-related transcripts such as TRPV1, ASIC3, and CGRP than control small interfering ribonucleic acid-transfected cells. Conversely, the treatment of RD cells with ADIPOQ induced a substantial reduction in the expressions of pain-related transcripts, suggesting a potential therapeutic role of ADIPOQ supplementation in sensitive skin.

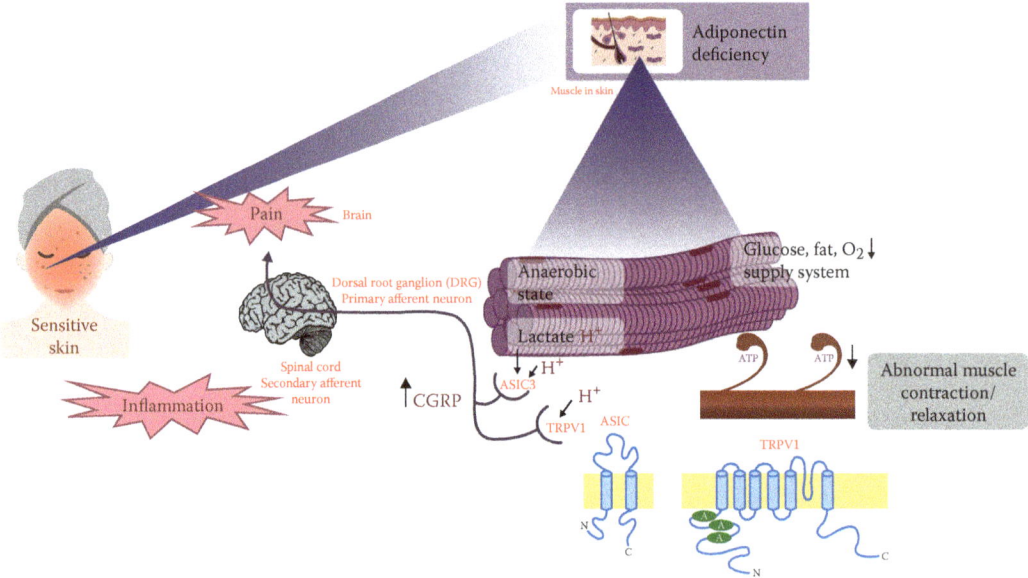

FIGURE 6.4 A schematic model of putative pathway from reduced adiponectin to sensitive skin.

The disruption of metabolic homeostasis can cause variable diseases such as obesity, diabetes, and metabolic syndrome, which are closely associated with reduced ADIPOQ production (78). Little is known about the relationship between sensitive skin and metabolic disorders. Sensitive skin is also linked to ADIPOQ deficiency (Figure 6.4), and reduced ADIPOQ in sensitive skin may influence metabolic disorders or vice versa. Further preclinical and clinical studies are required to confirm its role in the treatment of sensitive skin in vivo.

REFERENCES

1. Farage MA, Maibach HI. Sensitive skin: Closing in on a physiological cause. *Contact Dermatitis*. 2010;62:137–149.
2. Kueper T, Krohn M, Haustedt LO, Hatt H, Schmaus G, Vielhaber G. Inhibition of TRPV1 for the treatment of sensitive skin. *Exp Dermatol*. 2010;19:980–986.
3. Stander S, Schneider SW, Weishaupt C, Luger TA, Misery L. Putative neuronal mechanisms of sensitive skin. *Exp Dermatol*. 2009;18:417–423.
4. Kim SJ, Lim SU, Won YH, An SS, Lee EY, Moon SJ et al. The perception threshold measurement can be a useful tool for evaluation of sensitive skin. *Int J Cosmet Sci*. 2008;30:333–337.
5. Querleux B, Dauchot K, Jourdain R, Bastien P, Bittoun J, Anton JL et al. Neural basis of sensitive skin: An fMRI study. *Skin Res Technol*. 2008;14:454–461.
6. Primavera G, Berardesca E. Sensitive skin: Mechanisms and diagnosis. *Int J Cosmetic Sci*. 2005;27:1–10.
7. Boulais N, Misery L. The epidermis: A sensory tissue. *Eur J Dermatol*. 2008;18:119–127.
8. Roosterman D, Goerge T, Schneider SW, Bunnett NW, Steinhoff M. Neuronal control of skin function: The skin as a neuroimmunoendocrine organ. *Physiol Rev*. 2006;86:1309–1379.
9. McGlone F, Reilly D. The cutaneous sensory system. *Neurosci Biobehav Rev*. 2010;34:148–159.
10. Steinhoff M, Stander S, Seeliger S, Ansel JC, Schmelz M, Luger T. Modern aspects of cutaneous neurogenic inflammation. *Arch Dermatol*. 2003;139:1479–1488.
11. Chiu IM, von Hehn CA, Woolf CJ. Neurogenic inflammation and the peripheral nervous system in host defense and immunopathology. *Nat Neurosci*. 2012;15:1063–1067.
12. Hendrix S, Peters EM. Neuronal plasticity and neuroregeneration in the skin—The role of inflammation. *J Neuroimmunol*. 2007;184:113–126.

13. Bayliss WM. On the origin from the spinal cord of the vaso-dilator fibres of the hind-limb, and on the nature of these fibres. *J Physiol*. 1901;26:173–209.

14. Gouin O, Lebonvallet N, L'Herondelle K, Le Gall-Ianotto C, Buhe V, Plee-Gautier E et al. Self-maintenance of neurogenic inflammation contributes to a vicious cycle in skin. *Exp Dermatol*. 2015.

15. Xanthos DN, Sandkuhler J. Neurogenic neuroinflammation: Inflammatory CNS reactions in response to neuronal activity. *Nat Rev Neurosci*. 2014;15:43–53.

16. Zegarska B, Lelinska A, Tyrakowski T. Clinical and experimental aspects of cutaneous neurogenic inflammation. *Pharmacol Rep*. 2006;58:13–21.

17. Richardson JD, Vasko MR. Cellular mechanisms of neurogenic inflammation. *J Pharmacol Exp Ther*. 2002;302:839–845.

18. Harvima IT, Nilsson G, Naukkarinen A. Role of mast cells and sensory nerves in skin inflammation. *G Ital Dermatol Venereol*. 2010;145:195–204.

19. Siebenhaar F, Magerl M, Peters EM, Hendrix S, Metz M, Maurer M. Mast cell-driven skin inflammation is impaired in the absence of sensory nerves. *J Allergy Clin Immunol*. 2008;121:955–961.

20. Quatresooz P, Pierard-Franchimont C, Pierard GE. Vulnerability of reactive skin to electric current perception—A pilot study implicating mast cells and the lymphatic microvasculature. *J Cosmet Dermatol*. 2009;8:186–189.

21. Reilly DM, Parslew R, Sharpe GR, Powell S, Green MR. Inflammatory mediators in normal, sensitive and diseased skin types. *Acta Derm Venereol*. 2000;80(3):171–174.

22. Nilius B, Owsianik G, Voets T, Peters JA. Transient receptor potential cation channels in disease. *Physiol Rev*. 2007;87:165–217.

23. Kuner R. Central mechanisms of pathological pain. *Nat Med*. 2010;16:1258–1266.

24. Sandkuhler J. Models and mechanisms of hyperalgesia and allodynia. *Physiol Rev*. 2009;89:707–758.

25. Holzer P. Local effector functions of capsaicin-sensitive sensory nerve endings: Involvement of tachykinins, calcitonin gene-related peptide and other neuropeptides. *Neuroscience*. 1988;24:739–768.

26. Brain SD, Williams TJ. Interactions between the tachykinins and calcitonin gene-related peptide lead to the modulation of oedema formation and blood flow in rat skin. *Br J Pharmacol*. 1989;97:77–82.

27. Brain SD, Tippins JR, Morris HR, MacIntyre I, Williams TJ. Potent vasodilator activity of calcitonin gene-related peptide in human skin. *J Invest Dermatol*. 1986;87:533–536.

28. Saria A. Substance P in sensory nerve fibres contributes to the development of oedema in the rat hind paw after thermal injury. *Br J Pharmacol*. 1984;82:217–222.

29. Kim EJ, Lee DH, Kim YK, Kim MK, Kim JY, Lee MJ et al. Decreased ATP synthesis and lower pH may lead to abnormal muscle contraction and skin sensitivity in human skin. *J Dermatol Sci*. 2014;76:214–221.

30. Peters EM, Ericson ME, Hosoi J, Seiffert K, Hordinsky MK, Ansel JC et al. Neuropeptide control mechanisms in cutaneous biology: Physiological and clinical significance. *J Invest Dermatol*. 2006;126:1937–1947.

31. Madva EN, Granstein RD. Nerve-derived transmitters including peptides influence cutaneous immunology. *Brain Behav Immun*. 2013;34:1–10.

32. Mikami N, Fukada S, Yamamoto H, Tsujikawa K. Neuronal derivative mediators that regulate cutaneous inflammations. *Crit Rev Immunol*. 2012;32:307–320.

33. Cevikbas F, Steinhoff A, Homey B, Steinhoff M. Neuroimmune interactions in allergic skin diseases. *Curr Opin Allergy Clin Immunol*. 2007;7:365–373.

34. Gonzalez-Rey E, Chorny A, Delgado M. Regulation of immune tolerance by anti-inflammatory neuropeptides. *Nat Rev Immunol*. 2007;7:52–63.

35. Aubdool AA, Brain SD. Neurovascular aspects of skin neurogenic inflammation. *J Investig Dermatol Symp Proc*. 2011;15:33–39.

36. Gutwald J, Goebeler M, Sorg C. Neuropeptides enhance irritant and allergic contact dermatitis. *J Invest Dermatol*. 1991;96:695–698.

37. Misery L. Atopic dermatitis and the nervous system. *Clin Rev Allergy Immunol*. 2011;41:259–266.

38. Bak H, Lee WJ, Lee YW, Chang SE, Choi JH, Kim MN et al. Expression of neuropeptides and their degrading enzymes in ACD. *Clin Exp Dermatol*. 2010;35:318–323.

39. Yin S, Luo J, Qian A, Du J, Yang Q, Zhou S et al. Retinoids activate the irritant receptor TRPV1 and produce sensory hypersensitivity. *J Clin Invest*. 2013;123:3941–3951.

40. Riol-Blanco L, Ordovas-Montanes J, Perro M, Naval E, Thiriot A, Alvarez D et al. Nociceptive sensory neurons drive interleukin-23-mediated psoriasiform skin inflammation. *Nature*. 2014;510:157–161.

41. Scholzen TE, Brzoska T, Kalden DH, O'Reilly F, Armstrong CA, Luger TA et al. Effect of ultraviolet light on the release of neuropeptides and neuroendocrine hormones in the skin: Mediators of photodermatitis and cutaneous inflammation. *J Investig Dermatol Symp Proc*. 1999;4:55–60.

42. Farage MA, Katsarou A, Maibach HI. Sensory, clinical and physiological factors in sensitive skin: A review. *Contact Dermatitis*. 2006;55:1–14.

43. Caterina MJ, Schumacher MA, Tominaga M, Rosen TA, Levine JD, Julius D. The capsaicin receptor: A heat-activated ion channel in the pain pathway. *Nature*. 1997;389:816–824.

44. Szallasi A, Cortright DN, Blum CA, Eid SR. The vanilloid receptor TRPV1: 10 years from channel cloning to antagonist proof-of-concept. *Nat Rev Drug Discov*. 2007;6:357–372.

45. Patapoutian A, Tate S, Woolf CJ. Transient receptor potential channels: Targeting pain at the source. *Nat Rev Drug Discov*. 2009;8:55–68.

46. Veldhuis NA, Poole DP, Grace M, McIntyre P, Bunnett NW. The G protein-coupled receptor-transient receptor potential channel axis: Molecular insights for targeting disorders of sensation and inflammation. *Pharmacol Rev*. 2015;67:36–73.

47. Ramsey IS, Delling M, Clapham DE. An introduction to TRP channels. *Annu Rev Physiol*. 2006; 68:619–647.

48. Song MY, Yuan JX. Introduction to TRP channels: Structure, function, and regulation. *Adv Exp Med Biol*. 2010;661:99–108.

49. Clapham DE. TRP channels as cellular sensors. *Nature*. 2003;426:517–524.

50. Kim SJ, Lee SA, Yun SJ, Kim JK, Park JS, Jeong HS et al. Expression of vanilloid receptor 1 in cultured fibroblast. *Exp Dermatol*. 2006;15:362–367.

51. Stander S, Moormann C, Schumacher M, Buddenkotte J, Artuc M, Shpacovitch V et al. Expression of vanilloid receptor subtype 1 in cutaneous sensory nerve fibers, mast cells, and epithelial cells of appendage structures. *Exp Dermatol*. 2004;13:129–139.

52. Inoue K, Koizumi S, Fuziwara S, Denda S, Inoue K, Denda M. Functional vanilloid receptors in cultured normal human epidermal keratinocytes. *Biochem Biophys Res Commun*. 2002;291:124–129.

53. Denda M, Fuziwara S, Inoue K, Denda S, Akamatsu H, Tomitaka A et al. Immunoreactivity of VR1 on epidermal keratinocyte of human skin. *Biochem Biophys Res Commun*. 2001;285:1250–1252.

54. Planells-Cases R, Garcia-Sanz N, Morenilla-Palao C, Ferrer-Montiel A. Functional aspects and mechanisms of TRPV1 involvement in neurogenic inflammation that leads to thermal hyperalgesia. *Pflugers Arch*. 2005;451:151–159.

55. Caterina MJ, Leffler A, Malmberg AB, Martin WJ, Trafton J, Petersen-Zeitz KR et al. Impaired nociception and pain sensation in mice lacking the capsaicin receptor. *Science*. 2000;288:306–313.

56. Davis JB, Gray J, Gunthorpe MJ, Hatcher JP, Davey PT, Overend P et al. Vanilloid receptor-1 is essential for inflammatory thermal hyperalgesia. *Nature*. 2000;405:183–187.

57. Prescott ED, Julius D. A modular PIP2 binding site as a determinant of capsaicin receptor sensitivity. *Science*. 2003;300:1284–1288.

58. Premkumar LS, Ahern GP. Induction of vanilloid receptor channel activity by protein kinase C. *Nature*. 2000;408:985–990.

59. Chuang HH, Prescott ED, Kong H, Shields S, Jordt SE, Basbaum AI et al. Bradykinin and nerve growth factor release the capsaicin receptor from PtdIns(4,5)P2-mediated inhibition. *Nature*. 2001;411:957–962.

60. Waldmann R, Champigny G, Bassilana F, Heurteaux C, Lazdunski M. A proton-gated cation channel involved in acid-sensing. *Nature*. 1997;386:173–177.

61. Bhave G, Zhu W, Wang H, Brasier DJ, Oxford GS, Gereau RWt. cAMP-dependent protein kinase regulates desensitization of the capsaicin receptor (VR1) by direct phosphorylation. *Neuron*. 2002;35:721–731.

62. Lee YM, Kang SM, Chung JH. The role of TRPV1 channel in aged human skin. *J Dermatol Sci*. 2012;65:81–85.

63. Lee YM, Kang SM, Lee SR, Kong KH, Lee JY, Kim EJ et al. Inhibitory effects of TRPV1 blocker on UV-induced responses in the hairless mice. *Arch Dermatol Res*. 2011;303:727–736.

64. Lee YM, Kim YK, Kim KH, Park SJ, Kim SJ, Chung JH. A novel role for the TRPV1 channel in UV-induced matrix metalloproteinase (MMP)-1 expression in HaCaT cells. *J Cell Physiol*. 2009;219:766–775.

65. Lee YM, Kim YK, Chung JH. Increased expression of TRPV1 channel in intrinsically aged and photo-aged human skin in vivo. *Exp Dermatol.* 2009;18:431–436.

66. Li WH, Lee YM, Kim JY, Kang S, Kim S, Kim KH et al. Transient receptor potential vanilloid-1 mediates heat-shock-induced matrix metalloproteinase-1 expression in human epidermal keratinocytes. *J Invest Dermatol.* 2007;127:2328–2335.

67. Pinto P, Rosado C, Parreirao C, Rodrigues LM. Is there any barrier impairment in sensitive skin?: A quantitative analysis of sensitive skin by mathematical modeling of transepidermal water loss desorption curves. *Skin Res Technol.* 2011;17:181–185.

68. Kim EJ, Lee DH, Kim YK, Eun HC, Chung JH. Adiponectin deficiency contributes to sensitivity in human skin. *J Invest Dermatol.* 2015;135:2331–2334.

69. Yus ES, Simon P. Striated muscle: A normal component of the dermis and subcutis in many areas of the face. *Am J Dermatopathol.* 2000;22:503–509.

70. Kho AL, Perera S, Alexandrovich A, Gautel M. The sarcomeric cytoskeleton as a target for pharmacological intervention. *Curr Opin Pharmacol.* 2012;12:347–354.

71. van Loon LJ, Greenhaff PL, Constantin-Teodosiu D, Saris WH, Wagenmakers AJ. The effects of increasing exercise intensity on muscle fuel utilisation in humans. *J Physiol.* 2001;536(Pt 1):295–304.

72. MacIntosh BR, Holash RJ, Renaud JM. Skeletal muscle fatigue—Regulation of excitation-contraction coupling to avoid metabolic catastrophe. *J Cell Sci.* 2012;125(Pt 9):2105–2114.

73. Issberner U, Reeh PW, Steen KH. Pain due to tissue acidosis: A mechanism for inflammatory and ischemic myalgia? *Neurosci Lett.* 1996;208:191–194.

74. Molliver DC, Immke DC, Fierro L, Pare M, Rice FL, McCleskey EW. ASIC3, an acid-sensing ion channel, is expressed in metaboreceptive sensory neurons. *Mol Pain.* 2005;1:35.

75. Holzer P. Acid-sensitive ion channels and receptors. *Handb Exp Pharmacol.* 2009;194:283–332.

76. Goldstein BJ, Scalia R. Adiponectin: A novel adipokine linking adipocytes and vascular function. *J Clin Endocrinol Metab.* 2004;89:2563–2568.

77. Hardie DG, Hawley SA, Scott JW. AMP-activated protein kinase—Development of the energy sensor concept. *J Physiol.* 2006;574(Pt 1):7–15.

78. Kadowaki T, Yamauchi T, Kubota N, Hara K, Ueki K, Tobe K. Adiponectin and adiponectin receptors in insulin resistance, diabetes, and the metabolic syndrome. *J Clin Invest.* 2006;116:1784–1792.

7

Itch and Sensitive Skin

Martin Schmelz

Specific Neurons for Itch: Pruriceptors

Afferent nerve fibers dedicated to pain (nociceptors) and to itch (pruriceptors) have been hypothesized in the late nineteenth and early twentieth centuries (1). Unmyelinated primary afferents that responded to histamine iontophoresis in parallel to the itch ratings of subjects were finally discovered among the group of mechano-insensitive C fibers (2). In contrast, the most common C fibers, mechanoheat nociceptors (*polymodal nociceptors*), are either insensitive to histamine or only weakly activated by this stimulus (3). Hence, this fiber type cannot account for the prolonged itch induced by the iontophoretic application of histamine.

In accordance with the existence of dedicated histamine-sensitive primary afferents, cat spinal cord recordings provided evidence for a specific class of dorsal horn neurons projecting to the thalamus, which strongly respond to histamine administered to the skin by iontophoresis (4). The itch-selective units in lamina I of the spinal cord form a distinct pathway projecting to the posterior part of the ventro-medial thalamic nucleus, which projects to the dorsal insular cortex (5), a region which has been shown to be involved in a variety of interoceptive modalities such as thermoception, visceral sensations, thirst, and hunger. Thus, the combination of dedicated peripheral and central neurons with a unique response pattern to pruritogenic mediators and anatomically distinct projections to the thalamus provides the basis for a specific neuronal pathway for itch.

Molecular Markers for Pruriceptors

Functional classes of primary afferent neurons are defined primarily on the basis of their response characteristics. However, functional markers are required to identify the neuronal classes also in vitro. For the separation of functional classes among primary afferents, marker proteins that are involved in sensory transduction such as transient receptor potential (TRP) sensors (TRPV1, TRPA1) and purinergic receptors (purinergic receptor P2X3) have been established. Moreover, not only neuropeptides such as SP and CGRP receptors for growth factors, but also receptors of yet unknown function such as the family of Mas-related G protein-coupled receptors (Mrgprs) are used. Markers that have been used to characterize the neurons involved in itch processing (6) include histamine H1 receptors, the neuropeptides gastrin-releasing peptide and B-type natriuretic peptide, and the several members of the Mrgpr family (A3, D, C11) (7–9). Unfortunately, there are only a few examples for a convincing link between the rodent marker and the functional neuronal class in primates.

In the realm of itch processing, however, we do not have such convincing ties between molecular markers used in rodents and fiber classes in the primate. There is evidence that cowhage induces itch via the activation of proteinase-activated receptors (10). Thus, the activation of a subtype of mechanosensitive nociceptors by cowhage (11) might be possibly linked to MrgprC11 (6). Beta alanine, the activator of MrgprD, does provoke itch in humans (12–14) and activates this subtype of mechanosensitive nociceptors in the monkey (15), but the corresponding fiber type in humans is yet unclear. This is similarly true for the cleavage product of proenkephalin bovine adrenal medulla 8-22, an activator of MrgprC11, that

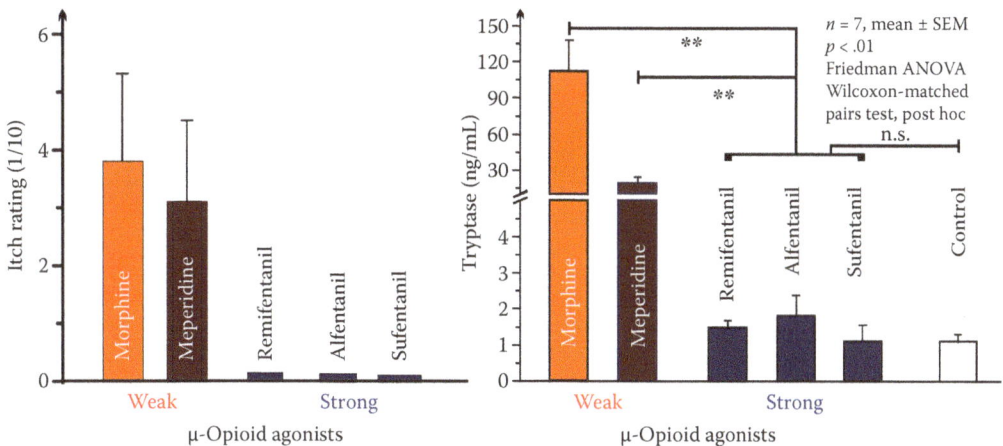

FIGURE 7.1 Weak and strong μ-opioids were applied in the volar forearm of volunteers by dermal microdialysis. The intensity of opioid-induced maximum itch is shown in the left panel (visual analog scale: 0–10; mean ± SEM). Peak mast cell tryptase release during stimulation with the opioids is shown in the right panel (mean ± SEM). Only low-affinity opioids meperidine (40.4 mM) and morphine (3.11 mM) caused tryptase release from mast cells. The potent opioids alfentanil (1.2 mM), sufentanil (0.12 mM), and remifentanil (2.65 mM) provoked neither itch nor tryptase release. (Modified from Blunk, J. A, Schmelz, M., Zeck, S., Skov, P., Likar, R., and Koppert, W., *Anesth Analg*, 98, 364–370, 2004.)

also provokes histamine-independent itch in humans (16) probably via activating MrgprX1, the human homologue of rodent MrgprC11.

Opioid Effects in Neurons and Keratinocytes

Opioid-induced itch has often been linked to peripheral release of histamine from mast cells as intradermally injected opioids can activate mast cells by a non-receptor-mediated mechanism (17). Accordingly, weak opioids, such as codeine, have been used as a positive control in skin prick tests. The opioid-induced release of histamine and mast cell tryptase can be specifically monitored by measuring tryptase concentration with dermal microdialysis following intraprobe delivery (18). In contrast to morphine, the highly potent μ-opioid agonist fentanyl does not provoke any mast cell degranulation, even if applied at concentrations having μ-agonistic effects exceeding those of morphine (Figure 7.1) (19). Thus, only high local concentrations of opioids are sufficient to degranulate mast cells and to induce itching regardless of their affinity to μ-opioid receptors. Therefore, local μ-opioid activation in the skin is not sufficient to provoke acute itch.

However, local opioid signaling in the skin has been identified as an important factor for epidermal homeostasis and including modulation of keratinocyte differentiation, skin barrier function, inflammation, and wound healing (20–22). Thus, therapeutic approaches using modulators of opioid signaling in the skin are not primarily directed toward neuronal effects but use these homeostatic interactions such as delta-opioids for improving skin barrier repair (23). Based on the close interactions between keratinocytes and sensory nerve endings in the epidermis, the cross talk between them (24–26) changes in keratinocyte differentiation, and mediator release based on changes in opioid signaling appears sufficient to cause sensitization and activation of the sensory nerves and thus underlie skin symptoms of itch and pain reported in sensitive skin.

Itch Induced by Nociceptors

Cowhage spicules inserted into the human skin produce itch in an intensity which is comparable to that following histamine application (27,28) but is not accompanied by an axon reflex erythema and is unresponsive to histamine (H1) blocker (29). The active compound cysteine protease muconain has been

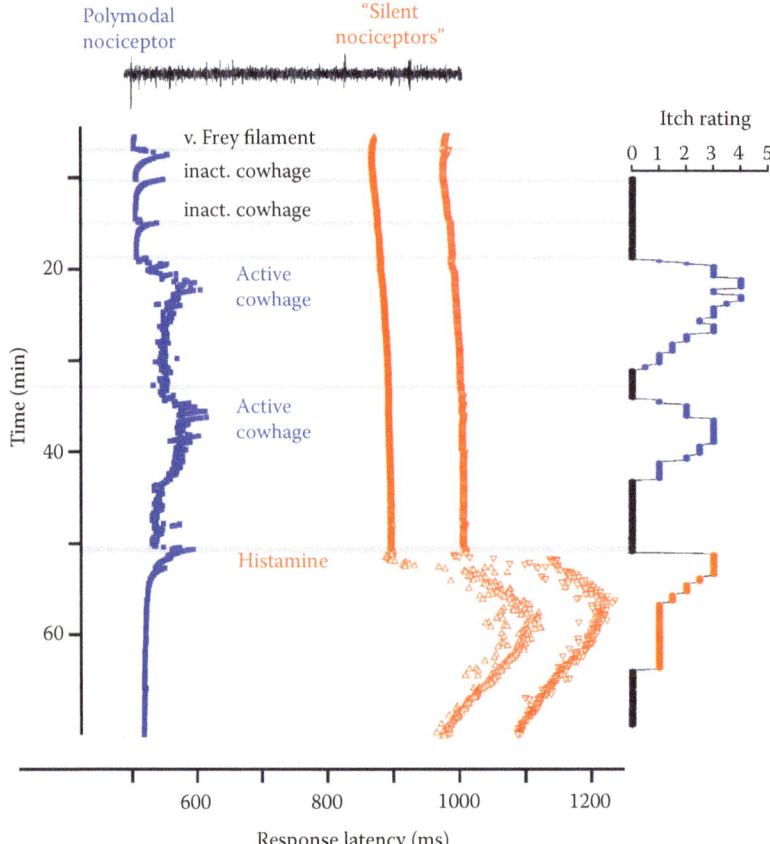

FIGURE 7.2 Specimen of a microneurography recording from the peroneal nerve in humans (raw signal with marked action potentials on *top*) showing action potential responses to electrical stimulation to successive electrical stimulation in the receptive field plotted from top to bottom. Mechanical stimuli (von Frey filament, inactivated cowhage spicules) only activate the polymodal nociceptor (blue squares) as seen by irregular increases of response latency, whereas the two mechano-insensitive *silent* nociceptors (orange-red symbols) are not activated. The polymodal nociceptor is activated by the application of active cowhage in parallel to the itch rating of the subject shown on the right panel. In contrast, the silent nociceptors do not respond to cowhage stimulation but are activated following histamine ionotophoresis. Itch ratings are given on a numerical rating scale from 0 (0 = no itch) to 10 (10 = maximal imaginable itch). Active cowhage and histamine evoke similar itch; however, the first appears to be encoded by polymodal nociceptors whereas the latter by histamine-sensitive silent nociceptors. (Modified from Tominaga, M., and Takamori, K., *J Dermatol*, 41, 205–212, 2014.)

identified and has shown to activate proteinase-activated receptor 2 (PAR 2) and even more potently PAR 4 (10). Interestingly, mechanoresponsive *polymodal* C fiber afferents, the most common type of afferent C nociceptors in the human skin (30), can be activated by cowhage in the cat (31), in nonhuman primates (11,29), and in human volunteers (32) (Figure 7.2).

Given that cowhage spicules can activate a large proportion of polymodal nociceptors, we face a major problem to explain why the activation of these fibers by heat or by scratching actually inhibits itch, whereas the activation by cowhage produces it.

Encoding Itch by Subpopulations of Nociceptors

Considering nociceptors being involved in generating itch, a population code has been postulated (*pattern theory*) (1,6,33) in which only a subpopulation of nociceptors can also be activated by pruritic stimuli, whereas pure nociceptors are only responsive to algogens. Accordingly, itch will be felt when only the first subpopulation is responding but pain will be felt when both populations are active.

The encoding of itch by nociceptors has also been proposed to rely on a spatial code (34) based on the itch induced by capsaicin being locally applied on a cowhage spicule into the epidermis (28). The highly localized stimulation in the epidermis strongly activates some of the local nociceptors, while their immediate neighbors remain silent, resulting in a mismatch signal of activation and absence of activation from this site. It has thus been hypothesized that this mismatch might be perceived by the CNS as itch (32,34). Therefore, it needs to be pointed out that pruritus cannot only be explained by itch-specific or itch-selective neurons (7) along the specificity theory. In addition, the pure spatial pattern of activated nociceptors might similarly underlie the itch sensation without any requirement of itch-specific primary afferent neurons.

Peripheral Sensitization in Itch and Pain

Spontaneous itch and pain are of paramount clinical relevance, as they correlate with the main complaint of patients with chronic itch and pain. It is highly interesting that the patterns of sensitization linked to chronic pain and itch are remarkably similar.

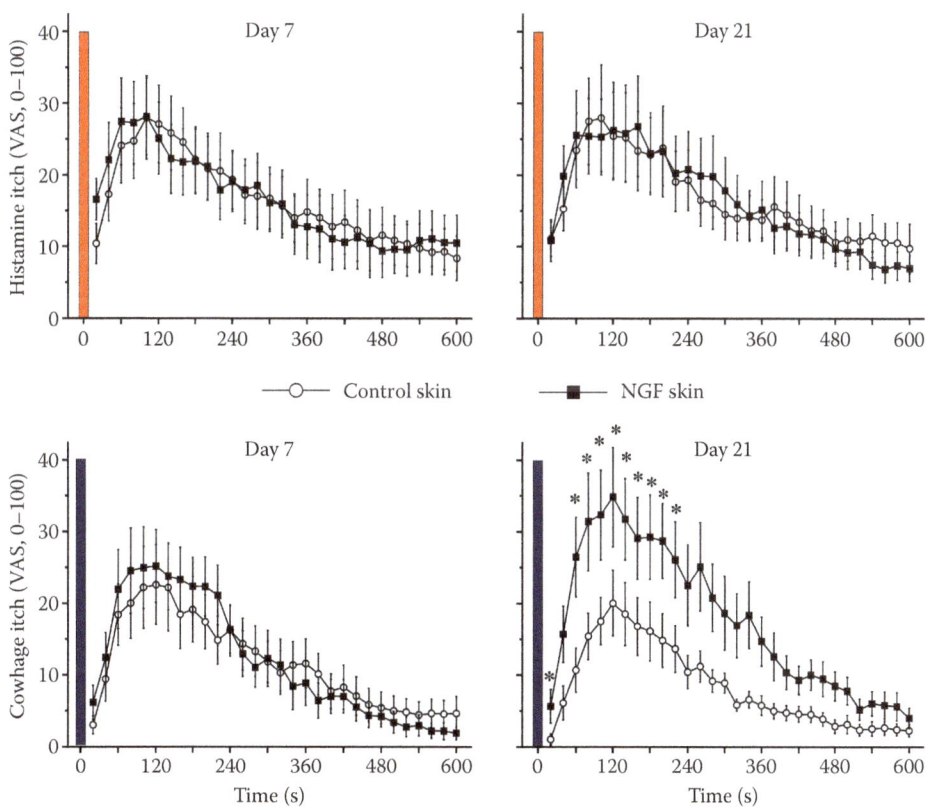

FIGURE 7.3 Itch ratings of human volunteers following stimulation with histamine (*upper panels*) and cowhage spicules (*lower panels*) are shown. The stimulations were applied in the forearm skin injected with saline (control) or NGF (1 µg in 50 µL) 7 days (*left panels*) or 21 days (*right panels*) after the injections. NGF injections did not sensitize histamine-induced itch, but cowhage-induced itch was increased by NGF at the maximum of the mechanical hyperalgesia (21 days; *right lower panel*). (Modified from Rukwied, R. R., Main, M., Weinkauf, B., and Schmelz, M., *J Invest Dermatol*, 133, 268–270, 2013.)

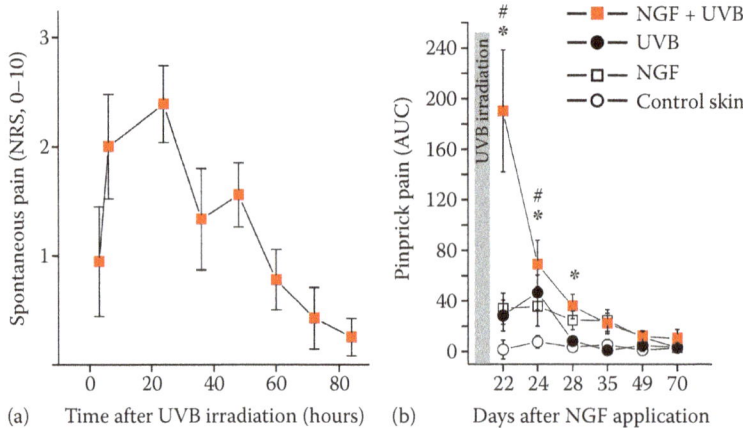

FIGURE 7.4 (a) Presensitization with NGF (1 μg) injected 3 weeks before UVB irradiation (threefold minimum erythema dose) provoked spontaneous pain in subjects with a time course matching the intensity of the UV-induced inflammation. (b) Hyperalgesia to pinprick stimuli develops following intradermal NGF injection and also for about 3 days after UVB irradiation. Combined sensitization with NGF and UVB irradiation causes a supraadditive increase of mechanical hyperalgesia. (Reprinted from *Biochimie*, 92, Okudaira, S., Yukiura, H., and Aoki, J., Biological roles of lysophosphatidic acid signaling through its production by autotaxin, 698–706, Copyright (2010), with permission from Elsevier.)

There is cumulative evidence for a prominent role of NGF-induced sensitization of primary afferents in both chronic itch and pain; increased levels of NGF were found in patients with chronic itch suffering from atopic dermatitis or psoriasis (35–38). Similarly, there is clear evidence for a major role of NGF in chronic inflammatory pain (39–41). Moreover, blocking NGF by specific antibodies proved to be analgesic in the patients with chronic pain (42,43). Anti-NGF strategies were also successful in animal models of chronic itch (44). It is therefore not surprising that intradermally injected NGF not only causes hyperalgesia to heat and mechanical stimuli in volunteers (45,46), but also sensitizes for cowhage-induced itch (47) (Figure 7.3).

Intracutaneous NGF injection does not induce visual inflammatory responses in humans (46), but interestingly, when combined with an inflammatory pain model (ultraviolet B [UVB] sunburn), the subjects report spontaneous pain (Figure 7.4) and pronounced hyperalgesia (48) that also includes axonal hyperexcitability (49). These results nicely match the analgesic effects of anti-NGF in chronic inflammatory pain that are not accompanied by reduced signs of inflammation (42). Therefore, it emerges that neurotrophic factors such as NGF can change expression patterns of primary afferent nociceptors such that their ability to signal pain or itch by local inflammatory mediators is increased. This increase might be based on higher discharge frequencies linked not only to sensitized transduction, but also to axonal hyperexcitability.

Links between Sensitization Mechanisms in Chronic Itch and Sensitive Skin

The structural damage of neurons can lead to hyperexcitability resulting in neuropathic itch and pain. The neuropathy of skin nerves can be quantified functionally by quantitative sensory testing or structurally by staining nerve fibers in skin biopsies (50). The correlation between structural loss of skin nerve fibers and reduced sensory function is well established (51). Unexpectedly, the degree of neuropathy does not predict the level of pain or itch symptoms (52,53). Functional and structural impairments are therefore essential to diagnose neuropathy (54). However, in most cases, neuropathy will simply lead to diminished sensory function without spontaneous pain or itch, for example, in diabetic neuropathy. Among patients with neuropathy, those with pain do not separate from those without pain based on the pattern or the degree of their neuropathy (52,55,56).

TABLE 7.1

Characteristics of Neuropathic and Inflammatory Pain as Compared to Sensitive Skin

		Neuropathic Pain and Itch	Inflammatory Pain and Itch	Sensitive Skin
Functional changes	Sensitized evoked responses	+	+++	+++
	Spontaneous symptoms	+++	+++	+++
	Quantitative sensory testing	Sensitization and desensitization	Sensitization	
		Mechanical hyperalgesia	Mechanical and heat hyperalgesia	?
Structural changes		Reduced nerve fiber density	Tendency to increased nerve fiber density	?
Biomarkers		Methylglyoxal	Autotaxin, lysophosphatidic acid	?
Successful new treatment options			Anti-NGF SP antagonists	

Recently, it has been suggested that small fiber neuropathy might contribute to sensitive skin (56) and could be regarded as similar to neuropathic pain (58). While questionnaires on neuropathic pain appear to be sensitive also for subjects with sensitive skin (58), it is unclear if sensitive skin is also linked to structural impairment of skin innervation. Measurements of epidermal innervation densities of sensitive skin in rosacea and its reduction following laser treatment (59) would suggest hyperinnervation rather than reduced fiber density in the epidermis as a correlate of increased sensitivity. Increased innervation density underlying skin hypersensitivity has been reported before in vulvodynia (60).

However, based on the experience from patients with neuropathic pain and neuropathic itch, it should be noted that levels of spontaneous pain and itch do not correlate with innervation density. Thus, measurements of innervation density in subjects with sensitive skin might not provide crucial pieces of information. The lack of correlation between evoked pain responses and occurrence of spontaneous pain in patients with neuropathic pain adds another key problem. In contrast, evoked and spontaneous symptoms are correlated and highly clinically relevant in chronic inflammatory hypersensitivity. In this respect, sensitive skin—when defined as increased sensitivity to evoked pain and itch—appears to be closely related to chronic inflammatory hypersensitivity (Table 7.1).

Biomarkers for Pain and Itch—Possible Overlap to Sensitive Skin?

Researchers have tried to identify biomarkers for pain and itch for decades. In more recent years, there has been some success as lysophosphatidic acid and its generating enzyme autotaxin have been found to correlate with the severity of pruritus in cholestatic pregnant women (61,62). Interestingly, lysophosphatidic acid has also been linked to the mechanisms of neuropathic pain (63). For neuropathic pain, there is evidence that methylglyoxal, a metabolite in the glucose metabolism, might serve as a biomarker for pain in painful diabetic neuropathy (64). Yet, there are no clinical trials that would use therapeutic approaches based on these two biomarkers. In terms of innovative mechanism-based therapies in the pain field, anti-NGF has proven to be clinically effective against chronic inflammatory pain (42,65). Interestingly, there are also suggestions to use the same approach in chronic itch (44). Antagonists of the neuropeptide SP have failed as a treatment for chronic pain (66) but appear promising as antipruritics (67,68). Thus, there are advances in itch and pain research that have resulted in the identification of first biomarkers and the successful development of therapies. The key question would be how this knowledge can be used for research in sensitive skin.

Perspectives

Our knowledge about mediators and mechanisms of chronic itch and pain has considerably increased in the last decade. In particular, specific markers for pruriceptors and first biomarkers for pain and itch have been found. It appears straightforward to simply use the functional and structural assessment tools validated for neuropathic and inflammatory conditions linked to chronic itch and pain also in subjects with sensitive skin. On the other hand, there are unsolved problems concerning the definition of sensitive skin. Moreover, the high percentage of around 50% of the population appears to be at odds with the assumption that the condition is a disease, unless one would assume that healthy subjects are a minority of the population. The dwindling percentage of healthy subjects as a consequence of the inflation of diagnoses has been criticized before, particularly in psychiatry (69). When based only on self-reports, it is questionable whether a sufficiently homogenous group of subjects that is suitable for mechanistic studies would evolve. Even in a seemingly homogeneous population of patients with neuropathic pain, current approaches try to cluster the patients according to sensory profiles as major mechanistic differences are assumed (70,71). Thus, for subjects reporting sensitive skin, even more heterogeneity is expected. It will be a highly interesting task in the future to define the path for the identification of those clusters for which identified mechanisms of chronic itch and pain are the underlying symptoms of sensitive skin.

REFERENCES

1. Handwerker HO. Itch hypotheses: From pattern to specificity and to population coding. In: Carstens E, Akiyama T, editors. *Itch: Mechanisms and Treatment*. Boca Raton, FL: Frontiers in Neuroscience; 2014.
2. Schmelz M, Schmidt R, Bickel A, Handwerker HO, Torebjörk HE. Specific C-receptors for itch in human skin. *J Neurosci*. 1997;17:8003–8008.
3. Schmelz M, Schmidt R, Weidner C, Hilliges M, Torebjörk HE, Handwerker HO. Chemical response pattern of different classes of C-nociceptors to pruritogens and algogens. *J Neurophysiol*. 2003;89:2441–2448.
4. Andrew D, Craig AD. Spinothalamic lamina 1 neurons selectively sensitive to histamine: A central neural pathway for itch. *Nature Neuroscience*. 2001;4:72–77.
5. Craig AD. How do you feel? Interoception: The sense of the physiological condition of the body. *Nat Rev Neurosci*. 2002;3:655–666.
6. Akiyama T, Carstens E. Neural processing of itch. *Neuroscience*. 2013;250:697–714.
7. LaMotte RH, Dong X, Ringkamp M. Sensory neurons and circuits mediating itch. *Nat Rev Neurosci*. 2014;15:19–31.
8. Bautista DM, Wilson SR, Hoon MA. Why we scratch an itch: The molecules, cells and circuits of itch. *Nat Neurosci*. 2014;17:175–182.
9. Braz J, Solorzano C, Wang X, Basbaum AI. Transmitting pain and itch messages: A contemporary view of the spinal cord circuits that generate gate control. *Neuron*. 2014;82:522–536.
10. Reddy VB, Iuga AO, Shimada SG, LaMotte RH, Lerner EA. Cowhage-evoked itch is mediated by a novel cysteine protease: A ligand of protease-activated receptors. *J Neurosci*. 2008;28:4331–4335.
11. Johanek LM, Meyer RA, Friedman RM, Greenquist KW, Shim B, Borzan J et al. A role for polymodal C-fiber afferents in nonhistaminergic itch. *J Neurosci*. 2008;28:7659–7669.
12. Qu L, Fan N, Ma C, Wang T, Han L, Fu K et al. Enhanced excitability of MRGPRA3- and MRGPRD-positive nociceptors in a model of inflammatory itch and pain. *Brain*. 2014; 137(Pt 4):1039–1050.
13. Han L, Ma C, Liu Q, Weng HJ, Cui Y, Tang Z et al. A subpopulation of nociceptors specifically linked to itch. *Nat Neurosci*. 2012;16:174–182.
14. Liu Q, Sikand P, Ma C, Tang Z, Han L, Li Z et al. Mechanisms of itch evoked by beta-alanine. *J Neurosci*. 2012;32:14532–14537.
15. Wooten M, Weng HJ, Hartke TV, Borzan J, Klein AH, Turnquist B et al. Three functionally distinct classes of C-fibre nociceptors in primates. *Nat Commun*. 2014;5:4122.
16. Sikand P, Dong X, LaMotte RH. BAM8–22 peptide produces itch and nociceptive sensations in humans independent of histamine release. *J Neurosci*. 2011;31:7563–7567.

17. Ferry X, Brehin S, Kamel R, Landry Y. G protein-dependent activation of mast cell by peptides and basic secretagogues. *Peptides.* 2002;23:1507–1515.

18. Blunk JA, Seifert F, Schmelz M, Reeh PW, Koppert W. Injection pain of rocuronium and vecuronium is evoked by direct activation of nociceptive nerve endings. *Eur J Anaesthesiol.* 2003;20:245–253.

19. Blunk JA, Schmelz M, Zeck S, Skov P, Likar R, Koppert W. Opioid-induced mast cell activation and vascular responses is not mediated by mu-opioid receptors: An in vivo microdialysis study in human skin. *Anesth Analg.* 2004;98:364–370.

20. Slominski AT. On the role of the endogenous opioid system in regulating epidermal homeostasis. *J Invest Dermatol.* 2015;135:333–334.

21. Bigliardi PL, Neumann C, Teo YL, Pant A, Bigliardi-Qi M. Activation of the delta-opioid receptor promotes cutaneous wound healing by affecting keratinocyte intercellular adhesion and migration. *Br J Pharmacol.* 2015;172:501–514.

22. Neumann C, Bigliardi-Qi M, Widmann C, Bigliardi PL. The delta-opioid receptor affects epidermal homeostasis via ERK-dependent inhibition of transcription factor POU2F3. *J Invest Dermatol.* 2015;135:471–480.

23. Chajra H, Amstutz B, Schweikert K, Auriol D, Redziniak G, Lefevre F. Opioid receptor delta as a global modulator of skin differentiation and barrier function repair. *Int J Cosmet Sci.* 2015;37:386–394.

24. Lebonvallet N, Boulais N, Le Gall C, Pereira U, Gauche D, Gobin E et al. Effects of the re-innervation of organotypic skin explants on the epidermis. *Exp Dermatol.* 2012;21:156–158.

25. Pereira U, Boulais N, Lebonvallet N, Lefeuvre L, Gougerot A, Misery L. Development of an in vitro coculture of primary sensitive pig neurons and keratinocytes for the study of cutaneous neurogenic inflammation. *Exp Dermatol.* 2010;19:931–935.

26. Roggenkamp D, Falkner S, Stab F, Petersen M, Schmelz M, Neufang G. Atopic keratinocytes induce increased neurite outgrowth in a coculture model of porcine dorsal root ganglia neurons and human skin cells. *J Invest Dermatol.* 2012;132:1892–1900.

27. LaMotte RH, Shimada SG, Green BG, Zelterman D. Pruritic and nociceptive sensations and dysesthesias from a spicule of cowhage. *J Neurophysiol.* 2009;101:1430–1443.

28. Sikand P, Shimada SG, Green BG, LaMotte RH. Similar itch and nociceptive sensations evoked by punctate cutaneous application of capsaicin, histamine and cowhage. *Pain.* 2009;144:66–75.

29. Johanek LM, Meyer RA, Hartke T, Hobelmann JG, Maine DN, LaMotte RH et al. Psychophysical and physiological evidence for parallel afferent pathways mediating the sensation of itch. *J Neurosci.* 2007;27:7490–7497.

30. Schmidt R, Schmelz M, Forster C, Ringkamp M, Torebjörk HE, Handwerker HO. Novel classes of responsive and unresponsive C nociceptors in human skin. *J Neurosci.* 1995;15:333–341.

31. Tuckett RP, Wei JY. Response to an itch-producing substance in cat. II. Cutaneous receptor populations with unmyelinated axons. *Brain Res.* 1987;413:95–103.

32. Namer B, Carr R, Johanek LM, Schmelz M, Handwerker HO, Ringkamp M. Separate peripheral pathways for pruritus in man. *J Neurophysiol.* 2008;100:2062–2069.

33. McMahon SB, Koltzenburg M. Itching for an explanation. *Trends Neurosci.* 1992;15:497–501.

34. Schmelz M, Handwerker HO. *Itch.* Philadelphia, PA: Elsevier; 2013.

35. Toyoda M, Nakamura M, Makino T, Hino T, Kagoura M, Morohashi M. Nerve growth factor and substance P are useful plasma markers of disease activity in atopic dermatitis. *Br J Dermatol.* 2002;147:71–79.

36. Tominaga M, Tengara S, Kamo A, Ogawa H, Takamori K. Psoralen-ultraviolet A therapy alters epidermal Sema3A and NGF levels and modulates epidermal innervation in atopic dermatitis. *J Dermatol Sci.* 2009;55:40–46.

37. Toyoda M, Nakamura M, Makino T, Morohashi M. Localization and content of nerve growth factor in peripheral blood eosinophils of atopic dermatitis patients. *Clin Exp Allergy.* 2003;33:950–955.

38. Yamaguchi J, Aihara M, Kobayashi Y, Kambara T, Ikezawa Z. Quantitative analysis of nerve growth factor (NGF) in the atopic dermatitis and psoriasis horny layer and effect of treatment on NGF in atopic dermatitis. *J Dermatol Sci.* 2009;53:48–54.

39. Chevalier X, Eymard F, Richette P. Biologic agents in osteoarthritis: Hopes and disappointments. *Nat Rev Rheumatol.* 2013;9:400–410.

40. Watanabe T, Inoue M, Sasaki K, Araki M, Uehara S, Monden K et al. Nerve growth factor level in the prostatic fluid of patients with chronic prostatitis/chronic pelvic pain syndrome is correlated with symptom severity and response to treatment. *BJU Int.* 2011;108:248–251.

41. Barcena de Arellano ML, Arnold J, Vercellino GF, Chiantera V, Ebert AD, Schneider A et al. Influence of nerve growth factor in endometriosis-associated symptoms. *Reprod Sci*. 2011;18:1202–1210.
42. Lane NE, Schnitzer TJ, Birbara CA, Mokhtarani M, Shelton DL, Smith MD et al. Tanezumab for the treatment of pain from osteoarthritis of the knee. *N Engl J Med*. 2010;363:1521–1531.
43. Sanga P, Katz N, Polverejan E, Wang S, Kelly KM, Haeussler J et al. Efficacy, safety, and tolerability of fulranumab, an anti-nerve growth factor antibody, in treatment of patients with moderate to severe osteoarthritis pain. *Pain*. 2013;154:1910–1919.
44. Tominaga M, Takamori K. Itch and nerve fibers with special reference to atopic dermatitis: Therapeutic implications. *J Dermatol*. 2014;41:205–212.
45. Hirth M, Rukwied R, Gromann A, Turnquist B, Weinkauf B, Francke K et al. NGF induces sensitization of nociceptors without evidence for increased intraepidermal nerve fiber density. *Pain*. 2013;154:2500–2511.
46. Rukwied R, Mayer A, Kluschina O, Obreja O, Schley M, Schmelz M. NGF induces non-inflammatory localized and lasting mechanical and thermal hypersensitivity in human skin. *Pain*. 2010;148:407–413.
47. Rukwied RR, Main M, Weinkauf B, Schmelz M. NGF sensitizes nociceptors for cowhage—But not histamine-induced itch in human skin. *J Invest Dermatol*. 2013;133:268–270.
48. Rukwied R, Weinkauf B, Main M, Obreja O, Schmelz M. Inflammation meets sensitization—An explanation for spontaneous nociceptor activity? *Pain*. 2013:10.
49. Rukwied R, Weinkauf B, Main M, Obreja O, Schmelz M. Axonal hyperexcitability after combined NGF sensitization and UV-B inflammation in humans. *Eur J Pain*. 2014;18:785–793.
50. Haanpaa M, Attal N, Backonja M, Baron R, Bennett M, Bouhassira D et al. NeuPSIG guidelines on neuropathic pain assessment. *Pain*. 2011;152:14–27.
51. Lauria G, Hsieh ST, Johansson O, Kennedy WR, Leger JM, Mellgren SI et al. European Federation of Neurological Societies/Peripheral Nerve Society Guideline on the use of skin biopsy in the diagnosis of small fiber neuropathy: Report of a joint task force of the European Federation of Neurological Societies and the Peripheral Nerve Society. *Eur J Neurol*. 2010;17:903–909.
52. Martinez V, Uceyler N, Ben Ammar S, Alvarez JC, Gaudot F, Sommer C et al. Clinical, histological and biochemical predictors of post-surgical neuropathic pain. *Pain*. 2015.
53. Uceyler N, Zeller D, Kahn AK, Kewenig S, Kittel-Schneider S, Schmid A et al. Small fibre pathology in patients with fibromyalgia syndrome. *Brain*. 2013;136:1857–1867.
54. Mellgren SI, Nolano M, Sommer C. The cutaneous nerve biopsy: Technical aspects, indications, and contribution. *Handb Clin Neurol*. 2013;115:171–188.
55. Kalliomaki M, Kieseritzky JV, Schmidt R, Hagglof B, Karlsten R, Sjogren N et al. Structural and functional differences between neuropathy with and without pain? *Exp Neurol*. 2011;231:199–206.
56. Wildgaard K, Ringsted TK, Hansen HJ, Petersen RH, Werner MU, Kehlet H. Quantitative sensory testing of persistent pain after video-assisted thoracic surgery lobectomy. *Br J Anaesth*. 2012;108:126–133.
57. Misery L, Bodere C, Genestet S, Zagnoli F, Marcorelles P. Small-fibre neuropathies and skin: News and perspectives for dermatologists. *Eur J Dermatol*. 2014;24:147–153.
58. Saint-Martory C, Sibaud V, Theunis J, Mengeaud V, Lauze C, Schmitt AM et al. Arguments for neuropathic pain in sensitive skin. *Br J Dermatol*. 2015;172:1120–1121.
59. Lonne-Rahm S, Nordlind K, Edstrom DW, Ros AM, Berg M. Laser treatment of rosacea: A pathoetiological study. *Arch Dermatol*. 2004;140:1345–1349.
60. Tympanidis P, Terenghi G, Dowd P. Increased innervation of the vulval vestibule in patients with vulvodynia. *Br J Dermatol*. 2003;148:1021–1027.
61. Kremer AE, Martens JJ, Kulik W, Rueff F, Kuiper EM, Van Buuren HR et al. Lysophosphatidic acid is a potential mediator of cholestatic pruritus. *Gastroenterology*. 2010;139:1008–1018.
62. Kremer AE, Feramisco J, Reeh PW, Beuers U, Oude Elferink RP. Receptors, cells and circuits involved in pruritus of systemic disorders. *Biochim Biophys Acta*. 2014;1842:869–892.
63. Okudaira S, Yukiura H, Aoki J. Biological roles of lysophosphatidic acid signaling through its production by autotaxin. *Biochimie*. 2010;92:698–706.
64. Bierhaus A, Fleming T, Stoyanov S, Leffler A, Babes A, Neacsu C et al. Methylglyoxal modification of Na(v)1.8 facilitates nociceptive neuron firing and causes hyperalgesia in diabetic neuropathy. *Nat Med*. 2012;18:926–933.
65. Lewin GR, Lechner SG, Smith ES. Nerve growth factor and nociception: From experimental embryology to new analgesic therapy. *Handb Exp Pharmacol*. 2014;220:251–282.

66. Hill R. NK1 (substance P) receptor antagonists—Why are they not analgesic in humans? *Trends Pharmacol Sci.* 2000;21:244–246.

67. Stander S, Luger TA. NK-1 antagonists and itch. *Handb Exp Pharmacol.* 2015;226:237–255.

68. Stander S, Siepmann D, Herrgott I, Sunderkotter C, Luger TA. Targeting the neurokinin receptor 1 with aprepitant: A novel antipruritic strategy. *PloS One.* 2010;5:e10968. DOI: 10.1371/journal.pone.0010968.

69. Frances A. ICD, DSM and the Tower of Babel. *Aust N Z J Psychiatry.* 2014;48:371–373.

70. von Hehn CA, Baron R, Woolf CJ. Deconstructing the neuropathic pain phenotype to reveal neural mechanisms. *Neuron.* 2012;73:638–652.

71. Baron R, Forster M, Binder A. Subgrouping of patients with neuropathic pain according to pain-related sensory abnormalities: A first step to a stratified treatment approach. *Lancet Neurol.* 2012;11:999–1005.

Section III

Investigative Methods

8

Challenges of Investigation

Lidia Maroñas-Jiménez, Elena González-Guerra, and Aurora Guerra-Tapia

Facing Sensitive Skin

Traditionally known as *reactive* or *overreactive skin* or intolerant or irritable skin, the concept of *sensitive skin* still remains under discussion (1,2). Nowadays, it is generally considered a complex syndrome characterized by the occurrence of unpleasant temporary sensations of varying intensity in response to physical, chemical, and even psychological or hormonal factors (3–5). Different triggers, such as type of clothing and environmental conditions, also seem to play a major pathogenic role (6).

Patients experiencing sensitive skin typically report exaggerated tingling, burning, itching, tightness, or pain when their skin is in contact with commonly used personal care products, such as soaps, cosmetics, and sun creams. Although erythema, dryness, and inflammatory rashes can be present, visible lesions are usually absent (3,7,8). Thus, facing these patients may become a great challenge in daily practice.

The wide spectrum of differential diagnosis, along with the lack of objective clinical signs and solid scientific tests that guarantee an accurate diagnosis of sensitive skin, is an issue of special concern for dermatologists (9). This chapter provides an overview of the currently available workups for evaluation and diagnosis of patients with sensitive skin from a practical clinical approach (Figure 8.1).

Objective Evaluation

During the last years, important efforts are being made trying to develop standardized measurement methods that accurately reflect the severity of sensitive skin (10). However, quantifying reactive skin with objective tests continues to be difficult due to the broad range of possible symptoms, the absence of evident clinical signs, and the common multifactorial character of this condition (11,12). Therefore, diagnosis is mainly based on a detailed history taking, which represents the most reliable diagnosing method currently used (13).

Clinical Investigation

A thorough clinical evaluation should include a detailed personal and familial history; hygienic habits and topical products of daily use; hobbies; occupational factors; and potential environmental, hormonal, and psychological triggers (4–6,14). Likewise, a complete physical examination is recommended to identify both subtle signs of cutaneous inflammation and presence of other underlying skin barrier problems, such as atopic dermatitis, rosacea, seborrheic dermatitis, and contact dermatitis (14).

Self-Assessment Questionnaires

Because tests for sensitive skin are generally based on the report of sensation induced by topically applied chemicals, the use of self-assessment scales is the best method to identify *hyperreactors* and a valuable tool for irritancy assessment of cosmetics (15,16). Unfortunately, no robust validated questionnaires exist. Gougerot et al. (17) proposed the *Score d'Irritabilité Global Local* as a useful clinical

Step 1: Clinical assessment
• History taking: Familial and personal history, hygienic habits, topical products, hobbies, occupational factors, and triggers (environmental, hormonal, and psychological) • Physical exam: Signs of skin inflammation; rule out specific diseases (atopic dermatitis, rosacea, seborrheic dermatitis, and contact dermatitis)

Step 2: Self-assessment questionnaires
• *Score d'Irritabilité Global Local* (Gougerot et al. (17)) • Scales for sensitive skin specifically related to cosmetic or environmental factors (Querleux et al. (18)) • Scales for specialized locations: *3S* questionnaire for sensitive scalps (Misery et al. (21))

Step 3: Testing methods
• Sensory reactivity tests: To investigate neurosensory response • Irritant reactivity tests: To evaluate visible cutaneous signs of irritation • Dermal function tests: To measure structural and physiological parameters

Step 4: Contact allergy test	Step 5: Psychological assessment
• Patch test: Standard, cosmetics, and own • Open test • Repeated application test • Photopatch test • Type 1 hypersensitivity tests	Refer patients to mental health specialists when there are no signs suggestive of sensitive skin in previous steps.

FIGURE 8.1   Practical approach to sensitive skin.

TABLE 8.1

Overview of Testing Methods for Sensitive Skin

	Sensory Reactivity Tests	**Irritant Reactivity Tests**	**Dermal Function Tests**
Goal	To evaluate cutaneous neurosensory response to the application of different chemical substances, or physical stimuli	To assess objective signs of skin irritation after the application of SLS or other known irritants	To measure structural or physiological cutaneous changes after the application of topical irritants
Tests	• Self-assessment questionnaires • Stinging test: 10% lactic acid (or capsaicin, ethanol, menthol, benzoic acid) • Thermal sensation test (QST) • Evaluation of itching response • Washing and exaggerated immersion test	Assessment of cutaneous irritation by the following: • Colorimetry (visual erythema) • Laser Doppler velocimetry (nicotinate test) • Electrical capacitance • Corneometry (skin hydration) • Reflectance	Parameters evaluated: • TEWL (basal or dynamic desorption curves) • Cutaneous pH • Epidermal thickness (measured by US, OM, or CM) • Skin penetrability (measured by UV light)
Advantages	Fast and easy to perform	Objective and noninvasive	Quantitative and accurate
Disadvantages	Subjective, intraindividual variability, and lack of predictive value	Indirect measurement and specialized complex tools	Time consuming, specialized, and expensive

Source: Primavera, G., and Beradesca, E., *Int J Cosmet Sci*, 27, 1–10, 2005; *Piel*, 28, Rodrigues-Barata, R., and Conde Salazar-Gómez, L., Sensitive skin, 520–530, Copyright (2013), with permission from Elsevier; Escalas-Taberner, J., González-Guerra, E., and Guerra-Tapia, A., *Actas Dermosifiliogr*, 102, 563–571, 2011.

Note: CM: confocal microscopy; OM: optical microscopy; QST: quantitative sensory test; US: ultrasonography.

evaluation method for sensitive skin. The questionnaire developed by Querleux et al. (18) assesses a specific subgroup of patients with sensitive skin, in whom symptoms are primarily related to cosmetic and environmental factors. Although the face has demonstrated to be the most common site of skin sensitivity, significant numbers of individuals experience sensitivity of the scalp, feet, neck, torso, and back (19,20). These specialized locations ideally require specific self-assessment scales, such as the *3S* questionnaire for sensitive scalps, proposed by Misery et al. (21).

Testing Methods

To evaluate and quantify the severity of sensitive skin objectively, reproducible and noninvasive tests are absolutely necessary. According to Farage et al. (22,23), testing methods can be divided into three main groups depending on the biophysical factor assessed: those that investigate neurosensory response (sensory reactivity tests), those that evaluate visible cutaneous signs of irritation (irritant reactivity tests), and those that measure structural and physiological parameters of the skin as a consequence of the irritant effect (dermal function tests) (24). Table 8.1 represents an overview of the currently available testing methods.

Sensory Reactivity Tests

Because almost half of patients with sensitive skin report uncomfortable symptoms without accompanying visible signs of inflammation, new tools of sensory testing have been increasingly utilized to provide definite information (13).

These methods evaluate cutaneous neurosensory response to the application of different chemical substances or other physical stimuli (7). Of them, the stinging test of Frosch and Kligman (25), which consists of the application of 0.5 mL of 10% lactic acid to the nasolabial fold with subsequent assessment of the severity of the subjective symptoms, has traditionally been considered to be the most suitable, fast, and easy to perform (26). However, nasolabial stinging seems to be a poor predictor of general skin sensitivity (27). Marriott et al. (27) tested four chemicals commonly used to induce different sensory effects (lactic acid, stinging; capsaicin, burning; menthol, cooling; and ethanol, a mixture of burning and stinging), reporting a high number of variations in reactivity to the tested substances and a lack of predictive value of increased reactivity among the different materials (27). In addition, an important intraindividual variability has been demonstrated comparing the responses to only two chemicals (28).

Irritant Reactivity Tests

Irritant reactivity tests measure objective signs of skin irritation after the application of a known irritant substance (13). They are based on the topical application of sodium lauryl sulfate (SLS), or other chemicals, followed by the assessment of cutaneous irritation through several procedures, such as colorimetry (visual erythema after the application of varying concentrations of methyl nicotinate or SLS to the forearm), laser Doppler velocimetry (vasodilatory effect following nicotinate test), electrical capacitance or corneometry (skin hydration), and reflectance (14).

These methods are suitable noninvasive tools to objectively quantify sensitive skin but may occasionally require robust specialized appliances.

Dermal Function Tests

These types of tests relies on the measurement of structural or physiological cutaneous changes after the application of topical irritants, such as SLS or others. TEWL, cutaneous pH, and epidermal thickness, measured by ultrasonography, optical microscopy, or confocal microscopy, as well as skin penetrability, assessed with UV light, are the parameters most commonly used (13,14,24).

Although dermal function tests are highly accurate quantitative methods, their use is mainly limited to the investigation field, as they are especially very time consuming and require expensive and specialized tools to be carried out in daily clinical practice (14,29,30).

TEWL assessment is the most frequent procedure performed to evaluate and quantify the function of stratum corneum (24). The basal evaluation of TEWL is able to measure preclinical disease without altering the underlying skin condition by a noninvasive estimation of water pressure gradient above the skin surface (13,24). Some studies have proposed a combined assessment of desorption curves of TEWL and plastic occlusion test to quantify the severity of sensitive skin objectively. Most investigators already prefer this new approach, as changes on skin barrier can be dynamically assessed (26,31).

Contact Tests

To conclude the diagnosing process of sensitive skin properly, Pons-Guiraud (12) recommends performing patch tests in order to find out any sources of allergic contact dermatitis and advise the patient accordingly. In addition to standard series, these patients should be tested with their own products of daily use and specific batteries that include the most common allergens present in cosmetic and personal care products (24,26). Likewise, open and repeated application tests must be performed before making a final diagnosis (32). When photoallergic contact dermatitis or contact urticaria is suspected, workup should include photopatch and hypersensitivity test type 1, respectively (14).

Other Evaluations

Finally, if the whole complementary exams do not reveal any underlying signs suggestive of sensitive skin, the patient should be referred to mental health care providers (14,24).

Conclusion

The high prevalence and complex physiopathological origin of sensitive skin represent a challenge for dermatologists who face an increasing demand for the management of this condition. Because the manifestations of skin sensitivity are mainly subjective and transient, symptoms self-reported by the patients through self-assessment questionnaires, along with an accurate clinical evaluation, remain the best methods of diagnosis. Developing standardized and reproducible testing methods that let physicians objectively quantify the severity of the disease to advise and treat patients properly remains a real need not yet covered.

REFERENCES

1. Kligman AM, Sadiq I, Zhen Y, Crosby M. Experimental studies on the nature of sensitive skin. *Skin Res Technol* 2006; 12: 217–222.
2. Slodownik D, Williams J, Lee A, Tate B et al. Controversies regarding the sensitive skin syndrome. *Expert Rev Dermatol* 2007; 2: 579–584.
3. Kamide R, Misery L, Perez-Cullell N, Sibaud V et al. Sensitive skin evaluation in the Japanese population. *J Dermatol* 2013; 40: 177–181.
4. Misery L, Myon E, Martin N, Consoli S et al. Sensitive skin: Psychological effects and seasonal changes. *J Eur Acad Dermatol Venereol* 2007; 21: 620–628.
5. Farage MA, Katsarou A, Maibach HI. Sensory, clinical and physiological factors in sensitive skin: A review. *Contact Derm* 2006; 55: 1–14.
6. Misery L. How the skin reacts to environmental factors. *J Eur Acad Dermatol Venereol* 2007; 21: 5–8.
7. Berardesca E, Farage M, Maibach H. Sensitive skin: An overview. *Int J Cosmet Sci* 2013; 35: 2–8.
8. Simion FA, Rau AH. Sensitive skin. *Cosmet Toilet* 1994; 109: 43–50.
9. Richters R, Falcone D, Uzunbajakava N, Verkruysse W et al. What is sensitive skin? A systematic literature review of objective measurements. *Skin Pharmacol Physiol* 2015; 28: 75–83.
10. Diogo L, Papoila AL. Is it possible to characterize objectively sensitive skin? *Skin Res Technol* 2010; 16: 30–37.
11. Misery L, Sibaud V, Merial-Kieny C, Taïeb C. Sensitive skin in the American population: Prevalence, clinical data, and role of the dermatologist. *Int J Dermatol* 2011; 50: 961–967.
12. Pons-Guiraud A. Sensitive skin: A complex and multifactorial syndrome. *J Cosmet Dermatol* 2004; 3: 145–148.
13. Primavera G, Beradesca E. Sensitive skin: Mechanisms and diagnosis. *Int J Cosmet Sci* 2005; 27: 1–10.
14. Rodrigues-Barata R, Conde Salazar-Gómez L. Sensitive skin. *Piel* 2013; 28: 520–530.
15. Willis CM, Shaw S, De Lacharrière O, Baverel M et al. Sensitive skin: An epidemiological study. *Br J Dermatol* 2001; 145: 258–261.
16. Simion FA, Rhein LD, Morrison BM Jr, Scala DD et al. Self-perceived sensory responses to soaps and synthetic detergent bars correlate with clinical signs of irritation. *J Am Acad Dermatol* 1995; 32: 205–207.
17. Gougerot A, Vigan M, Bourrain SL. Le SIGL: Un outil d'évaluation clinique des peaux réactives? *Nouv Dermatol* 2007; 26: 13–15.
18. Querleux B, Dauchot K, Jourdain R, Bastien P et al. Neural basis of sensitive skin: An fMRI study. *Skin Res Technol* 2008; 14: 454–461.
19. Misery L, Sibaud V, Ambronati M, Macy G et al. Sensitive scalp: Does this condition exist? An epidemiological study. *Contact Dermatitis* 2008; 58: 234–238.
20. Saint-Martory C, Roguedas-Contios AM, Sibaud V, Degouy A et al. Sensitive skin is not limited to the face. *Br J Dermatol* 2008; 158: 130–133.
21. Misery L, Rahhali N, Ambonati M, Black D et al. Evaluation of sensitive scalp severity and symptomatology by using a new score. *J Eur Acad Dermatol Venereol* 2011; 25: 1295–1298.
22. Farage MA, Katsarou A, Maibach HI. Sensory, clinical and physiological factors in sensitive skin: A review. *Contact Dermatitis* 2006; 55: 1–14.

23. Farage MA, Maibach HI. Sensitive skin syndrome: Methodological approaches. *Cosmet Toil* 2008; 123: 28–33.
24. Inamadar A, Palit A. Sensitive skin: An overview. *Indian J Dermatol Venereol Leprol* 2013; 79: 9–16.
25. Frosch PJ, Kligman AM. A method of appraising the stinging capacity of topically applied substances. *J Soc Cosmet Chem* 1977; 28: 197–209.
26. Escalas-Taberner J, González-Guerra E, Guerra-Tapia A. Sensitive skin: A complex syndrome. *Actas Dermosifiliogr* 2011; 102: 563–571.
27. Marriott M, Holmes J, Peters L, Cooper K et al. The complex problem of sensitive skin. *Contact Derm* 2005; 53: 93–99.
28. Green BG, Shaffer GS. Psychophysical assessment of the chemical irritability of human skin. *J Soc Cosmet Chem* 1992; 43: 131–147.
29. Farage MA, Maibach HI. Sensitive skin: Closing in on a physiological cause. *Contact Dermatitis* 2010; 62: 137–149.
30. Farage M, Robinson M. Sensitive skin: Intrinsic and extrinsic contributors. In: Lode´n M, Maibach HI, editors. *Treatment of Dry Skin Syndrome*. Berlin–Heidelberg: Springer-Verlag 2012; 95–109.
31. Pinto P, Rosado C, Parreirão C, Rodrigues LM. Is there any barrier impairment in sensitive skin?: A quantitative analysis of sensitive skin by mathematical modeling of transepidermal water loss desorption curves. *Skin Res Technol* 2011; 17: 181–185.
32. Lev-Tov H, Maibach H. The sensitive skin syndrome. *Indian J Dermatol* 2012; 57: 419–423.

9

Self-Assessment of Sensitive Skin

Charles Taïeb and Laurent Misery

Introduction

The International Forum for the Study of Itch has defined *sensitive skin* as the "occurrence of unpleasant sensations (stinging, burning, pain, pruritus, and tingling sensations) in response to stimuli which normally should not provoke such sensations. These symptoms may be accompanied by erythema or not. Sensitive skin is not only limited to the face."

The assessment of sensitive skin can be helped by many sensory testing methods, from a stinging test with lactic acid (or capsaicin or dimethyl sulfoxide) and other tests (occlusion tests, behind-the-knee test, washing and exaggerated immersion tests) to the evaluation of itching or QST (1). In all cases, there is a need to get the perceptions of the patients. Because sensitive skin is defined by abnormal sensations in response to a variety of factors, the best method to diagnose sensitive skin is the use of scales (2). To our knowledge, the first questionnaire was the *Score d'Irritabilité Global Local*, but there is no translation in other languages than French (3).

The Sensitive Scale is a new scale with a 14-item and a 10-item version (Figure 9.1) that was tested in 11 countries in different languages on 2966 participants (4). The aim of this study was to validate the pertinence of using the Sensitive Scale to measure the severity of sensitive skin. The internal consistency was high. Correlations with the dry skin type, higher age, female gender, fair phototypes, and the Dermatology Quality of Life Index (DLQI) were found. DLQI is a tool to evaluate the quality of life in patients with skin disorders (5). Using the 10-item version appeared to be preferable because it was quicker and easier to complete, with the same internal consistency, and the four items that were excluded were very rarely observed in patients. The mean initial scores were around 44/140 and 37/100.

Among localizations of sensitive skin, the scalp is more and more well known. An opinion poll was conducted on 2117 persons, which were representative of the French population, and a new questionnaire was validated: the 3S questionnaire (6) (Table 9.1). The total score was obtained by multiplying the score severity of abnormal sensations by the number of these sensations. About one-third of the population declared to suffer from a sensitive scalp. It was increasingly frequent with age. The 3S questionnaire allowed for discrimination between subjects with slightly sensitive, sensitive, and very sensitive scalps. Itching and prickling were the most frequent symptoms. Sensitive scalp was sometimes associated with some scalp diseases. Dandruff cannot be considered as a symptom of sensitive scalp. The 3S questionnaire is a convenient and effective tool for investigating the severity and symptomatology of the sensitive scalp.

These scales for the self-assessment of sensitive skin are very useful for a self-diagnosis and also for the evaluation of the severity of skin sensitivity and the effects of treatments of skin sensitivity.

Degree of overall skin irritation during the past 3 days

Using a vertical line, indicate the symptoms felt during the past 3 days on the horizontal line (0 = absence of irritation, 10 = intolerable irritation)

⚠ Important: To be completed by the patient.

Skin irritation   0   10
                         Min ├──────────────────────────┤ Max

Severity of skin condition during the past 3 days

Please indicate the intensity of each of the following symptoms during the past 3 days. 0 = zero intensity, 10 = intolerable intensity; darken one number between 0 and 10.

⚠ Important: To be completed by the patient.

Skin condition felt:

Tingling   ⓪ ① ② ③ ④ ⑤ ⑥ ⑦ ⑧ ⑨ ⑩
Burning   ⓪ ① ② ③ ④ ⑤ ⑥ ⑦ ⑧ ⑨ ⑩
Sensations of heat ⓪ ① ② ③ ④ ⑤ ⑥ ⑦ ⑧ ⑨ ⑩
Tautness   ⓪ ① ② ③ ④ ⑤ ⑥ ⑦ ⑧ ⑨ ⑩
Itching   ⓪ ① ② ③ ④ ⑤ ⑥ ⑦ ⑧ ⑨ ⑩
Pain   ⓪ ① ② ③ ④ ⑤ ⑥ ⑦ ⑧ ⑨ ⑩
General discomfort ⓪ ① ② ③ ④ ⑤ ⑥ ⑦ ⑧ ⑨ ⑩
Hot flashes   ⓪ ① ② ③ ④ ⑤ ⑥ ⑦ ⑧ ⑨ ⑩

Visible skin conditions:

Redness   ⓪ ① ② ③ ④ ⑤ ⑥ ⑦ ⑧ ⑨ ⑩

FIGURE 9.1   Ten-item questionnaire for assessing sensitive skin (Sensitive Scale). (From Misery, L., Jean-Decoster, C., Mery, S., Goergescu, V., and Sibaud, V., *Acta Derm Venereol*, 94, 635–639, 2014. With permission.)

TABLE 9.1

The 3S Questionnaire

For Each of the Five Following Symptoms (Do You Feel Itching, Prickling, Tightness, Pain, or Burning on Your Scalp?), Which of the Following Statements Best Describes How It Affects You?
No, I do not feel it.
Yes, but it is not troublesome.
Yes, and it is slightly troublesome.
Yes, and it is sufficiently troublesome to alter my lifestyle.
Yes, and it is unbearable.

Source: Misery, L., Rahhali, N., Ambonati, M., Black, D., Saint-Martory, C., Schmitt, A. M., and Taïeb, C.: Evaluation of sensitive scalp severity and symptomatology by using a new score. *J Eur Acad Dermatol Venereol.* 2011. 25. 1295–1298. Copyright Wiley-VCH Verlag GmbH & Co. KGaA. Reproduced with permission.

REFERENCES

1. Berardesca E, Farage M, Maibach H. Sensitive skin: An overview. *Int J Cosmet Sci* 2013; 35: 2–8.
2. Misery L. Sensitive skin. *Expert Rev Dermatol* 2013; 8: 631–637.
3. Gougerot A, Vigan M, Bourrain JL, Mathelier-Fusade P, Tennstedt D, Pons-Guiraud A, Chapalain V, Zourabichvili O. Le SIGL: Un outil d'évaluation clinique des peaux réactives? *Nouv Dermatol* 2007; 26: 13–15.
4. Misery L, Jean-Decoster C, Mery S, Goergescu V, Sibaud V. A new ten-item questionnaire for assessing sensitive skin: The Sensitive Scale-10. *Acta Derm Venereol* 2014; 94: 635–639.
5. Finlay AY, Khan GK. Dermatology Life Quality Index (DLQI)—A simple practical measure for routine clinical use. *Clin Exp Dermatol* 1994; 19: 210–216.
6. Misery L, Rahhali N, Ambonati M, Black D, Saint-Martory C, Schmitt AM, Taïeb C. Evaluation of sensitive scalp severity and symptomatology by using a new score. *J Eur Acad Dermatol Venereol* 2011; 25: 1295–1298.

10

Confocal Raman Microspectroscopy: A New Paradigm in the Diagnosis of Sensitive Skin?

Denise Falcone, Natallia E. Uzunbajakava, Piet E. J. van Erp,
and Peter C. M. van de Kerkhof

Introduction

Sensitive skin, a condition of subjective cutaneous hyperreactivity to various factors, is widespread in the industrialized world but still far from being well defined and completely understood (1). An impairment of the skin barrier function, located primarily in the stratum corneum (SC), is one of the key pathomechanisms considered to be involved in sensitive skin (2). Decreased thickness, imbalanced intercellular lipids, and decreased hydration have been associated with the SC of subjects with sensitive skin or hyperreactors (3,4). A causal pathway between the impairment of the skin barrier function, causing higher transcutaneous penetration of water-soluble chemicals, and skin hyperreactivity has been hypothesized (5).

Over the last three decades, skin barrier function was mainly described in terms of its water holding capacity and hydration and has been extensively evaluated by means of transepidermal water loss (TEWL) and electrical methods such as capacitance and conductance, respectively (6,7). These noninvasive biophysical techniques, although well established and widely accepted by scientists, only provide indirect assessments of the skin barrier, since the molecular composition of the SC is not directly measured. Increased TEWL is associated with an impaired skin barrier while lower capacitance and conductance with decreased SC hydration. Several studies used such biophysical techniques to detect differences between subjects with sensitive skin and nonsensitive skin (NSS); while significantly higher TEWL and lower capacitance were reported in some cases, other studies found only trends or no difference at all (4,8,9). This diversity of outcomes could be not only due to differences in study setup and inclusion criteria (2), but also due to the fact that inherent changes in barrier function properties in sensitive skin might not be detectable with indirect traditional biophysical techniques or variations in individual components could mask the total integral outcome.

In the last 10 years, confocal Raman microspectroscopy (CRS) has emerged as a tool for the in vivo, noninvasive, and direct measurement of the molecular composition of the skin and, in particular, of the SC (10,11). CRS is an optical technique that combines inelastic (Raman) photon scattering with the principle of confocal signal acquisition. The collected signal originates from a small and spatially defined volume of tissue, allowing for the so-called *optical sectioning* of the skin, and carries information on its molecular composition. The measurement principle is schematically shown in Figure 10.1 (12). CRS, being able to detect differences at the molecular level, could allow determining whether the barrier function in subjects with sensitive skin is impaired with respect to subjects with NSS in terms of changes in molecular composition and distribution. This would ultimately leverage new insights that traditional biophysical methods were not able to deliver until now.

The following section describes the most frequently used technical implementations based on the principle of CRS for in vivo skin analysis. Subsequently, an overview of possible applications of CRS in the study of barrier function involvement in sensitive skin is presented. Finally, we put CRS in a perspective of applying it not only for diagnosis of sensitive skin but also for evaluation of potential treatment modalities aimed at restoring, or improving, skin barrier function, both for cosmetic and for medical applications.

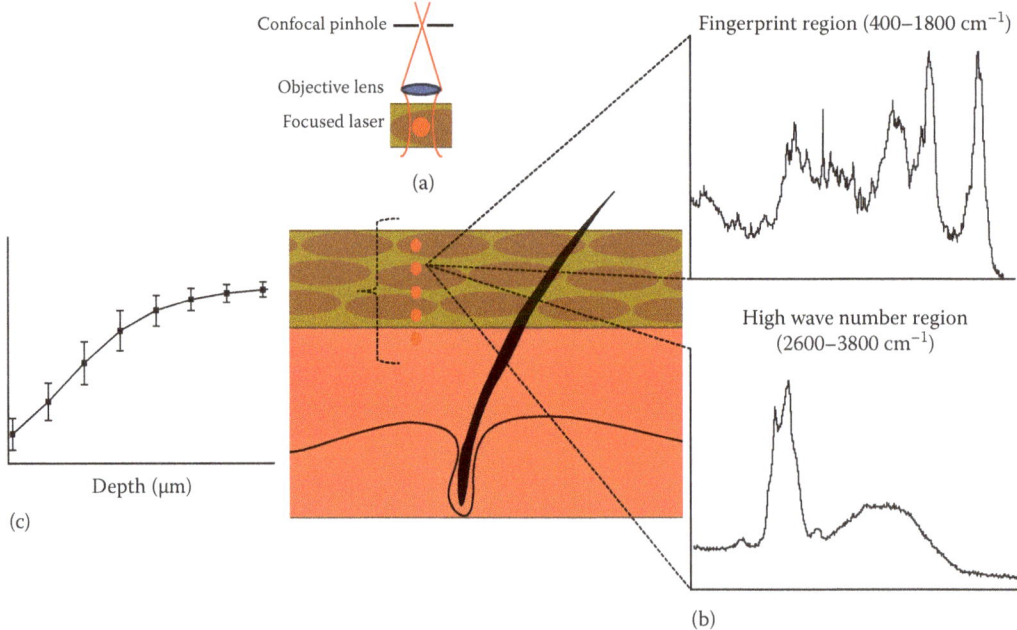

FIGURE 10.1 Principle of measurement of CRS. (a) Monochromatic laser light is focused in the SC in a volume of about 5 μm length (axial resolution) and 1 μm width (dimension of the laser spot). Photons interact with the molecules, releasing some of their energy. Of the photons that exit the skin, only the ones coming from the focus region are detected thanks to the presence of a confocal pinhole. (b) The photons which underwent frequency shifts due to the release of energy to molecules during interaction are used to obtain Raman spectra. The position and the intensity of each peak are representative of the different molecules and their amounts, respectively. Raman spectra can be obtained in a low-(fingerprint) as well as high-energetic region; each region contains different information about the molecular composition of the SC. (c) By focusing the laser light at different depths, concentration profiles of molecules are obtained. The minimum measurement time for acquiring a spectrum ranges from 1 to 3 s according to the energetic region. (Modified from Falcone et al. (12).)

Technical Implementations

The first commercially available confocal Raman instrumentation for in vivo measurements on human subjects was introduced on the market in 2004 (model 3510 skin composition analyzer, RiverD International B.V., the Netherlands) (13). The device consists of an inverted microscope coupled to a Raman microspectrometer assembled on a top-table configuration (10). Laser light is transmitted from the source to the sample through a flat fused silica window. The skin of the volunteer has to be placed in contact with the window, and laser light is focused at different depths by means of a precision translation table. While this top-table implementation allows obtaining an excellent refractive index matching, leading to maintenance of a good depth resolution and of a high signal-to-noise ratio, it limits the body locations that can be measured (14).

An alternative technical implementation overcoming this inconvenience is based on coupling the Raman microspectrometer with fiber optic probes for sample irradiation and scattered light collection (15). While this design allows easier handling of the probe with access to more body locations, technical issues linked to the fiber optic design arise, such as lower depth-resolving power in the SC and strong background signal in the fingerprint region given by the fused silica used in the fiber construction (14).

In vivo confocal Raman instruments may typically employ one or two laser sources in the visible or near infrared range (10,11); the choice of the wavelength depends on the application, since shorter wavelengths allow faster collection of Raman spectra but generate higher tissue autofluorescence in the fingerprint region, while longer wavelengths generate less autofluorescence but require longer exposure times (13).

Characterization of SC Molecular Composition and Structure

Water

Water content measured with CRS is usually expressed as the ratio of the Raman signal intensity of water band (due to OH-stretching vibrations) integrated from 3350 to 3550 cm^{-1} to that of protein (due to CH$_3$ symmetric stretching vibrations) integrated from 2910 to 2965 cm^{-1} (10). Normalization by the protein band serves to compensate for signal losses taking place at increasing depths. A typical water concentration profile obtained with CRS is shown in Figure 10.2. The validity of this method of water measurement was demonstrated by comparison with the Karl Fisher titration method in an ex vivo study (16). Decreased capacitance values, as well as subjective assessment of dry skin, have been reported for sensitive skin in experimental and epidemiological studies, respectively (4,17). As CRS is validated and gives water concentration as a function of depth in the skin, we recommend benchmarking of subjective assessments as well as of traditional biophysical measurements with the direct measurement of the water content in the SC by means of CRS. Besides measuring water concentration at baseline, the water holding properties of the SC could be evaluated dynamically following, for example, exogenous water application (18,19). Changes in water holding properties could be due to an interplay of factors linked to barrier function structure and composition (such as corneocyte maturity, lipid amount and organization, surface path length (19)), water binding to hygroscopic substances (natural moisturizing factor [NMF]) (20), and water diffusion in SC due to different mobilities of water molecules. Many of these factors can be measured by CRS, as described in the following paragraphs. For what concerns water diffusion in SC, a study showed that CRS can distinguish the contributions of three different water-binding states (unbound, partially bound, and totally bound), determined by the strength of hydrogen bonds between the water molecules and other SC components (21).

As a last remark, one study reported that two distinct groups of subjects could be identified based on the difference in water profiles measured with CRS before and after repetitive tape stripping: one group with almost no changes in the water profile and a group in which considerable changes were present (22).

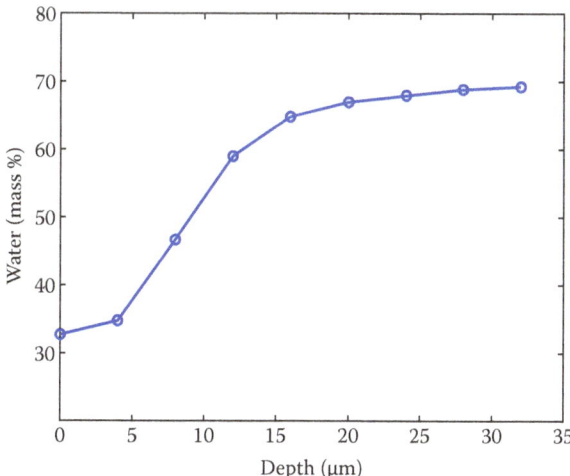

FIGURE 10.2 Water concentration profile measured on the volar forearm of a healthy volunteer. Water concentration shows a steep gradient across the SC and reaches a plateau in the upper epidermis. The determination of water concentration is quantitative (i.e., expressed in grams of water per 100 g of wet tissue or mass percentage) because of the addition of a *calibration factor* based on a solution of protein in water (see data in Caspers et al. (10)).

The difference in water influx from the viable epidermis following tape stripping could reflect differences in SC composition and be possibly linked to sensitive skin.

Natural Moisturizing Factor

NMF is a hygroscopic mixture of several substances, including amino acids and their derivatives, mainly derived from the degradation of the epidermal protein filaggrin (FLG), as well as components such as urea, lactate, sodium, and potassium, derived from eccrine sweat (23). NMF is an efficient humectant, helping to bind water within the cells and to maintain skin hydration and flexibility (24). It could therefore be another parameter of interest in the evaluation of water-handling properties in the SC of subjects with sensitive skin. The relation between the amount of (bound) water and the NMF content across the SC could also be explored (25). NMF information in Raman spectra can be extracted from the fingerprint region, and a semiquantitative method based on least square fitting with good agreement with in vitro results has been described (10). A typical NMF concentration profile obtained with CRS is shown in Figure 10.3.

Less clear is the role of NMF content on the impairment of skin barrier. Previous studies have shown that patients with atopic dermatitis (AD) carrying mutations in the FLG gene have significantly lower NMF content with respect to wild-type AD patients; at the same time, no significant differences could be found in the impairment of the skin barrier evaluated with TEWL (26,27). Similarly, sensitive skin could be characterized by a decrease in NMF, explaining the frequent association with dryness symptoms, and yet no detectable difference at the level of skin barrier impairment measured by TEWL.

Intercellular Lipids

The lipid matrix surrounding the corneocytes in the SC plays an essential role in the skin barrier function by preventing loss of water and other electrolytes and by blocking the entry of exogenous compounds (28). The lipid matrix is composed of a mixture of ceramides, cholesterol, and fatty acids arranged in parallel layers (lamellae) between the corneocytes; within the lamellae, lipids are present in three different lateral organizations, ranging from a very dense to a disordered liquid phase (29). An imbalance

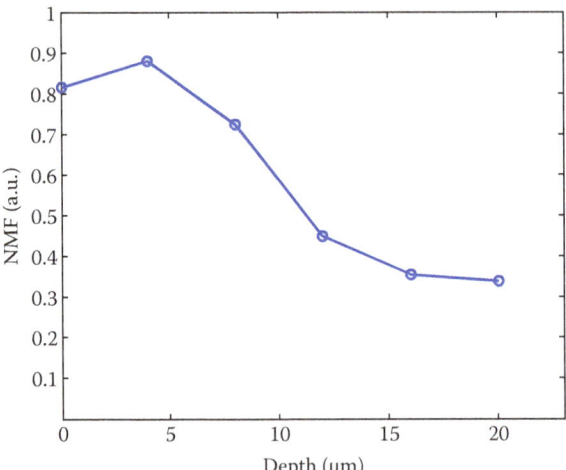

FIGURE 10.3 NMF concentration profile measured on the volar forearm of a healthy volunteer. Increase of NMF from the bottom of the SC is in correspondence with the degradation process of FLG. The characteristic depletion near the skin surface has been associated with washing-out processes, for example, due to daily cleansing (24). NMF is expressed here as the weighted sum of the dominant constituents pyrrolidone carboxylic acid, ornithine, serine, proline, glycine, histidine, and alanine. The determination of NMF concentration is semiquantitative (i.e., expressed in arbitrary units, relative to the concentration of keratin) (see data in Caspers et al. (10)).

of the intercellular lipids has been suggested among the mechanisms leading to an impaired barrier function in sensitive skin (3). In addition, a study demonstrated decreased ceramide levels in the face of subjects with sensitive skin (30). Several spectral features providing direct information on the lateral organization and the conformational order of the lipid chains have been identified in both the fingerprint and high wave number regions (31). In addition, the same semiquantitative method developed for NMF can be used to differentiate cholesterol from ceramides/fatty acid contribution (10). Finally, lipid content can be expressed as the ratio of the Raman signal of lipids (due to CH_2 asymmetric stretching) integrated from 2866 to 2900 cm^{-1} to that of protein (due to CH_3 symmetric stretching vibrations) integrated from 2910 to 2965 cm^{-1} (32).

Besides the diagnosis of sensitive skin, lipid measurement with CRS could be beneficial for studies of the adverse effects of psychological stress on sensitive skin and on other skin disorders. In fact, stress resulted as one of the main triggering stimuli of sensitive skin in an epidemiological study (33) and an association with the exacerbation of several skin disorders is recognized (34). Epidermal lipid synthesis was shown to decrease following acute psychological stress, possibly due to increased glucocorticoid levels; this, in turn, would decrease the production and secretion of lamellar bodies, necessary for the recovery of barrier function following perturbation (34). Such mechanism would explain the delayed recovery of barrier function following tape stripping in the presence of various types of stress (35,36).

Stratum Corneum Thickness

The high end of the steep water concentration profile measured with CRS has been identified as the boundary between the SC and the stratum granulosum (10,37). Several algorithms to determine the SC thickness have been developed and validated against other techniques with similar spatial resolution (38–40).

A thinner SC had been hypothesized in sensitive skin (3). Also, it is evident that daily activities as well as personal care treatments subject the skin to mild mechanical trauma (e.g., shaving, exfoliating, scratching, rubbing, clothing). The high spatial resolution afforded by CRS might help determine

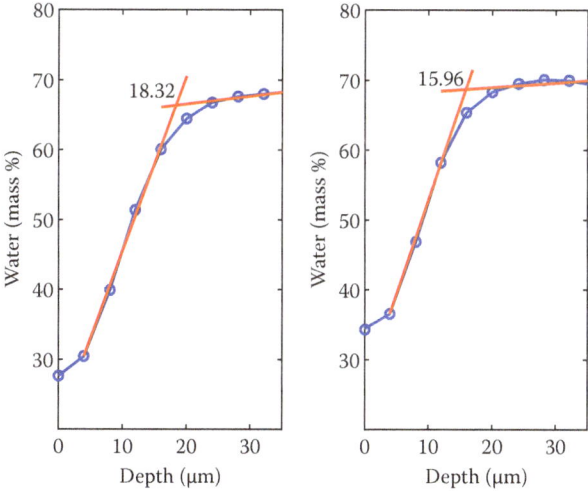

FIGURE 10.4 Examples of SC thickness calculated from the water concentration profile as the intersection of two straight lines in the SC and upper epidermis (38). The fit with a linear model in the SC follows the assumption of validity of Fick's first law of diffusion (38). Both water concentration profiles represent the average profile measured on the volar forearm of six volunteers, where subjects with sensitive skin and NSS were included. *Left*, baseline (SC thickness = 18.32 μm); *right*, following a mild skin MDA treatment using a Philips VisaCare home use device (SC thickness = 15.96 μm). The sensitivity of measurements with CRS allows for the monitoring of small changes in thickness of the superficial layers of the SC, such as those occurring after a mild abrasion. Hydration in the deeper layers stays constant, indicating that the skin barrier function remains intact.

whether changes between the SC thickness of subjects with sensitive skin and NSS are present and how these subjects respond to mild mechanical trauma. An example of how CRS allows for the monitoring of small changes in thickness of the SC is shown in Figure 10.4. Here, we compared the SC thickness calculated at baseline and following a mild skin microdermabrasion (MDA) treatment using a Philips VisaCare* home use device, which shows gentle removal of the outmost cells composing the SC. Further evaluation of the water profile with CRS also confirms that hydration in the deeper layers stays constant, indicating that the skin barrier function stays intact after MDA. This is an important parameter to consider when evaluating the impact of personal care treatments on the skin and, in particular, on subjects with sensitive skin.

Transcutaneous Penetration of Substances

CRS can be used to investigate the transcutaneous penetration of topically applied substances, provided that these have a distinct Raman signature and are applied in sufficient amounts to be detected by currently available spectrophotometers (41). In addition to the kinetics of penetration, the effects of different vehicles on the delivery of active ingredients into the skin can be distinguished (42). Good agreement between in vivo measurement with CRS and in vitro measurements with Franz-type diffusion cells has been found for different substances (43,44).

Sensory testing methods based on the report of sensations induced by topically applied substances have been utilized in the diagnosis of sensitive skin for years (3,5). Despite being quick, easy, and inexpensive to perform, these methods lack objective criteria (5). The concomitant measurement of the topically applied substance with CRS would allow correlation of the subjective assessments of intensity and time to onset of the sensation with the objective measurements of amount and penetration kinetics of the substance in the skin. With CRS, transcutaneous penetration of substances can also be evaluated in light of the biomolecular composition and structure of the skin barrier. It would thus be possible to determine whether the hyperreactivity of sensitive skin to exogenous substances is more linked to an impairment of the barrier function, to an acceleration of the neurosensory system, or to a concomitant effect of both.

Evaluation of Treatments for Barrier Function Repair and Improvement

As no consensus on definition and pathophysiology of sensitive skin has been reached at this point in time, no standardized and validated treatments for sensitive skin have been proposed so far (3). Yet as the current evidence suggests an impairment of the skin barrier function, solutions aimed at its improvement and, if necessary, repair, might be the first ones to consider as remedies for sensitive skin treatment.

Previous studies have elucidated the repair mechanisms that lead to the restoration of the skin barrier following damage due to mechanical (tape stripping) or chemical (solvent, detergent) perturbations (45). Within the first minutes after damage, preformed lamellar bodies containing epidermal lipid precursors and enzymes involved in the extracellular processing of lipids are released from keratinocytes in the stratum granulosum, situated at the boundary with the SC. Subsequently, new lamellar bodies are formed and secreted in an accelerated fashion sustained by an increased activity of enzymes responsible for de novo lipid synthesis. The precursors of epidermal lipids are processed by the enzymes in the extracellular space of the SC, leading to the formation of ceramides, fatty acids, and cholesterol, ultimately contributing to the restoration of the barrier function.

Interestingly, several physical modalities with the ability to accelerate or delay this barrier repair process have been found, among which temperature, electric potential and visible light (46). For example, exposure of tape-stripped human and murine skins at temperature between 36°C and 40°C accelerated barrier recovery, while exposure at 42°C delayed recovery. These effects were attributed to the cation-permeable channels TRPV4 and TRPV1, present in epidermal keratinocytes and activated by

---

* Philips and VisaCare are registered trademarks in the name of Koninklijke Philips N.V.

temperatures at and above 35°C and 42°C, respectively. The influx of calcium ions into epidermal keratinocytes, previously shown to delay lamellar body secretion, could explain the delaying effects of TRPV1 but not the accelerating effects of TRPV4 (47). Other signaling systems regulating lamellar body secretion might play a role here and remain to be elucidated. As another example, exposure of tape-stripped murine skin to red light (550–670 nm) accelerated barrier recovery, while exposure to blue light (430–510 nm) delayed recovery. These results suggest the presence of a sensory system for visible radiation in the epidermis. This hypothesis is supported by the discovery of the expression of an opsin-like protein, a photosensitive protein found in the retina, in human epidermal cells (46). Next to this, the application of blue light to human epidermal keratinocytes and fibroblasts resulted in a dose-dependent reduction in proliferation due to an increased differentiation, as shown in in vitro studies (48,49). This effect laid a base for the treatment of hyperproliferative skin conditions; promising results in clinical trials involving patients with psoriasis vulgaris and atopic eczema have already been reported (50,51).

Temperature, electrical potential, visible light, and other physical factors shown to accelerate barrier function recovery could constitute innovative treatments for the restoration of skin barrier homeostasis in sensitive skin following acute perturbations. Their long-term use might also determine an overall improvement of the barrier function, leading to decreased transcutaneous penetration of irritants and consequent soothed sensory hyperreactivity (4). CRS, with its biomolecular discrimination capacity, high spatial and temporal resolution, and nondestructive nature, could provide valuable insights into such mechanisms, when applied during skin barrier studies. This is supported by a recent study where acute increase of ceramide levels attributed to increased lamellar body secretion was measured with CRS following skin barrier perturbation with sodium lauryl sulfate (SLS) (52).

Summary and Conclusion

Although sensitive skin has been investigated for years, a clear and consistent picture of the pathomechanisms involved in this condition is still lacking. Indirect assessments of barrier function and hydration by means of TEWL and electrical methods such as capacitance lack specificity and sensitivity if barrier function impairment in sensitive skin is subtle. CRS, being able to detect differences at the molecular level, could provide a breakthrough in the evaluation of barrier function involvement in sensitive skin. The underlying causes of impaired skin barrier, such as changes in molecular composition, could be directly measured in a depth-resolved, in vivo, and noninvasive way. The subjective assessment of cutaneous hyperreactivity involved in sensitive skin could be linked to the objective measurement of increased transcutaneous penetration of a topically applied substance. In addition to sensitive skin diagnosis, CRS could start playing a leading role in the evaluation of innovative treatments for barrier function restoration, not only for sensitive skin but also for hyperproliferative skin conditions such as psoriasis and atopic dermatitis.

In conclusion, CRS could open the way to more focused diagnosis of skin conditions involving the barrier function, helping to pave the path toward personalized treatments based on differences in molecular composition of individual subjects.

REFERENCES

1. Primavera G, Berardesca E. Sensitive skin: Mechanisms and diagnosis. *Int J Cosmet Sci.* 2005;27:1–10.
2. Richters R, Falcone D, Uzunbajakava N, Verkruysse W, van Erp P, van de Kerkhof P. What is sensitive skin? A systematic literature review of objective measurements. *Skin Pharmacol Physiol.* 2015;28:75–83.
3. Berardesca E, Farage M, Maibach H. Sensitive skin: An overview. *Int J Cosmet Sci.* 2013;35:2–8.
4. Seidenari S, Francomano M, Mantovani L. Baseline biophysical parameters in subjects with sensitive skin. *Contact Dermatitis.* 1998;38:311–315.
5. Farage M, Katsarou A, Maibach H. Sensory, clinical and physiological factors in sensitive skin: A review. *Contact Dermatitis.* 2006;55:1–14.

6. Nilsson GE. Measurement of water exchange through skin. *Med Biol Eng Comput.* 1977;15:209–218.

7. Tagami H, Ohi M, Iwatsuki K, Kanamaru Y, Yamada M, Ichijo B. Evaluation of the skin surface hydration in vivo by electrical measurement. *J Invest Dermatol.* 1980;175:500–507.

8. Diogo L, Papoila AL. Is it possible to characterize objectively sensitive skin? *Skin Res Technol.* 2010;16:30–37.

9. Distante F, Rigano L, D'Agostino R, Bonfigli A, Berardesca E. Intra- and inter-individual differences in sensitive skin. *Cosmet Toiletries.* 2002;117:39–46.

10. Caspers PJ, Lucassen GW, Carter EA, Bruining HA, Puppels GJ. In vivo confocal Raman microspectroscopy of the skin: Noninvasive determination of molecular concentration profiles. *J Invest Dermatol.* 2001;116:434–442.

11. Chrit L, Hadjur C, Morel S, Sockalingum G, Lebourdon G, Leroy F et al. In vivo chemical investigation of human skin using a confocal Raman fiber optic microprobe. *J Biomed Opt.* 2005;10:44007.

12. Falcone D, Uzunbajakava NE, Varghese B, de Aquino Santos GR, Richters RJ, van de Kerkhof PC et al. Micro-spectroscopic confocal Raman and macroscopic biophysical measurements in the in vivo assessment of the skin barrier: Perspective for dermatology and cosmetic sciences, *Skin Pharmacol Physiol.* 2015;28(6):307–317.

13. Sieg A. Raman Spectroscopy. In: Berardesca E, Maibach HI, Wilhelm K-P, editors. *Non Invasive Diagnostic Techniques in Clinical Dermatology*: Springer, Berlin–Heidelberg; 2014. 217–223.

14. Pudney PD, Bonnist EY, Caspers PJ, Gorce JP, Marriot C, Puppels GJ et al. A new in vivo Raman probe for enhanced applicability to the body. *Appl Spectrosc.* 2012;66:882–891.

15. Santos L, Wolthuis R, Koljenovic S, Almeida R, Puppels G. Fiber-optic probes for in vivo Raman spectroscopy in the high wavenumber region. *Anal Chem.* 2005;77:6747–6752.

16. Wu J, Polefka T. Confocal Raman microspectroscopy of stratum corneum: A pre-clinical validation study. *Int J Cosmet Sci.* 2008;30:47–56.

17. Willis C, Shaw S, De Lacharriere O, Baverel M, Reiche L, Jourdain R et al. Sensitive skin: An epidemiological study. *Br J Dermatol.* 2001;145:258–263.

18. Egawa M, Kajikawa T. Changes in the depth profile of water in the stratum corneum treated with water. *Skin Res Technol.* 2009;15:242–249.

19. Nikolovski J, Stamatas GN, Kollias N, Wiegand BC. Barrier function and water-holding and transport properties of infant stratum corneum are different from adult and continue to develop through the first year of life. *J Invest Dermatol.* 2008;128:1728–1736.

20. Rawlings AV, Arding CRH. Moisturization and skin barrier function. *Dermatol Ther.* 2004;17:43–48.

21. Vyumvuhore R, Tfayli A, Duplan H, Delalleau A, Manfait M, Baillet-Guffroy A. Effects of atmospheric relative humidity on stratum corneum structure at the molecular level: Ex vivo Raman spectroscopy analysis. *Analyst.* 2013;138:4103–4111.

22. Boncheva M, de Sterke J, Caspers PJ, Puppels GJ. Depth profiling of stratum corneum hydration in vivo: A comparison between conductance and confocal Raman spectroscopic measurements. *Exp Dermatol.* 2009;18:870–876.

23. Watabe A, Sugawara T, Kikuchi K, Yamasaki K, Sakai S, Aiba S. Sweat constitutes several natural moisturizing factors, lactate, urea, sodium, and potassium. *J Dermatol Sci.* 2013;72:177–182.

24. Crowther JM, Matts PJ, Kaczvinsky JR. Changes in stratum corneum thickness, water gradients and hydration by moisturizers. In: Loden M, Maibach HI, editors. *Treatment of Dry Skin Syndrome*: Springer, Berlin–Heidelberg; 2012. 545–560.

25. Boireau-Adamezyk E, Baillet-Guffroy A, Stamatas GN. Mobility of water molecules in the stratum corneum: Effects of age and chronic exposure to the environment. *J Invest Dermatol.* 2014;134: 2046–2049.

26. Kezic S, O'Regan GM, Lutter R, Jakasa I, Koster ES, Saunders S et al. Filaggrin loss-of-function mutations are associated with enhanced expression of IL-1 cytokines in the stratum corneum of patients with atopic dermatitis and in a murine model of filaggrin deficiency. *J Allergy Clin Immunol.* 2012;129:1031–1039.el.

27. O'Regan GM, Kemperman PM, Sandilands A, Chen H, Campbell LE, Kroboth K et al. Raman profiles of the stratum corneum define 3 filaggrin genotype-determined atopic dermatitis endophenotypes. *J Allergy Clin Immunol.* 2010;126:574–580.el.

28. Feingold KR, Elias PM. Role of lipids in the formation and maintenance of the cutaneous permeability barrier. *Biochim Biophys Acta.* 2014;1841:280–294.

29. van Smeden J, Janssens M, Gooris GS, Bouwstra JA. The important role of stratum corneum lipids for the cutaneous barrier function. *Biochim Biophys Acta*. 2014;1841:295–313.

30. Cho HJ, Chung BY, Lee HB, Kim HO, Park CW, Lee CH. Quantitative study of stratum corneum ceramides contents in patients with sensitive skin. *J Dermatol*. 2012;39:295–300.

31. Tfayli A, Guillard E, Manfait M, Baillet-Guffroy A. Raman spectroscopy: Feasibility of in vivo survey of stratum corneum lipids, effect of natural aging. *Eur J Dermatol*. 2012;22:36–41.

32. Janssens M, van Smeden J, Puppels GJ, Lavrijsen AP, Caspers PJ, Bouwstra JA. Lipid to protein ratio plays an important role in the skin barrier function in patients with atopic eczema. *Br J Dermatol*. 2014;170:1248–1255.

33. Saint-Martory C, Roguedas-Contios AM, Sibaud V, Degouy A, Schmitt AM, Misery L. Sensitive skin is not limited to the face. *Br J Dermatol*. 2008;158:130–133.

34. Choi E, Brown B, Crumrine D, Chang S, Man M, Elias P et al. Mechanisms by which psychologic stress alters cutaneous permeability barrier homeostasis and stratum corneum integrity. *J Invest Dermatol* 2005;124:587–595.

35. Altemus M, Rao B, Dhabhar F, Ding W, Granstein R. Stress-induced changes in skin barrier function in healthy women. *J Invest Dermatol* 2001;117:309–317.

36. Muizzuddin N, Matsui M, Marenus K, Maes D. Impact of stress of marital dissolution on skin barrier recovery: Tape stripping and measurement of trans-epidermal water loss (TEWL). *Skin Res Technol*. 2003;9:34–38.

37. Caspers P, Lucassen GW, Puppels GJ. Combined in vivo confocal Raman spectroscopy and confocal microscopy of human skin. *Biophys J*. 2003;85:572–580.

38. Bohling A, Bielfeldt S, Himmelmann A, Keskin M, Wilhelm KP. Comparison of the stratum corneum thickness measured in vivo with confocal Raman spectroscopy and confocal reflectance microscopy. *Skin Res Technol*. 2014;20:50–57.

39. Crowther JM, Sieg A, Blenkiron P, Marcott C, Matts PJ, Kaczvinsky JR et al. Measuring the effects of topical moisturizers on changes in stratum corneum thickness, water gradients and hydration in vivo. *Br J Dermatol*. 2008;159:567–577.

40. Egawa M, Hirao T, Takahashi M. In vivo estimation of stratum corneum thickness from water concentration profiles obtained with Raman spectroscopy. *Acta Derm Venereol*. 2007;87:4–8.

41. Lademann J, Meinke MC, Schanzer S, Richter H, Darvin ME, Haag SF et al. In vivo methods for the analysis of the penetration of topically applied substances in and through the skin barrier. *Int J Cosmet Sci*. 2012;34:551–559.

42. Melot M, Pudney PD, Williamson AM, Caspers PJ, Van Der Pol A, Puppels GJ. Studying the effectiveness of penetration enhancers to deliver retinol through the stratum cornum by in vivo confocal Raman spectroscopy. *J Control Release*. 2009;138:32–39.

43. Mateus R, Moore DJ, Hadgraft J, Lane ME. Percutaneous absorption of salicylic acid—In vitro and in vivo studies. *Int J Pharm*. 2014;475:471–474.

44. Mohammed D, Matts PJ, Hadgraft J, Lane ME. In vitro-in vivo correlation in skin permeation. *Pharm Res*. 2014;31:394–400.

45. Feingold KR, Denda M. Regulation of permeability barrier homeostasis. *Clin Dermatol*. 2012;30:263–268.

46. Denda M. Physical and chemical factors that improve epidermal permeability barrier homeostasis. In: Esparza-Gordillo J, editor. *Atopic Dermatitis—Disease Etiology and Clinical Management*: Available from http://www.intechopen.com/books/atopic-dermatitis-disease-etiology-and-clinical-management /chemical-and-physical-factors-that-improve-epidermal-permeability-barrier-homeostasis; 2012.

47. Denda M, Sokabe T, Fukumi-Tominaga T, Tominaga M. Effects of skin surface temperature on epidermal permeability barrier homeostasis. *J Invest Dermatol*. 2007;127:654–659.

48. Liebmann J, Born M, Kolb-Bachofen V. Blue-light irradiation regulates proliferation and differentiation in human skin cells. *J Invest Dermatol*. 2010;130:259–269.

49. Oplander C, Deck A, Volkmar CM, Kirsch M, Liebmann J, Born M et al. Mechanism and biological relevance of blue-light (420–453 nm)-induced nonenzymatic nitric oxide generation from photolabile nitric oxide derivates in human skin in vitro and in vivo. *Free Radic Biol Med*. 2013;65:1363–1377.

50. Becker D, Langer E, Seemann M, Seemann G, Fell I, Saloga J et al. Clinical efficacy of blue light full body irradiation as treatment option for severe atopic dermatitis. *PLoS One*. 2011;6:e20566.

51. Weinstabl A, Hoff-Lesch S, Merk HF, von Felbert V. Prospective randomized study on the efficacy of blue light in the treatment of psoriasis vulgaris. *Dermatology* 2011;223:251–259.
52. Hoffman DR, Kroll LM, Basehoar A, Reece B, Cunningham CT, Koenig DW. Immediate and extended effects of sodium lauryl sulphate exposure on stratum corneum natural moisturizing factor. *Int J Cosmet Sci.* 2014;36:93–101.

11

Dynamic Quantification of the Human Skin Barrier in Sensitive Skin Syndrome

Luís M. Rodrigues, Henrique Silva, and Catarina Rosado

Introduction

Some studies regarding the prevalence of sensitive skin syndrome (SSS) clearly reveal values as high as 60% among women and 45% among men (1–6) which, beyond the evidence of the magnitude of this health problem, explains the remarkable boom of a rapidly growing market, especially among industrialized countries. This market, somewhere between cosmetics and medicines, evidenced by some well-known fantasy designations (e.g., cosmeceutics), have led to more discussion and controversy around these subjects (7,8).

The huge amount of research published in the last years has tried to relate this (subjective) often vague, variable syndromes with proper (objective) data, mostly resulting in considerable frustration when taking into account the disproportion between effort/limited study design and quality of results (5,9,10). Although they are repeated many times, special efforts should be directed to reach a consensus on the definition of sensitive skin syndromes (or definition of this condition), including admissible designations, and to harmonize diagnostic procedures and evaluation methods. These are crucial to promote a new quality level of research on this subject. In a systematic review on the literature published between 2000 and 2012 focused on sensitive skin, only 93 papers were designated as noteworthy from 3267 previously identified (9). Selection involved the application of criteria related to definition, epidemiology, demography, and diagnostics, and the main exclusion criterion was the absence of description(s) or evaluation of perceptions.

The mechanism(s) involved with the syndrome present another difficulty. Common SSS symptoms are often reported in association with atopic disorders (including rosacea), dermatitis (also perioral), acne, and psoriasis (3,5,9). Thus, in addition to the individual's neurosensory hyperreactivity, on the basis of which sensations of discomfort are self-perceived (9–11), an impaired skin barrier function favoring the intervention of inflammatory mediators is consistently expected (1,12,13). In fact, several studies have shown higher TEWL values, although nonsignificant in most cases, related to this syndrome (8,14–16). An impaired barrier seems to be linked to lactic acid sting test (LAST) scores (9,17) so that the LAST has been useful in detecting sensitive individuals where higher TEWL values were measured. Higher baseline TEWL seems to correlate with SSS, in particular in the face (18,19). Closer relationships with stingers (compared to nonstingers) are known, but again, only a few studies demonstrated this clearly (14,18,20).

Other biometrical variables are also referred as complementary indicators of impaired barrier function, such as SC hydration, sebum, pH, biomechanics, and microcirculation (including biochemical markers) (5,7,10). Data are scarce, however, and often unrelated. Despite the recognized criticisms, TEWL is still the most relevant variable to consider when trying to characterize barrier impairment in the sensitive skin context.

Two factors should be highlighted:

- Most of the studies ignore the patient's symptoms with reference to its body site. In fact, SSS symptoms are rarely referred to the whole body if not to a specific anatomical area or region. Even so, some specific forms of irritancy are underestimated (e.g., vulvar) (3,5,21), and the most frequently referred sites are the face, the volar forearm, the scalp, and the hands (6,9). Thus, unless there is clear evidence of a generalized impairment of skin physiology, it is important to focus research efforts and means at the anatomical area(s) referred with the symptoms by the patient.

- Although regarded as the most reliable indicator of human epidermal barrier, TEWL assessment suffers from several limitations (8,19,22). The technology provides instantaneous, highly variable (anatomical, climatic, circadian, sweat gland activity) data, and this might explain the difficulties experienced by researchers attempting to detect often discrete changes such as those associated with sensitive skin.

This latter factor is a known problem which has also motivated other quantification approaches (23–31). Skin surface water loss has been presented as the area under the curve (AUC) of a TEWL curve registered between 0 and 30 minutes (23–26), typically showing an asymptotic distribution gradually declining over time. It has been applied in a few studies (26,31), but its great dependency on psychophysiological factors, including glandular activity, and the absence of a clear definition about its nature, impossible to differentiate from true TEWL, dramatically reduced its interest.

The plastic occlusion stress test (POST) is another strategy developed to study in vivo water dynamics following a predetermined skin occlusion (usually 24 hours) with proper material (23,25,26). After patch removal, the water desorption curves were treated with biexponential regression analysis and the AUC was calculated to thoroughly describe the phenomena. This rather simplistic way to describe the complex water balance between the different layers of the skin motivated other approaches while using this POST methodology as a stress test, becoming the origin of extensively studied mathematical modeling of the TEWL curves to enable a detailed quantitative characterization of the dynamic water balance between skin structures (27,28).

In the present chapter, we specially focus this very precise method to quantitatively describe human in vivo TEWL from a dynamical perspective.

Method

The Model

This model was inspired by classical pharmacokinetic/pharmacodynamic models applied to drugs, consisting of a bicompartmental model designed to describe the in vivo mechanisms of water distribution (14,27,28) where compartment 1 represents the skin barrier with the lowest water content and compartment 2 represents the fully hydrated deeper layers of the skin (Figure 11.1). One should note that there are no direct relationships between these compartments and the histological components of human skin.

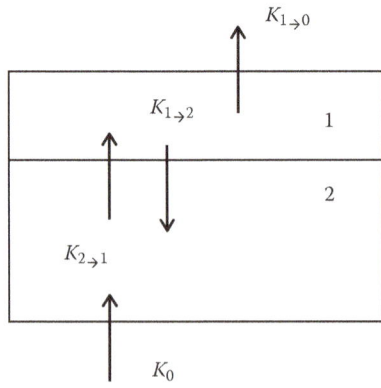

FIGURE 11.1 The experimental TEWL decay curves data have been analyzed using a bicompartmental model. This model simulates the barrier and the inner layers of the skin as two spaces with different water contents. Compartment 1 represents the skin barrier with poor water content, and compartment 2 represents the deeper layers of the skin.

The POST method allows to modify the in vivo water balance between these two compartments so that, from the water flux described by Fick's first law of diffusion and this model, the TEWL can be modulated by two linear first-order differential equations (27) from which an algebraic sum of two exponential terms is deduced,

$$\text{TEWL} = B + I\left(e^{-K_{\text{evap}}t} - e^{-K_{\text{hydr}}t}\right), \tag{11.1}$$

where
  B is the baseline effect.
  I is the multiplicative parameter common to both exponentials.
  K_{evap} is the evaporation rate constant (used to evaluate the barrier function).
  K_{hydr} is the hydration rate constant related to the distribution of the water through both compartments.

These two exponentials are affected by the macroconstants K_{evap} and K_{hydr}. The latter is related to the occlusion period and to the water retention capacity of the SC, while K_{evap} describes the evaporation process to the exterior and is affected by changes to the barrier function. So we suggested a simplification of K_{evap} as follows:

$$t_{1/2\text{evap}} = \frac{\ln(2)}{K_{\text{evap}}}, \tag{11.2}$$

where $t_{1/2\text{evap}}$ represents the evaporation half-life period—the time the system takes to reduce its water loss to half.

Dynamic water mass (DWM) represents the relevant water mass involved in the desorption process. The AUC from t_{max} measures this parameter until the end of the process.

Experimental

These methods have already been explored and published and may be applied as a *barrier* quantification strategy in SSS patients (15,27,28).

A group of female individuals ($n = 15$) with self-perceived sensitive skin, ranging from 23–64 years old, (mean 54 ± 10 years old) was enrolled following specifically predefined inclusion/noninclusion criteria and compared with a normal control group ($n = 18$), age range 20–58 years old (mean 34 ± 10 years old). All procedures complied with the applicable ethical requirements and relevant guidelines.

Subjective sensitive skin complaints focused the hands as the anatomical area of interest. Therefore, we selected a site in the dorsal aspect of each volunteer's hand, between the thumb and the index finger, to register TEWL values with a Tewameter TM 300® (CK Electronics, GmbH, Germany) after applying a POST methodology as a stress test. As previously described (32,33), a standard patch was applied (Figure 11.2). After a 24-hour occlusion period, TEWL desorption curve data points were obtained, to

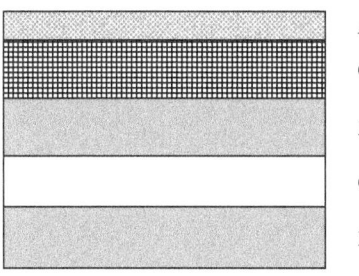
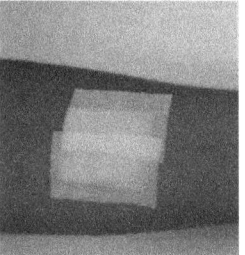

Adhesive

Gauze

Parafilm

Cling film

Parafilm

FIGURE 11.2 Scheme of the occlusive patch used in the study.

which the mathematical model was applied in order to obtain the relevant parameters used to describe each individual's barrier dynamics under these circumstances.

Nonparametric comparative analysis (Wilcoxon signed-rank test) was used, and a 0.05 significance level was adopted.

Results and Discussion

These individuals, consistently complaining of sensitive skin of their hands, presented higher mean basal TEWL values than the control group, but no statistically significant differences could be found ($P = 0.059$), as shown in Figure 11.3. After the patch removal following a 24-hour occlusion, TEWL desorption curves were obtained and data were fitted by the model (Figure 11.4). The continuous lines represent the calculated data obtained by the application of the model to the median individual values. These points are within the range of standard deviation of the mean experimental results, indicating a good adjustment of the model to the raw data. As shown, these curve decays exhibit very different profiles, signifying that subjects with normal skin recover faster than the subjects with sensitive skin. In sequence, this normal skin group shows a smaller AUC.

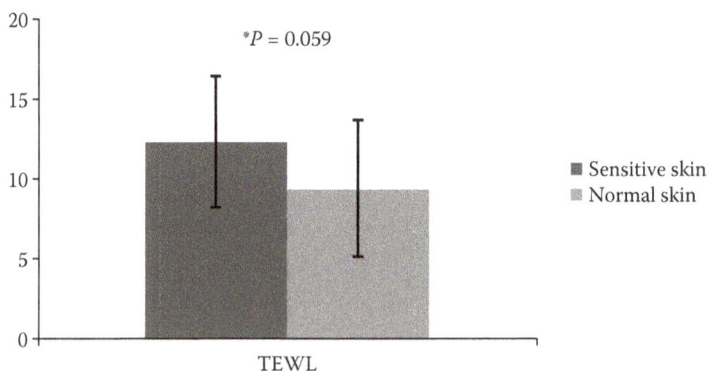

FIGURE 11.3   Comparison between the TEWL values obtained in sensitive skin with those of normal skin (mean ± SD).

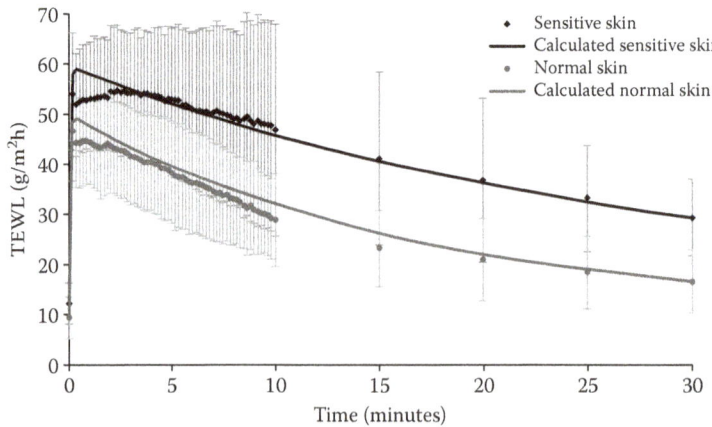

FIGURE 11.4   POST desorption curves obtained after 24 hours of occlusion (mean ± SD); the continuous lines represent the calculated data obtained by application of the model to the median individual parameters.

TABLE 11.1

Evaporation Half-Life ($t_{1/2evap}$) and DWM Values Obtained in the Study (Mean ± SD)

Group	$t_{1/2evap}$ (min)		DWM (g/m²)	
Sensitive skin ($n = 15$)	25.28 ± 22.91	$P = .005$	1216.45 ± 299.83	$P = .0001$
Normal skin ($n = 18$)	10.15 ± 5.34		787.51 ± 196.98	

Calculating the model's dynamical parameters obtained after adjustment (Table 11.1), statistically significant differences between the two groups were immediately found, indicating a higher $t_{1/2evap}$ and DWM in the sensitive skin group.

Some degree of barrier impairment and higher than normal TEWL measurements were expected in the sensitive skin group. In particular, this was expected because all selected patients stated a regular (daily), often unprotected (no gloves) contact with detergents as part of their jobs (lab personnel). However, as reported in other studies, no matter the clear symptoms and clinical evidence, TEWL changes seemed to be discrete, and statistical differences between groups could not be detected.

The application of our method to these same patients revealed statistically significant differences between the kinetic parameters obtained in the normal and sensitive skin groups in the same experimental conditions. Higher values of $t_{1/2evap}$ and DWM indicate that the kinetics of desorption profiles obtained in the subjects with sensitive skin are due to a slower decay in the TEWL values and a higher water mass released after the removal of occlusion. This increase in both parameters can be explained by an impaired barrier function which causes more water accumulation during the occlusion. Thus, once the patch is removed, a higher mass of water is involved in the entire recovery process, with a higher half-life time.

Conclusion

Some key aspects, previously mentioned, should be taken in to special account:

First, the patient's inclusion criteria involved the application of the original *sensitive skin* proposed by Kligman et al. (7), that is, the propensity to develop abnormal reactions such as stinging, prickling, burning, itching, and discomfort to cosmetics and exogenous environmental factors. Clear definition is crucial for diagnostic purposes, in particular when the purpose is to find objective proof of concepts. Vague concepts will always be present (32), but should be recognized and strongly avoided. Second, it is important to focus research efforts and means at the anatomical area related by the patient with the symptoms, as in the study presented in this chapter. If there is clear evidence of a generalized impairment of skin physiology, other options for analysis will then be possible, depending on the clinical investigative criteria adopted. Finally, regarding objective measurements, TEWL seems to be the most reliable indicator to measure an eventual barrier change related to SSS. There are other relevant indicators such as epidermal cohesion (although rarely referred), while for other indicators (e.g., hydration, sebum, pH, biomechanics), direct relationships with TEWL and TEWL's contribution to the epidermal barrier function is still poorly understood, particularly in this context. Nevertheless, taking into account the discrete nature of most of the changes involved, more precise methods, developed with these dynamical concerns, as it happens in the model used in this study, are especially applicable.

REFERENCES

1. Willis CM, Shaw S, de Lacharriere O, Baverel M, Reiche L, Jourdain R et al. Sensitive skin—An epidemiological study. *Br J Dermatol.* 2001; 145: 258–263.
2. Misery L, Myron E, Martin N, Verriere F, Nocera T, Taïeb C. Sensitive skin in France: An epidemiological approach (in French). *Ann Dermatol Venereol.* 2005; 132: 425–429.
3. Farage MA. How do perceptions of sensitive skin differ at different anatomical sites? An epidemiological study. *Clin. Exp Dermatol.* 2009; 34: e521–e530.

4. Rodrigues LM, Diogo L. Sensitive Skin Syndrome in Portugal—A concise (social and demographic) caracterization of the Portuguese reality. *IFSCC Mag.* 2009; 12 (2): 107–110.
5. Berardesca E, Farage M, Maibach H. Sensitive skin: An overview. *Int J Cosmet Sc.* 2013; 35: 2–8.
6. Misery L, Sibaud V, Merial-Kieny C, Taïeb C. Sensitive skin in the American population: Prevalence, clinical data and role of the dermatologist. *Int J Dermatol.* 2011; 50(8): 961–967.
7. Kligman a M, Sadiq I, Zhen Y, Crosby M. Experimental studies on the nature of sensitive skin. *Skin Res Technol.* 2006; 12(4): 217–222.
8. Rodrigues LM. Discussing cosmetics through a functional scope—A potential contribution to facilitate decisions and procedures. In *Advances in the Dermatological Sciences*, ed., Brain KR and Chilcott RP, Royal Society of Chemistry "Issues in Toxicology," series eds, Anderson D, Marrs TC, Waters MD and Wilks M. 2014.
9. Richters R, Falcone D, Uzunbajakava N, Verkruysse W, van Erp P, de Kerkhof P. What is sensitive skin? A systematic literature review of objective measurements. *Skin Pharmacol Physiol.* 2015; 28: 75–83.
10. Rodrigues-Barata AR, Gomez LC. Sensitive skin (in Spanish). *Piel.* 2013; 28(9): 520–530.
11. Pons-Guiraud A. Sensitive skin: A complex and multifactorial syndrome. *J Cosmet Dermatol.* 2004; 3(3): 145–148.
12. Kligman AM, Sadiq I, Zhen Y, Crosby M. Experimental studies on the nature of sensitive skin. *Skin Res Technol.* 2006; 12(4): 217–222.
13. Pinto P, Rosado C, Parreirão C, Rodrigues LM. Is there any barrier impairment in sensitive skin?: A quantitative analysis of sensitive skin by mathematical modeling of transepidermal water loss desorption curves. *Skin Res Technol.* 2011; 17(2): 181–185.
14. Darlenski R, Kazandjieva J, Fluhr J, Maurer M, Tsankov N. Lactic acid sting test does not differentiate between facial and generalized skin functional impairment in sensitive skin in atopic dermatitis and rosacea. *J Dermatol Sc.* 2014; 76: 151–153.
15. Otha M, Hikima R, Ogawa T. Physiological characteristics of sensitive skin classified by the sting test. *J Cosmet Sc Soc Jpn.* 2000; 23: 163–167.
16. Seidenari S, Francomano M, Mantovani L. Baseline biophysical parameters in subjects with sensitive skin. *Contact Dermat.* 1998; 38(6): 311–315.
17. Marriott M, Holmes J, Peters L, Cooper K, Rowson M, Basketter DA. The complex problem of sensitive skin. *Contact Dermat.* 2005; 53(2): 93–99.
18. An S, Lee E, Kim S, Nam G, Lee H, Moon S et al. Comparison and correlation between stinging responses to lactic acid and bioengineering parameters. *Contact Dermat.* 2007; 57: 157–162.
19. Wu Y, Wang X, Zhou Y, Tan Y, Chen D, Chen Y et al. Correlation between stinging TEWL and capacitance. *Skin Res Technol.* 2003; 9: 90–93.
20. Distante F, Rigano L, D Agostino R, Bonfigli A, Berardesca E. Intra and inter individual differences in sensitive skin. *Cosmet Toiletries.* 2002; 117: 39–46.
21. Farage MA. Vulvar susceptibility to contact irritants and allergens: A review. *Arch Gynecol Obstet.* 2005; 272: 167–172.
22. Pinnagoda J, Tupker RA, Agner TSJ. Guidelines for transepidermal water loss (TEWL) measurement: A report from the standardisation group of the European Society of Contact Dermatitis. *Contact Dermat.* 1990; 22: 164–172.
23. Tagami H, Kanamaru Y, Inoue K, Suehisa S, Inoue F, Iwatsuki K et al. Water sorption-desorption test of the skin in vivo for functional assessment of the stratum corneum. *J Invest Dermatol.* 1982 May; 78(5): 425–428.
24. Kligman AM. Regression method for assessing the efficacy of moisturizers. *Cosmet Toilet.* 1987; 93: 27–35.
25. Berardesca E, Maibach HI. Monitoring the water-holding capacity in visually non-irritated skin by plastic occlusion stress test (POST). *Clin Exp Dermatol.* 1990; 15(2): 107–110.
26. Berardesca E, Herbst R, Maibach H. Plastic occlusion stress test as a model to investigate the effects of skin delipidization on the stratum corneum water holding capacity in vivo. *Dermatology.* 1993; 187(2): 91–94.
27. Rodrigues L, Pinto P, Galego N, Silva PA, Pereira LM. Transepidermal water loss kinetic modeling approach for the parameterization of skin water dynamics. *Ski Res Technol.* 1999; 5(2): 72–82.
28. Rosado C, Pinto P, Rodrigues LM. Modeling TEWL-desorption curves: A new practical approach for the quantitative in vivo assessment of skin barrier. *Exp Dermatol.* 2005; 14(5): 386–390.

29. Gioia F, Celleno L. The dynamics of transepidermal water loss (TEWL) from hydrated skin. *Skin Res Technol.* 2002; 8: 178–186.

30. Endo K, Suzuki N, Yoshida O, Sato H, Fujikura Y. The barrier component and the driving force component of transepidermal water loss and their application to skin irritant tests. *Skin Res Technol.* 2007; 13: 425–435.

31. Warren R, Bauer A, Greif C, Wigger-Alberti W, Jones MB, Roddy MT et al. Transepidermal water loss dynamics of human vulvar and thigh skin. *Skin Pharmacol Physiol.* 2005; 18: 139–143.

32. Frosch PJ, Kligman AM. Recognition of chemically vulnerable and delicate skin. In *Principles of Cosmetics for the Dermatologist,* 1982: 287–296.

33. Haftek M, Coutanceau C, Taïeb C. Epidemiology of "fragile skin": Results from a survey of different skin types. *Clin Cosmet Investig Dermatol.* 2013; 6: 289–294.

12

Irritant Reactivity Tests

David A. Basketter

Introduction

To paraphrase Jane Austen, it is a truth universally acknowledged that sensitive skin in contact with an irritant must be in want of an overreaction. Therein lies the problem. In this book, which focuses specifically on sensitive skin, there is an obvious, albeit implicit, assumption that this skin type must react more aggressively to irritant and other noxious stimuli (in comparison to the responses seen in a normal population). This author remains fundamentally unconvinced that this is the case. Rather, in this chapter, it is hoped that he, and the reader, can set aside such preconceptions, examine the evidence, and draw evidence-based, scientifically rigorous conclusions. Central to such an analysis is the comparison of different human test groups (e.g., based on gender, age, ethnicity, and skin type). At least for some of the work that has been done, the test groups are evaluated in different locations, at different times of year, under different environmental conditions, and so forth. A properly controlled scientific experiment tests only a single variable and keeps all other variables constant. This is extremely difficult to achieve in human tests involving disparate groups and has always to be taken into account when apparent differences are observed—are they true differences or are they merely artifacts due to changes in humidity, use of different reaction scorers, cultural differences in question/response for sensory effects, and so on?

A consideration of irritant reactivity tests could be limited to the type of clinically obvious skin response, such as that which occurs to the anionic surfactant sodium lauryl sulphate (SLS); alternatively, it could encompass the broader spectrum of nonimmunologic reactions, including not only acute and cumulative irritation, but also nonimmunological immediate skin reactions (urticaria) and the panoply of sensory responses, such as burning, stinging, and itching. For the purposes of this chapter, the latter seems much more appropriate and will be adopted. What will not be included are detailed protocol instructions for any type of test; instead, basic principles will be identified in an effort to permit the user to develop a method best suited to their specific purpose. Nor will the work consider studies directed toward regulatory classification and labeling. However, any testing requires a test population, which is where we should start.

The Test Population

The possibility of using nonclinical approaches will be mentioned in the relevant sections that follow this one. However, irritant responses in the skin are highly diverse and best assessed in a human volunteer population (1). The identification of a suitable panel has been previously reviewed (2). Therefore, what follows are the essential elements.

It is always necessary to assemble a panel of sufficient size to provide appropriate discrimination. Little specific advice can be given except to consult a statistician prior to the establishment/finalization of the protocol. As a guide, however, even the simplest of questions is likely to require at least 15 panelists, and more commonly a minimum of 30 may well be appropriate. Frequently, the end point measures may be rather subtle, further increasing the need for higher numbers of volunteers.

Consideration must also be given to the matter of gender and age balance. Many of the responses considered in this chapter, indeed in this book, do not fluctuate dramatically in association with these variables, but it is nevertheless prudent to endeavor to match the panel to the question, keeping in mind the target population. Perhaps the most common misconception is that skin which is more sensitive than the average to one end point will also be more responsive to (all of) the others. To build an optimal sensitive skin panel, it is necessary to decide which end points are to be examined (stinging, burning, acute irritation, and so on) and then recruit individuals who are more reactive to the end point, or end points, which are to be tested. It is worth remembering that finding subjects who are broad spectrum high reactors to all the end points is rather like finding a needle in a haystack (2,3).

An interesting example to consider is lactic acid stinging, which despite much evidence to the contrary, is frequently taken as a general marker of sensitive skin. Almost 40 years ago, a method for assessing stinging capacity was detailed (4). The observation that 10% aqueous lactic acid in the nasolabial fold could evince a stinging reaction led to a quiet revolution in which many became convinced that this was the way to identify a *sensitive skin panel*. For example, in a study of 8 adult women (from a test group of 74) who were *stingers*, there was a greater history of intolerance to cosmetic products; evidence increased the response to urticants, but there was no enhanced irritant reaction (5). The absence of any difference in irritant responses between stingers and nonstingers was confirmed a few years later in two larger studies involving 50 and 58 volunteers, respectively (1,6). Interestingly, a decade after the original observation, the relationship between stinging and urticaria was reexamined. On this occasion, in a balanced panel of 44 stingers and 42 nonstingers, no relationship could be discerned between stinging and urticant susceptibility (3). The same study also showed that there was no relationship between a variety of sensory effects, the response to urticants and to irritants. In 2010, a study compared 15 stinger and nonstinger responses to two lipophilic irritants (7). No difference was found in the acute irritation response, whereas the cumulative irritant response was significantly higher in the stinger group. The sensory irritation arising from the two substances (cumene and octane) were identical in the stinger and nonstinger groups (8).

The message from the work is quite clear. A panel of volunteers has to be selected with due consideration for the key end point of interest. Of course, that may not be practicable for a number of reasons, including that the goal of the test is to seek out any unexpected skin reactions—which will likely lead to the need for a larger group size to increase the power of the study. All these matters will be explored in more detail in the sections that follow.

One final matter for consideration is the skin type and/or ethnic makeup of a test panel. This topic has been extensively reviewed elsewhere (9,10). These suggest that overall, there is a heightened response in Asians compared to Caucasians, who, in turn, may be a little more reactive than Blacks. More recent data are consistent with this trend (11). However, all authors agree that a variety of skin responses is equal in self-reported sensitive skin compared to normal skin.

Acute and Cumulative Irritations

Acute and cumulative irritations are the most obvious end points to consider given the title of this chapter, so let us lay down some basics: firstly, the acute skin irritant response does not always predict the cumulative irritant response, and second, a heightened responsiveness to one irritant does not imply increased reactivity to irritants in general. Thus, the choice of protocol and panel needs to carefully address the primary question of the investigation. For example, a single patch test has the capacity to provide an insight into the acute response, and if done with occlusion, it can provide a stringent assessment of hazard associated with single exposure to the substance (e.g., the study by Basketter et al. (12)). However, it might not deliver any useful insights into the response to repeated exposure—see Figure 12.1. Consider the two irritant substances A and B. A has a greater acute irritant response than B, and that response is both quicker to develop and to decay. Consequently, if the exposure is repeated at a relatively low frequency, whereas the response to B has the chance to accumulate, making, at least under these hypothetical exposure conditions, substance A the weaker cumulative irritant. Although this may seem theoretical, it is also, at least in terms of the outcome, consistent with the clinical experimental data

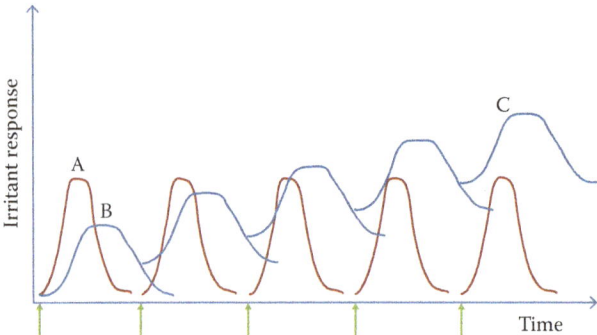

FIGURE 12.1   Acute versus cumulative irritation—a thought starter.

published two decades ago (13). Thus, where exposure to a material (substance or formulation) is repetitive, it makes good sense to design a protocol which mimics the typical mode of skin contact.

So what should be done in practice? Firstly, it is appropriate to adopt a protocol in which the skin exposure bears some resemblance to real-life exposure. Exposure may need to be repetitive, carried out for days, or even weeks. Next, it is essential to ensure that there is sufficient sensitivity built into the study to gain a meaningful response—a wholly negative set of skin reactions means nothing in isolation. Therefore, what is required is a panel with a sufficient number of volunteers and/or selection of panelists known to react with greater vigor to the type of irritancy problem associated with test material. It is almost always necessary to include a positive control material—a common choice is the anionic surfactant SLS, but it should generally be a last resort, since a better positive control is a related chemical or product formulation, relevant to the test material. For example, a clinical study of a new hand wash detergent formulation could involve several short exposures per day, with rinsing on one skin site, compared to a positive control site in which a product known to produce skin irritation in the exposed population is deployed. This study can then compare both the time to develop a cumulative irritant response, the nature and the degree of the irritant response, and as with all clinical studies, any observations on other aspects of the skin reaction, including sensory events. Ultimately, the question is "Does my clinical study have scientific integrity?"

There is one additional general question that has to be considered—how should any irritant reactions be assessed/measured? An argument can be made that properly trained skin assessors are more than sufficient to the task (14). However, and notwithstanding the additional time and expense, a good case can be made for use of one or (more usually) more instrumental assessment techniques (reviewed in the study by Berardesca and Maibach (15)).

Urticaria

In the preceding sections, it has been documented that urticaria has little relationship to skin irritation. This should hardly be a surprising statement. The mechanisms driving the two reactions are not at all the same (even if we do not necessarily always know what those mechanisms are!). Irritation is largely some combination of damage to the skin barrier function together with the activation of inflammatory pathways and, even with the acute response, occurs over a time period measured in hours/days (16). Skin contact urticaria on the other hand (we are not speaking here of systemic disease types classed as urticaria) arises within a few minutes and typically fades over an hour or so. Commonly, two types of contact urticaria are described (17). Here, we will focus only on the nonimmunologic variety, avoiding the complexity of immunoglobulin E-mediated protein allergic responses.

Nonimmunologic contact urticaria is perhaps not only particularly common, but also relatively easy to screen for. A good number of common chemical urticants are known, and from these, valuable insights have been derived, if not into the precise mechanism(s) of action, at least into the general characteristics of the response (18). Firstly, almost all individuals will produce a typical erythematous response, perhaps with a wheal, a few minutes after skin contact with a strong urticant (e.g., ethyl nicotinate, dimethylsul phoxide [DMSO]). Weaker urticants (e.g., benzoic acid, sorbic acid) do not produce any reaction in many subjects, particularly at lower concentrations (17). However, the use of a range of urticants shows that an individual giving a strong reaction to one urticant is in no way predictive of the reaction of that individual to a different urticant (19). The use of these benchmarks may permit the identification and calibration of a suitable volunteer panel.

So what should be done in practice? Skin contact urticaria is an acute response to a single contact (although of course it may be experienced repetitively). Thus, the use of a test panel, perhaps comprised of individuals who are known to have a greater level of response to a range of weaker urticants, can be exposed to the test agents, for example, on volar forearm skin sites, for 10–20 minutes, with assessment of responses from initial contact up to 60 minutes (longer if the reaction has not subsided). Occlusion may be used to enhance the sensitivity of the study (e.g., the study by Basketter and Wilhelm (19)).

Sensory Effects

As has already been mentioned earlier, any study involving human volunteers offers the benefit that those same volunteers can inform on any dermal effects that they perceive. However, although that aspect of clinical studies is extremely valuable in its own right, there is also the possibility of undertaking specifically directed assessment of sensory effects. Again, mention has already been made of the LAST (10). Unfortunately, a common error made has been to assume that individuals who are more susceptible to lactic acid-induced stinging are also more likely to experience other sensory responses, such as burning or itching. The most compelling demonstration of the problem arises from a study using DMSO (3). This substance generates many responses (including urticaria and, later, irritation), but the experiment reported using 86 volunteers also noted that stinging, tingling, itching, and burning triggered by DMSO was more or less equal in lactic acid stingers and nonstingers, with the latter if anything a little higher. Importantly, the stinging status was confirmed contemporaneously with the DMSO application.

Conclusions

Sensitive skin is an elusive entity (20). A heightened reactivity to one aspect of nonimmune skin responses is in no way indicative of a generally elevated sensitivity to any type of skin insult. The simple message therefore is that a test panel has to be selected according to the specific end point of interest. This cannot be achieved by using a lactic acid stinging screen on the nasolabial fold or an SLS patch test for acute irritancy any more than by using subjects with self-reported sensitive skin. Where human testing is conducted on sensitive skin in an attempt to use higher reactors as an enhanced indicator for a wider consumer population, the chance of achieving a scientifically defensible outcome is at best poor. However, where the testing is established with panels suitably screened for the particular end point of concern, where it employs sufficient numbers of individuals and contains concurrent positive and negative control materials, it can offer the optimum strategy for the identification and management of potentially adverse skin effects in a susceptible population.

REFERENCES

1. Marriott M, Basketter DA, Cooper K. Complex problem of sensitive skin. In: Berardesca E, Fluhr J, Maibach HI, editors. *Sensitive Skin Syndrome*. Boca Raton, FL: Taylor & Francis; 2006a. p. 61–65.
2. Marriott M, Basketter DA, Cooper K, Peters L. Identification of a sensitive skin panel. In: Berardesca E, Fluhr J, Maibach HI, editors. *Sensitive Skin Syndrome*. Boca Raton, FL: Taylor & Francis; 2006b. p. 107–119.
3. Coverly J, Peters L, Whittle E, Basketter DA. Susceptibility to skin stinging, non-immunologic contact urticaria and skin irritation—Is there a relationship? *Contact Dermat.* 1998; 38:90–95.

4. Frosch P, Kligman AM. Method for appraising the sting capacity of topically applied substances. *J Soc Cosmet Chem.* 1977; 28:197–209.
5. Lammintausta K, Maibach HI, Wilson D. Mechanisms of subjective (sensory) irritation: Propensity to non-immunologic contact urticaria and objective irritation in stingers. *Dermatosen.* 1988; 36:45–49.
6. Basketter DA, Griffiths HA. A study of the relationship between susceptibility to skin stinging and skin irritation. *Contact Dermat.* 1993; 29:185–188.
7. Schliemann S, Antonov D, Manegold N, Elsner P. The lactic acid stinging test predicts susceptibility to cumulative irritation caused by two lipophilic irritants. *Contact Dermat.* 2010; 63:347–356.
8. Schliemann S, Antonov D, Manegold N, Elsner P. Sensory irritation caused by two organic solvents-short-time single application and repeated occlusive test in stingers and non-stingers. *Contact Dermat.* 2011; 65:107–114.
9. Modjtahedi SP, Maibach HI. Ethnicity as a possible endogenous factor in irritant contact dermatitis: comparing the irritant response among Caucasians, blacks and Asians. *Contact Dermatitis* 2002; 47: 272–278.
10. Robinson MK. Population differences in acute skin irritation responses: Race, sex, age, sensitive skin and repeat subject comparisons. *Contact Dermat.* 2002; 46:86–93.
11. Lee E, Kim S, Lee J, Cho SA, Shin K. Ethnic differences in objective and subjective skin irritation response: An international study. *Skin Res Technol.* 2014; 20:265–269.
12. Basketter DA, Jirova D, Kandarova H. Review of skin irritation/corrosion hazards on the basis of human data: A regulatory perspective. *Interdiscip Toxicol.* 2012; 5:98–104.
13. Hannuksela A, Hannuksela, M. Irritant effects of a detergent in wash and chamber tests. *Contact Dermat.* 1995; 32:163–166.
14. Basketter DA, Reynolds FS, Rowson M, Talbot C, Whittle E. Visual assessment of human skin irritation: A sensitive and reproducible tool. *Contact Dermat.* 1997; 37:218–220.
15. Berardesca E, Maibach NI. *Non-Invasive Diagnostic Techniques in Clinical Dermatology.* Berlin: Springer; 2014.
16. Chew AL, Maibach HI. *Irritant Dermatitis.* Berlin: Springer-Verlag; 2006.
17. Basketter DA, Lahti A. Immediate contact reactions. In: Johansen JD, Frosch PF, Lepoittevin JP, editors. *Contact Dermatitis.* 5th edition. Berlin: Springer; 2011. p. 137–154.
18. Gimenez-Arnau A, Maibach HI. *Contact Urticaria Syndrome.* Boca Raton, FL: CRC Press; 2014.
19. Basketter DA, Wilhelm KP. Studies on non-immune immediate contact reactions in an unselected population. *Contact Dermat.* 1996; 35:237–240.
20. Berardesca E, Fluhr JW, Maibach HI. *Sensitive Skin Syndrome.* New York: Informa Healthcare; 2006.

13

Neurosensory Assessment

Roland Jourdain

Introduction

As initially described by Thiers in 1962 (1), sensitive skin is a rather common condition in people in contact with dermatological, cosmetic, spiced food, and household products. This syndrome, however, lacks a clear consensual definition. Subjects with sensitive skin complain about variable discomfort sensations after topical applications or when confronted with certain environmental factors. Very often, these subjective complaints, especially those related to the face, are not associated with evident clinical signs. Despite decades of research on such a condition, its pathophysiology remains poorly understood, albeit some findings indicate both heightened cutaneous nervous reactivity and increased SC permeability as possible contributors to sensitive skin. The prerequisite for understanding such skin condition is to clearly identify subjects with sensitive skin and to measure their own level of skin sensitivity. As this self-declared condition often expresses itself without evident clinical traits, the traditional bioengineering techniques used in dermocosmetic field (corneometry, TEWL, colorimetry, sebumetry) are of little help. Although these techniques are efficient to assess visible, biophysical parameters such as color, relief, hydration, sebum, or epidermal thickness, they cannot assess the subjective sensations of discomfort. For that purpose, different psychophysical tests have been proposed. They were often inspired by the quantitative sensory testing methods used to functionally study peripheral neuropathy. They aim at studying the heightened neurosensory traits of sensitive skin. Some of them have already proven their ability to detect subjects with sensitive skin and contributed to a better understanding of the etiology of sensitive skin. The present chapter aims at reviewing the most used and promising neurosensory assessment tests for diagnosing and quantifying sensitive skin.

Rationale

A Challenging Issue

Sensitive skin condition is extensively described in previous chapters of this book (and also in its first edition). This nonpathological skin condition affecting especially the face is very common worldwide, although it still lacks a clear definition. This can be explained by its high variety of symptoms and triggering factors across ethnicities, for example. The ability to identify sensitive skin is of paramount importance both to dermatologists and to cosmetics companies. In fact, since the sensitive skin population is the target of products dedicated to this skin condition, it is obviously relevant to test them especially for safety purpose on subjects with clear sensitive skin attributes. The primary issue is how to specifically diagnose and quantify sensitive skin (2). Sensitive skin expresses itself by a variety of discomfort signs (stinging, burning, itching, tingling) associated or not with erythema and scaling (3) induced by a great variety of triggering factors (environment, topical products). The diagnosis of this complex entity is a challenging and problematic issue, considering the lack of consensual definition, constant clear visible signs, and objective assessments for evaluating discomfort symptoms. It mostly relies upon the way subjects report their sensations (4,5) through questionnaires or during a provocative test such as LAST (6). Diagnosing sensitive skin should obviously start with a thorough clinical examination to eliminate obvious as well as more subtle atypical dermatoses such as eczema, atopic dermatitis, and rosacea, which could be mistaken as sensitive skin (7).

Role of Questionnaires

Initially, studies dealing with sensitive skin used open questionnaires to collect information as exhaustive as possible on self-perception of sensitive skin. People were asked to describe what they felt, in what circumstance with their own words (8,9). All this information was then gathered to establish questionnaires used as appropriate methods for conducting epidemiological studies on sensitive skin condition worldwide by mail (10), phone surveys (11–14) or face-to-face interviews at home (15). These questionnaires, which allow mathematical analysis of collected information to being carried out, are relevant when used to obtain epidemiological data by comparing large groups of subjects. At an individual level, self-assessment through a questionnaire—whatever its relevance—is not always optimum for classifying the skin as sensitive or nonsensitive because the meaning of sensitive skin is quite individual for any given subject. Indeed, up to now, no questionnaire has been validated as a diagnosis tool perfectly relevant by itself despite some recent advances (6,16). To select people with sensitive skin, it is generally recommended to add a positive result to a relevant psychophysical test to the self-reported sensitive skin statement.

Psychophysical Tests

Sensitive skin expresses itself by a variety of discomfort signs (stinging, burning, itching, tingling) associated or not with erythema and scaling (3). These unpleasant sensations are, at least partly, mediated by unmyelinated C fibers. These nerve endings, particularly abundant in the facial skin (17), are equipped with sensory receptors activated by different chemical or physical agents (mechanical strain, pH, capsaicin/chili, heat, cold). Some of these receptors are also present and functional on keratinocytes which play a more and more evidenced role in the modulation of sensory skin function (18,19). This repertoire of varied receptors is certainly the physiological support to the great diversity of triggering factors linked to sensitive skin. There is a clear evidence of the involvement of the peripheral nervous system in that skin condition, although through an unknown mechanism. To date, little is known about a possible alteration or changes in cutaneous nerve ending density and a possible difference in the repertoire of sensory receptors in terms of density, distribution, or functionality. However, there is a broad consensus that subjects with sensitive skin react more strongly to a determined stimulus than people with nonsensitive skin or react to weaker stimuli. This property has been taken into account for developing psychophysical tests dedicated to diagnose people with sensitive skin by investigating the neurosensory aspects of the sensitive skin. These tests aiming to assess subjective irritation are complementary of the more traditional tests dedicated to assess objective irritation signs such as redness or barrier function impairment which could be associated with sensitive skin condition as well (6). Widely used in research on various senses (vision, audition, olfaction, taste, or touch), psychophysical tests quantitatively investigate the relationship between the stimuli and the sensations and perceptions they induce. In the sensitive skin domain, they generally rely upon the induction of discomfort sensations similar to those characterizing sensitive skin most often by a topically applied chemical such as lactic acid and capsaicin among the most frequently used (6). Assessment of the induced sensations is performed by the subjects themselves. The most common site of test is the nasolabial fold, a facial site richly innervated with sensory fibers, followed by the cheek and the forearm. But apart from chemicals, other stimuli such as electrical current or changes in temperature have been or could be investigated to assess the exacerbated neurosensory features linked to sensitive skin.

The Lactic Acid Stinging Test

The LAST, initially proposed in 1977, relies upon the intensity of stinging sensations induced by a lactic acid aqueous solution (5% or 10%) applied to the nasolabial folds. This test can be performed by two different methods. In the first method, the subjects first undergo a facial sauna treatment for 5–15 minutes or are conditioned to a state of profuse sweating in an environmental chamber at 110°F and 80% relative humidity. A 5% lactic acid solution is then applied with a cotton swab to the test site later to record the self-declared response by subjects (20). In the second method, a 10% aqueous solution of lactic acid at room temperature is rubbed with a cotton swab on the test site. An inert substance, such as saline solution, is applied to the contralateral test site, used as control. Stinging experience is rated on a 4-point scale by patient at 2.5, 5, and 8 minutes postapplication. Subjects with scores equal to or above 3 are considered stingers. This very simple test is very popular and largely performed by cosmetic manufacturers for the selection of stingers. This selected population prone to experience neurosensory problems with topical products is asked to test new products to substantiate claims indicating that they are appropriate for sensitive skin (3). Depending especially on the concentration used for lactic acid solution, the incidence of stingers greatly varies. For example, the latter was found to be 51% in 86 subjects (women and men) with 10% lactic acid (21) and only 17.4% in an Asian female population (22) assessed with a 5% solution. Other parameters explain these important variations such as the mode of lactic acid solution application and the criterion to classify subjects as stingers according to their reported level of stinging sensation (22).

As the LAST is based upon the reported sensations by the subject in terms of nature and intensity, it has raised controversies owing to the use of a subjective individual pain scale hard to tackle by the investigator. Indeed, there is no consensual scale for quantifying the intensity of the sensory response experienced (23). So the experience of pain reported by a subject can never be fully confirmed or invalidated by an external observer. Nevertheless, the relevance of the stinging sensations reported by the subjects has been shown by measuring cerebral responses to the LAST with fMRI (24). According to their answers to a self-assessment questionnaire, 18 subjects were divided into two balanced groups: severe sensitive skin and completely nonsensitive skin. Inclusion criteria involved the absence of any dermatological, neurological, or vascular condition affecting the face. Event-related fMRI was used to measure cerebral activation induced by split-face application of lactic acid and its vehicle (control) (Figure 13.1). In both groups, skin discomfort due to lactic acid increased activity in the primary sensorimotor cortex contralateral to the application site and in a bilateral frontoparietal network including the parietal cortex, the prefrontal areas around the superior frontal sulcus, and the supplementary motor area. However, activity was significantly larger in the sensitive skin group. Most remarkably, in the sensitive skin group only, activity spread into the ipsilateral primary sensorimotor cortex and the bilateral peri-insular secondary somatosensory area (Figure 13.2). These results demonstrated that compared with control subjects,

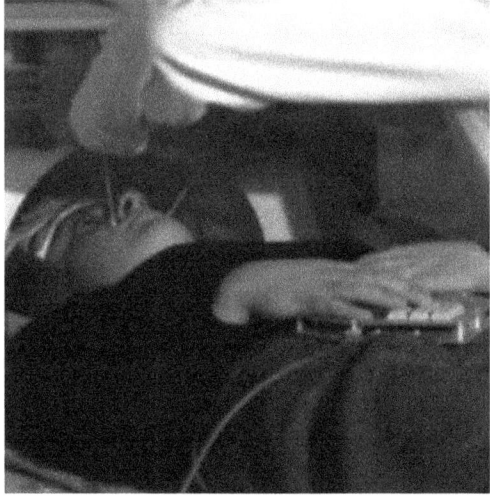

FIGURE 13.1 Split-face application of lactic acid and its vehicle (control) before measuring cerebral activation by fMRI. (From Querleux, B., Dauchot, K., Jourdain, R. et al., *Skin Res Technol*, 14, 454–461, 2008. With permission.)

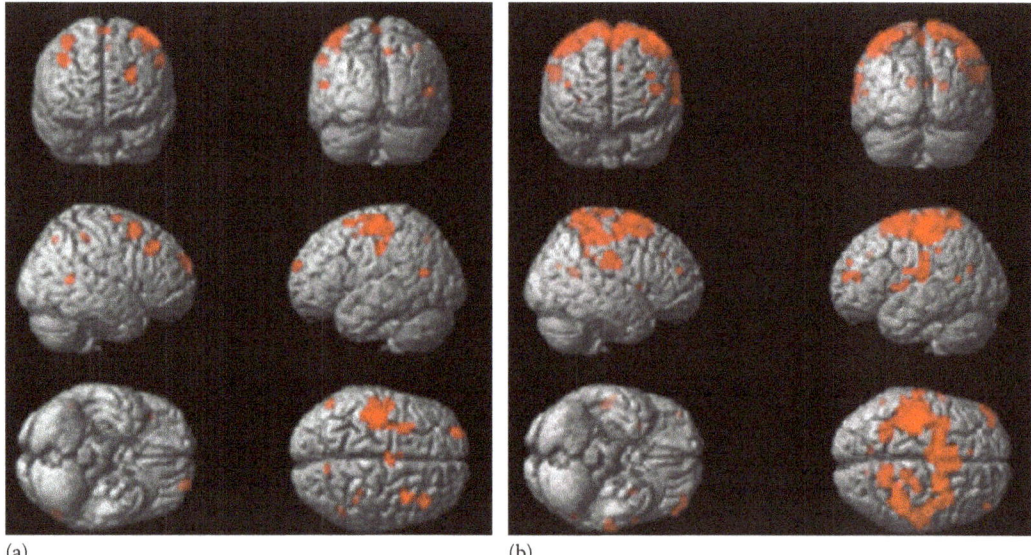

(a)   (b)

FIGURE 13.2   Evidence of SSS. Cerebral activity induced by lactic acid application is larger in sensitive skin subjects (a) than in nonsensitive skin subjects (b). (From Querleux, B., Dauchot, K., Jourdain, R. et al., *Skin Res Technol*, 14, 454–461, 2008. With permission.)

self-perceived sensitive skin subjects had a specific cerebral activation during LAST, which allowed the authors to hypothesize that self-perceived sensitive skin was intrinsically linked to a specific neurophysiologic pattern for these subjects. This study highly contributed to give evidence of the clinical reality of this syndrome and of the pertinence of the psychophysical approach.

Although very useful for assessing the product safety, the LAST does not fully render the complexity of self-assessed sensitive skin, as illustrated by the discrepancy between lactic acid response and self-perception of sensitive skin (25). In 2000, this difference was taken into account for the recommendation to include *stingers* with a concomitant self-declared sensitive skin as panelists for safety testing (26).

The Capsaicin Test

Owing to the great similarity of symptoms induced by topically applied capsaicin with those associated with sensitive skin (27), a new elicitation test using a 0.075% emulsion of this pungent compound extracted from chili peppers was proposed in the 1990s to identify people with sensitive skin (28). By activating TRPV1, the cutaneous application of capsaicin causes the appearance of uncomfortable sensations such as itching, burning, or stinging associated or not with redness at the application side (27,29). These unpleasant reactions are more frequent and more intense in self-declared sensitive skin subjects (28). Whether it is linked to difference in nerve ending density and/or TRPV1 functionality remains an open question. This initial capsaicin test was very promising as it presented a stronger link with self-declared sensitive skin than the LAST (30). But similar to the LAST, it could have been controversial since involving the use of a subjective individual pain scale as well and it induced too painful sensations in very sensitive skin subjects.

To overcome these issues, a second-generation test with capsaicin has been proposed. This test, called *capsaicin detection threshold* (CDT) test, combines the specific reactivity of sensitive skin to capsaicin confirmed by other studies (31), the application simplicity of the LAST, and a method of detection threshold. It does not rely anymore on the quantification of the intensity of the response but on the determination of detection thresholds of topically applied capsaicin. Five capsaicin concentrations are used in 10% ethanol aqueous solution ($3.16 \times 10^{-5}\%$, $1 \times 10^{-4}\%$, $3.16 \times 10^{-4}\%$, $1 \times 10^{-3}\%$, $3.16 \times 10^{-3}\%$).

The method used to attain the detection threshold consists of applying increasing concentrations of capsaicin onto the nasolabial folds (3-minute interval between each application). The vehicle is simultaneously applied following a split-face, single-blind plan. The test is stopped as soon as the subject reports a specific sensation on the capsaicin side. Its accuracy/reliability and its safety were first assessed in a random population of 150 healthy adult women (32). The CDT test allowed the test population to be classified according to six threshold levels corresponding to the sensitive reaction to one of the five capsaicin concentrations and to the absence of reaction to the highest concentration (Figure 13.3). The lowest capsaicin concentration was detected by 23.3% of the panelists, whereas almost the same proportion (27.3%) did not perceive even the highest concentration that is a hundred times more concentrated. This large distribution of the test population illustrated the very important interindividual differences concerning activity and/or density of cutaneous nerve endings, which is probably the major physiological feature explaining the phenomenon of sensitive skin. In addition, the distribution of the population was surprisingly not unimodal and revealed the existence of two different subgroups: individuals with low CDT and those with high threshold. These two subpopulations strongly differed in their respective self-perception of sensitive skin according to their responses to a sensitive skin questionnaire. The higher the self-declared sensitive skin incidence was, the lower the detection threshold was.

This difference is certainly due to an overactivation of TRPV1 receptor, which can be reduced by the selective antagonist *trans*-4-*tert*-butylcyclohexanol developed as a novel bioactive for the treatment of sensitive skin (33). In addition, the safety of the CDT test was judged as excellent by the panelists since all the reported sensations were considered as slightly or moderately perceptible, even in volunteers with the most sensitive skin. The total absence of pain is highly advantageous for testing routine in the cosmetic domain. The bilateral procedure with the simultaneous presentation of the vehicle on the contralateral side as control helps volunteers to differentiate background cutaneous sensations from those specifically caused by capsaicin (27), thus avoiding false-positive results (34). The single-blinded approach also helps to avoid false-positive results. The test based on the presence or absence of a sensation on the capsaicin side is easy to explain to the volunteers and, thus, far more reliable than those commonly used involving the highly variable individual pain scale. It was used to explore the controversial issue of ethnic variations in sensitive skin among 144 American women of three ethnicities: Asian, African, and Caucasian. Each ethnic group was split into six subgroups according to the threshold levels of sensitivity to capsaicin, and differences according to ethnic background appeared minimal (35). The test was used on 50 Caucasian women and 50 Caucasian men as well (to be published). There was no gender difference regarding the threshold levels of sensitivity to capsaicin. The only gender difference was the lower incidence of self-reported sensitive skin in the male population. Did males really understand what sensitive skin is? Or were they more reluctant than women to admit their skin sensitivity? These remain open questions. This test of facial skin neurosensitivity, which is simple, inexpensive, and

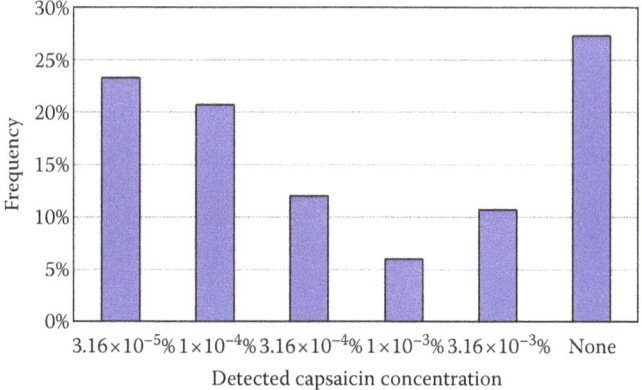

FIGURE 13.3 Distribution of 150 women in six subpopulations according to their CDT. (From Jourdain, R., Bastien, P., de Lacharrière, O., and Rubinstenn G., *J Cosmet Sci*, 56, 153–166, 2005. With permission.)

painless, appears to be a good prototype for the diagnosis of sensitive skin. Its sensitivity also allows modulators of skin neurosensitivity to be assessed as shown for a probiotic orally taken (36). The CDT test has inspired some research teams who used only one capsaicin concentration in ethanol aqueous concentration (37,38). Compared to the CDT test (32,35,36), both new proposed capsaicin tests with a unique concentration procedure presented an interesting reduction in the test duration, but as they were again based on the intensity of the perceived sensations, they probably lost some accuracy and certainly a high level of safety. Indeed, 4 females among 93 experienced painful burning sensations during the test proposed by Yu et al. (37) with a $1 \times 10^{-4}\%$ capsaicin solution.

Other Tests

Among other methods (clinical bedside examination, questionnaires, functional neuroimaging, skin biopsy), the assessment of patients with neuropathic disorders utilize several QST methods (39). These methods, aimed at studying the impairment of somatosensory function in neurologic diseases (i.e., diabetic neuropathy), are based on different stimuli: thermal (cold, warm), electrical, or mechanical. Some of them have been already assessed as possible diagnostic tools for studying the exacerbated neurosensory aspects of sensitive skin.

Cutaneous Thermal Sensation

In 1998, a psychophysical test based on the assessment of peripheral sensitivity to thermal stimuli was suggested as a possible diagnosis of sensitive skin. Thermal threshold is the function that can be measured most easily and conveniently (40). This test involved the use of a thermal testing instrument—for example, the Thermal Sensory Analyser (TSA 2001) manufactured by Medoc, Ramat Yishai, Israel—to assess the thermal functional components of cutaneous nerve endings. The device, called a *thermode*, delivered thermal stimuli capable of heating or cooling the skin. However, two studies showed that this promising test was of limited value in the diagnosis of sensitive skin. In a first study, the link between detection threshold to thermal stimuli assessed by the TSA and self-perceived sensitive skin was not as strong as that observed with skin reactivity to capsaicin and, to a lesser extent, with LAST (30). In another study, a significant difference in the mean of cold pain thresholds was reported between sensitive and nonsensitive self-assessed skin subjects (41). Unfortunately, this difference was too weak to consider this thermal parameter as a predictive indicator of sensitive skin. Medoc manufactures a new generation of the apparatus called TSA-II—NeuroSensory Analyzer integrating vibratory stimulus, which could be assessed for its relevance with sensitive skin as well.

Current Perception Threshold

Different teams have explored the interest of electrical stimuli for assessing the elevated neurosensory features of sensitive skin by using the Neurometer CPT® device (Neurotron Inc., Baltimore, Maryland, US). This neurodiagnostic portable device painlessly evaluates the functioning of cutaneous sensory nerve fibers (Figure 13.4). A pair of gel-type electrodes connected to the electric current generator and placed onto the skin randomly releases electric currents activating peripheral innervation. The device can deliver different wave stimuli to assess the different classes of sensory nerve fibers assuming that 5 Hz stimulation preferentially activates unmyelinated (C) fibers, 250 Hz would be optimum for small myelinated (A-δ) fibers, and 2000 Hz would be adequate for large myelinated (A-β) fibers. The results of this first study concerning a very small cohort of subjects indicated that the perception thresholds of sensitive skin subjects were low for the C fiber measurements at 5 Hz electric current stimulation. The authors concluded that the abnormal sensory perception in individuals with sensitive skin appeared to be related to neurological instability, where C fiber nociception plays a role, and that quantitative sensory perception threshold measurement was found to be a useful method for the identification of sensitive skin subjects (42). In a more recent study, the link between current perception threshold (CPT) and the response to the LAST has been established (43). Unlike the previous study, the link of the LAST response

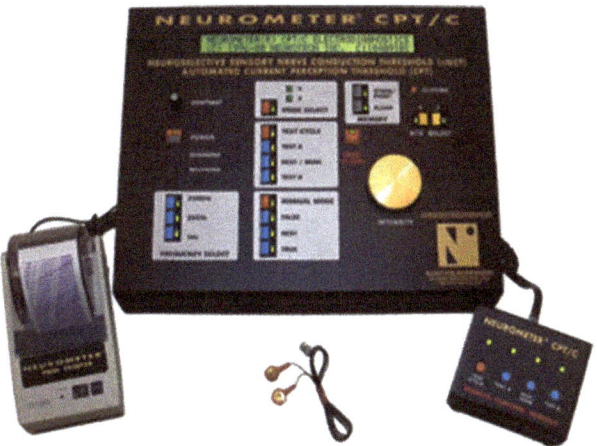

FIGURE 13.4 The Neurometer CPT.

was stronger with the response to 250 Hz than to 5 Hz stimuli suggesting a stronger role of A-δ fibers. As the LAST does not fully render the complexity of self-assessed sensitive skin (25), the interest of the CPT method would deserve to be confirmed for its ability to discriminate sensitive from nonsensitive subjects selected on a more predictive test.

Conclusion

SSS is a very common nonpathological skin condition detected in all countries where epidemiological surveys have been conducted. As this condition is merely expressed through subjective discomfort sensations such as stinging, burning, and itching, several psychophysical tests have been proposed to study the increased neurosensory traits of sensitive skin. The first tests used topical application of chemical probes such as lactic acid or capsaicin to induce discomfort sensations and measure their intensity. Despite a confirmation of the pertinence of this psychophysical approach by measuring cerebral activation during LAST, these tests remain a little bit controversial because of the very subjective individual pain scale. This weakness has been circumvented with the tests based on detection threshold. Subjects are subjected to an increasing signal until they feel a sensation irrespective of its nature and intensity. In such aspect, their pain scale is not solicited and the subjectivity of the test is reduced. The detection threshold method is a way to investigate the function of cutaneous nerves fully painlessly, and thus, it is of great interest for the cosmetic industry, which deeply cares about the comfort of the volunteers involved in clinical trials. For the time being, CDT is certainly the most pertinent method linked to self-declared sensitive skin. It allowed the role of TRPV1 receptor stimulation in the etiology of sensitive skin to be highlighted as well. Inspired by quantitative sensory testing procedures used to study peripheral neuropathy, other tests are based on physical stimuli (temperature, electrical current). Less employed until now than capsaicin, they need confirmation as effective diagnostic tool for sensitive skin. The efforts on that domain must be pursued to bring better products for sensitive subjects even though it is likely that no testing protocol will emerge as the unique gold standard diagnostic tool able to fully encompass the complexity of this self-diagnosed syndrome.

REFERENCES

1. Thiers H. Peau sensible. In *Les Cosmétiques*, second edn (Thiers H, ed). Paris: Masson, 1986: 266–8.
2. Marriott M, Basketter D, Cooper K, Peters L. Identification of a sensitive skin panel. In *Sensitive Skin Syndrome* (Berardesca E, Fluhr JW, Maibach HI, eds). New York: Taylor & Francis, 2006: 107–19.

3. Christensen M, Kligman AM. An improved procedure for conducting lactic acid stinging tests on facial skin. *J Soc Cosmet Chem* 1996; 47: 1–11.
4. Inamadar A, Palit A. Sensitive skin: An overview. *Indian J Dermatol Venereol Lepro* 2013; 79: 9–16.
5. Yosipovitch G. Evaluating subjective irritation and sensitive skin. *Cosmet Toiletries* 1999; 114: 41–2.
6. Richters R, Falcone D, Uzunbajakava N et al. What is sensitive skin? A systematic literature review of objective measurements. *Skin Pharmacol Physiol* 2015; 28: 75–83.
7. Lev-Tov H, Maibach HI. The sensitive skin syndrome. *Indian J Dermatol* 2012; 57: 419–23.
8. Kligman AM, Sadiq I, Zhen Y, Crosby M. Experimental studies on the nature of sensitive skin. *Skin Res Technol* 2006; 12: 217–22.
9. Johnson AW, Page DJ. Making sense of sensitive skin. Poster 78: 700–707. *Proceedings of the 17th IFSCC Congress 1992, Yokohama, Japan.*
10. Willis CM, Shaw S, De Lacharriere O et al. Sensitive skin: An epidemiological study. *Br J Dermatol* 2001; 145: 258–63.
11. Kamide R, Misery L, Perez-Cullell N et al. Sensitive skin evaluation in the Japanese population. *J Dermatol* 2013; 40: 177–81.
12. Misery L, Sibaud V, Merial-Keny C, Taïeb C. Sensitive skin in the American population: Prevalence, clinical data, and role of the dermatologist. *Int J Dermatol* 2011; 50: 961–7.
13. Jourdain R, De Lacharriere O, Bastien P, Maibach HI. Ethnic variations in self-perceived sensitive skin: Epidemiological survey. *Contact Dermat* 2002; 46: 162–9.
14. Misery L, Boussetta S, Nocera T et al. Sensitive skin in Europe. *J Eur Acad Dermatol Venereol* 2009; 23: 376–81.
15. Xu F, Yan S, Wu M et al. Self-declared sensitive skin in China: A community-based study in three top metropolises. *J Eur Acad Dermatol Venereol* 2013; 27: 370–5.
16. Misery L, Jean-Decoster C, Mery S et al. A new ten-item questionnaire for assessing sensitive skin: The Sensitive Scale-10. *Acta Derm Venereol* 2014; 94: 635–9.
17. Nolano M, Provitera V, Caporaso G et al. Cutaneous innervation of the human face as assessed by skin biopsy. *J Anat* 2013; 222: 161–9.
18. Denda M, Nakatani M, Ikeyama K et al. Epidermal keratinocytes as the forefront of the sensory system. *Exp Dermatol* 2007; 16: 157–61.
19. Ständer S, Schneider SW, Weishaupt C, Misery L. Putative neuronal mechanisms of sensitive skin. *Exp Dermatol* 2009; 18: 417–23.
20. Frosch P, Kligman AM. A method for appraising the stinging capacity of topically applied substances. *J Soc Cosmet Chem* 1977; 28: 197–209.
21. Coverly J, Peters L, Whittle E, Basketter DA. Susceptibility to skin stinging, non-immunologic contact urticaria and acute skin irritation; is there a relationship? *Contact Dermat* 1998; 38: 90–5.
22. An S, Lee E, Kim S, Nam G, Lee H, Moon S, Chang I. Comparison and correlation between stinging responses to lactic acid and bioengineering parameters. *Contact Dermat* 2007; 57: 158–62.
23. Slodownik D, Williams J, Lee A et al. Controversies regarding the sensitive skin syndrome. *Expert Rev Dermatol* 2007; 2: 579–84.
24. Querleux B, Dauchot K, Jourdain R et al. Neural basis of sensitive skin: A fMRI study. *Skin Res Technol* 2008; 14: 454–61.
25. Seidenari S, Francomano M, Mantovani L. Baseline biophysical parameters in subjects with sensitive skin. *Contact Dermat* 1998; 38: 311–5.
26. Bowman JP, Floyd AK, Znaniecki A et al. The use of chemical probes to assess the facial reactivity of women, comparing their self-perception of sensitive skin. *J Cosmet Sci* 2000; 51: 267–73.
27. Green BG, Bluth J. Measuring the chemosensory irritability of human skin. *J Toxicol Cutan Ocul Toxicol* 1995; 14: 23–48.
28. De Lacharrière O, Reiche L, Montastier C et al. Skin reaction to capsaicin: A new way for the understanding of sensitive skin. *19th World Congress of Dermatology (Sydney, Australia): Australas J Dermatol* 1997; 38(S2): 3.
29. Jessell TM, Iversen LL, Cuello AC. Capsaicin-induced depletion of substance P from primary sensory neurons. *Brain Research* 1978; 152: 183–8.
30. Jourdain R, de Lacharrière O, Willis C et al. Links between sensitive skin, sensitivity to thermal stimuli, lactic acid stinging test and capsaicin discomfort test. *20th World Congress of Dermatology (Paris, France). Ann Dermatol Venereol* 2002; 129: 1S594.

31. Robinson MK, Perkins MA. Evaluation of a quantitative clinical method for assessment of sensory skin irritation. *Contact Dermat* 2001; 45: 205–13.

32. Jourdain R, Bastien P, de Lacharrière O, Rubinstenn G. Detection thresholds of capsaicin: A new test to assess facial skin neurosensitivity. *J Cosmet Sci* 2005; 56: 153–66.

33. Kueper T, Krohn M, Haustedt L et al. Inhibition of TRPV1 for the treatment of sensitive skin. *Exp Dermatol* 2010; 19: 980–6.

34. Green BG. Regional and individual differences in cutaneous sensitivity to chemical irritants: Capsaicin and menthol. *J Toxicol Cutan Ocul Toxicol* 1996; 15: 277–95.

35. Jourdain R, Maibach HI, Bastien P et al. Ethnic variations in facial skin neurosensitivity assessed by capsaicin detection thresholds. *Contact Dermat* 2009; 61: 325–31.

36. Gueniche A, Philippe D, Bastien P et al. Randomised double-blind placebo-controlled study of the effect of Lactobacillus paracasei NCC 2461 on skin reactivity. *Benef Microbes* 2014; 5: 137–45.

37. Yu LL, Wang XM, Zou Y et al. Correlation between the capsaicin test and objective skin measurements in evaluating sensitive skin in Chinese females. *J Dermatol Sci* 2012; 68: 108–9.

38. Lee E, Kim S, Lee J et al. Ethnic differences in objective and subjective skin irritation response: An international study. *Skin Res Technol* 2014; 20: 265–9.

39. Rolke R, Magerl W, Campbell KA et al. Quantitative sensory testing: A comprehensive protocol for clinical trials. *Eur J Pain* 2006; 10: 77–88.

40. Yosipovitch G, Maibach HI. Thermal sensory analyzer, boon to the study of C and Aδ fibers. *Curr Probl Derm* 1998; 26: 84–89.

41. Saumonneau M, Black D, Bacle I et al. Cutaneous thermal reactivity and sensitive skin: A pilot study. *20th World Congress of Dermatology (Paris, France). Ann Dermatol Venereol* 2002; 129: 1S601.

42. Kim S, Lim S, Won Y et al. The perception threshold measurement can be a useful tool for evaluation of sensitive skin. *Int J Cosmet Sci* 2008; 30: 333–7.

43. Li S, Wang X, Gao Y et al. CPT, the main test method of skin neuronal sensitivity. *Cutan Ocul Toxicol* 2015; 34: 208–11.

Section IV

Clinical Considerations

14

Sensitive Skin: Is There a Link with Ethnicity?

Laurent Misery and Charles Taïeb

Ethnic groups are poorly defined, and the term *ethnicity* is frequently used as a synonym for *race*, especially in the United States. However, the American classical division of population into Caucasians, African Americans, Hispanics, Asians, and others is very well known to be not justified for scientific research, especially since the era of genomic studies that clearly demonstrates that these groups are not related to any genomic homogeneity (1). From the cultural point of view, there is also no reality. And from the medical point of view, especially dermatological, there is no interest to separate people into different ethnic groups because there is no relationship with their phenotype, their phototype, or any other characteristic of the body and especially the skin (2). Nonetheless, there are numerous studies about the differences between ethnic groups. Some of them were performed about skin sensitivity.

To examine possible ethnic variations in the perception of sensitive skin, an epidemiological survey was performed in the San Francisco area (3). Approximately 800 telephone interviews were conducted with women from four different ethnic groups (African Americans, Asians, Euro-Americans, Hispanics; approximately 200 women per group). There was no statistical difference between the ethnic groups in terms of sensitive skin prevalence. Nevertheless, some differences were noted between ethnic subgroups of sensitive skin. Euro-Americans were characterized by a higher skin reactivity to wind and tended to be less reactive to cosmetics. African Americans presented diminished skin reactivity to most environmental factors and a lower frequency of recurring facial redness. Asians appeared to have greater skin reactivity to spicy food, to sudden changes in temperature, and to wind and tended to suffer from itching more frequently. Hispanics presented a lower incidence of skin reactivity to alcohol. The differences in skin sensitivity between ethnic groups concerned mostly factors of skin reactivity and, to a lesser extent, its symptomatology. But taken together, the authors mainly noted the similarities in comparing how women of varying ethnic backgrounds perceive the sensitive skin condition.

The same authors performed a single-blind controlled study in 144 women from three ethnicities: Asian, African, and Caucasian (4). Five solutions with increasing capsaicin concentrations were successively applied to one side of the nasolabial folds, while the other side simultaneously received the vehicle as control. The test was discontinued when the volunteer reported a sensation on the capsaicin side whatever its nature. Otherwise, the experimenter continued the test, using the next solution with higher capsaicin content and so on, until the subject experienced a sensation on the capsaicin side. Each ethnic group was divided into six subgroups according to the level of sensitivity to capsaicin, that is, from detection of the lowest concentration up to no detection of the highest concentration, 100-fold higher. Asian women tended to have higher capsaicin detection thresholds than Caucasians, but lower thresholds than Africans. Nevertheless, the distribution did not greatly differ among the three ethnicities. The authors concluded that the capsaicin skin neurosensitivity test is painless and the changes across individuals of different ethnic backgrounds appear minimal.

In another study (5), 1039 individuals filled out standard questionnaires. About 53% stated that their skin had been sensitive for more than 5 years, and 31% claimed that their skin has become more sensitive. When asked to describe why they have sensitive skin, severe weather was the reason most commonly selected. Visual (redness/swelling) and sensory (burning/stinging) reactions to products was also selected as the reason. Caucasians more often claimed that products produced visual effects, whereas African Americans more often claimed that products produced sensory effects. The environmental factor most strongly associated with sensitive skin was stress.

TABLE 14.1

Prevalence of Sensitive Skin by Ethnicity

	Caucasians (%)	Blacks (%)	Hispanics (%)	Asians (%)	P Value χ^2
Sensitive	44.57	43.19	46.62	44.44	0
Not sensitive	55.43	56.81	53.38	55.56	0.352

TABLE 14.2

Prevalence of Sensitive Skin by Ethnicity in Terms of Climatic and Environmental Factors

	Caucasians (%)	Blacks (%)	Hispanics (%)	Asians (%)	P Value χ^2
To temperature shifts	48.16	45.76	54.24	25	0.31
To pollution	34.57	46.55	47.46	27.27	0.11
To air conditioning	11.45	20.97	21.31	8.33	0.07
To water	16.11	14.52	16.39	8.33	0.89
To cold climatic conditions	57.48	51.61	60.66	50	0.72
To warm climatic conditions	29.73	35	25	27.27	0.69
To windy climatic conditions	61.13	46.67	51.61	50	0.13
To dry air	63.09	50.85	54.84	66.67	0.24

TABLE 14.3

Prevalence of Sensitive Skin by Ethnicity in Terms of Emotion

	Caucasians (%)	Blacks (%)	Hispanics (%)	Asians (%)	P Value χ^2
Easily without any reason?	15.2	19.3	24.59	16.67	0.34
After each sun exposure?	36.73	25.86	41.67	36.36	0.32
After an emotion?	41.16	33.33	39.34	33.33	0.69

We found variations of prevalence according to different countries by using the same methodology for all these studies (6–13) (see Chapter 2) that could suggest that some variations could depend on ethnicity.

This is definitely a little quick shortcut if not foolhardy! These different factors are rather cultural, linguistic, climatic, industrial, and related to the level of pollution or lifestyle.

In any case, research is limited in these countries by the law, especially in France, which forbids to question a person about its skin or its ethnic group.*

We also performed a study in the United States (9) on a representative sample of the population (14), including ethnic groups.

With the help of an international polling institute (Paris, France), 1000 individuals from a national sample representative of the American population aged at least 18 years old were selected according to the quota method (sex, age, ethnic group, profession, area of living) (14) and interviewed via phone. There were 70% who declared themselves as "Caucasians"; 12%, "Blacks"; 13.5%, "Hispanics"; and 3%, "Asians."

The prevalence of sensitive skin was similar in the four ethnic groups; it varied slightly from 43.2% for Caucasian to 52.1% for African American individuals, 46.6% for Hispanic, and 44.4% for Asian without statistical significance ($P = .352$) (Table 14.1).

Likewise, no statistical difference was noted in terms of skin sensitivity to climatic and environmental factors among the different ethnic groups (Table 14.2). Skin reactivity to emotion was not significantly different in the four ethnic groups (Table 14.3).

---

* Article 8 of the Data Protection Act 1978 prohibits freedom "to collect or process personal data that reveals, directly or indirectly, the racial or ethnic origin."

Hence, we can conclude that there is no relationship of skin sensitivity and ethnicity. This is not surprising because the definition of these groups is not supported by scientific data and because there is no reason for differences in neuronal sensitivity according to these groups.

REFERENCES

1. Bryc K, Auton A, Nelson MR, Oksenberg JR, Hauser SL, Williams S, Froment A et al. Genome-wide patterns of population structure and admixture in West Africans and African Americans. *Proc Natl Acad Sci USA* 2010; 107: 786–791.
2. Verma SB. Proposing the demise of the terms "Asian skin" and "Asian skin type." *Int J Dermatol* 2015; 54: e48–e49.
3. Jourdrain R, de Lacharrière O, Bastien P, Maibach HI. Ethnic variations in self-perceived sensitive skin: Epidemiological survey. *Contact Dermat* 2002; 46: 162–169.
4. Jourdrain R, Maibach HI, Bastien P, de Lacharrière O, Breton L. Ethnic variations in facial skin neurosensitivity assessed by capsaicin detection thresholds. *Contact Dermat* 2009; 61: 325–331.
5. Farage MA. Perceptions of sensitive skin: Changes in perceived severity and associations with environmental causes. *Contact Dermat* 2008; 59: 226–232.
6. Misery L, Myon E, Martin N, Verrière F, Nocera T, Taïeb C. Sensitive skin in France: An epidemiological approach. *Ann Dermatol Venereol* 2005; 132: 425–972.
7. Misery L, Boussetta S, Nocera T, Perez-Cullell N, Taïeb C. Sensitive skin in Europe. *J Eur Acad Dermatol Venereol* 2009; 23: 376–381.
8. Misery L, Myon E, Martin N, Consoli S, Boussetta S, Nocera T, Taïeb C. Sensitive skin: Psychological effects and seasonal changes. *J Eur Acad Dermatol Venereol* 2007; 21: 620–628.
9. Misery L, Sibaud V, Taïeb C. Sensitive skin in the American population: Prevalence, clinical data and role of the dermatologist. *Int J Dermatol* 2011; 50: 961–967.
10. Kamide R, Misery L, Perez-Cullell N, Sibaud V, Taïeb C. Sensitive skin evaluation in the Japanese population. *J Dermatol* 2013; 40: 177–181.
11. Taïeb C, Auges M, Georgescu V, Perez-Cullell N, Misery L. Sensitive skin in Brazil and Russia: An epidemiological and comparative approach. *Eur J Dermatol* 2014; 24: 372–376.
12. Brenaut E, Misery L, Taïeb C, Sheth R. Sensitive skin in India: An epidemiological and comparative approach. In press.
13. Misery L, Taïeb C. *Sensitive Skin in Korea: An Epidemiological and Comparative Approach.* San Francisco: American Academy of Dermatology. 2015.
14. Hansen MH, Hurwitz WN, Madow WG. *Sample Survey Methods and Theory. Volume 1: Methods and Applications.* New York: John Wiley & Sons, Inc. 1993.

15

Gender and Age Influence on Sensitive Skin

Rosa M. Andersen

Subjective versus Objective Differences in Skin Reactivity

When interpreting data on differences in skin reactivity in various populations/subpopulations such as diverse ethnical and age groups along with gender, it is important to remember what type of response is being evaluated. Presently, when assessing the presence or the aspects of sensitive skin in populations, few responses are objective and can be measured by, for example, instrumental devices. Most parameters are entirely subjective including self-assessment of having sensitive skin or not, along with, for example, the severity (mild, moderate, or severe), quality of discomfort (stinging, burning, itching sensations) and triggering factors such as physical, emotional, chemical (products) or weather causes (1,2).

In the following sections, we study the objective age and gender differences in skin irritation and sensitization responses and move on to investigating differences in sensory irritation comparing it with results from studies on self-assessed perception of sensitive skin.

Objective Differences in Irritation and Sensitization Responses

Studies indicate that skin characteristics such as skin thickness, barrier function, and elasticity vary with age and gender (3,4). These characteristics potentially influence skin reactivity and perception.

Age Differences in Skin Irritation Responses

Further studies indicate that the elderly are less susceptible to skin irritants compared to younger people. When stimulating different age groups with a strong irritant stimulus such as SLS in different concentrations, a greater reactivity was seen in the young age group (5,6). A work (2002) compared results from nine studies on acute patch-test reactions to common irritants across different age groups (7). The oldest cohort showed significantly reduced reactivity to the two strongest irritants and also a tendency to have reduced reactivity to the weaker irritants in the test panel.

Gender Differences in Skin Irritation Responses

Because women are more exposed to wet work and detergents compared to men, they may present with greater amounts of irritant dermatitis of certain irritants. It does not apply, however, that women are generally more sensitive to skin irritants than men, which has otherwise been a long-standing perception (1). This conclusion is supported in multiple studies investigated in the study by Robinson (7), where results actually showed an increased reactivity in men to irritants (both significant and nonsignificant) compared to that in women.

Differences in Objective Skin Sensitization Responses

Sensitization requires, opposite to irritation, an immune response and therefore immune competence to carry out a skin response to allergens—allergic dermatitis.

It is difficult to explore if there is any difference in inherent immune competence or susceptibility comparing gender or various age groups. The big challenge is to separate gender-/age-related inherent susceptibility from gender-/age-related patterns of exposures/behavior. The only way to truly assess allergic sensitivity is thus to evaluate the induction of allergic contact sensitization in previously naive subjects, which nowadays, due to ethical aspects, is not conducted. This leaves us with difficult interpretations of retrospective studies of patch-testing cohorts and older studies investigating naive cohorts. A retrospective study from 1986 of 1873 persons who underwent patch-testing revealed significant increased sensitization in the elderly (<40 years old) compared to that in the young. This can be explained by repeated exposures during life (8). An older study from 1953 studied the induction of sensitization to a strong sensitizer (2,4-dinitrochlorobenzene) in 174 previously naive persons of various ages of which about half became sensitized (9). They did not find any significant difference in the incidence of sensitization with different age groups. From this, it appears that there is little age-related difference in allergic sensitivity, at least when it comes to very potent sensitizers.

The same issues and challenges apply when discussing gender. There seems, however, to be a tendency that women are slightly more sensitive than men when it comes to sensitization. Retrospective studies indicate that women have higher incidence of responses to certain allergens, for example, some metals, compared to men (10,11), whereas others do not find any differences in incidence of sensitization (8). In interpreting these results, one should keep in mind possible gender-specific patterns of allergen exposure. Few older studies have prospectively explored the induction of sensitization of both weaker and stronger sensitizers. These showed, not unanimously, a tendency for women to have stronger responses (12–14).

Differences in Sensory Perception

Few studies have investigated age and gender differences in sensory (chemical, thermal, mechanical) irritation, which is frequently the main symptom in patients complaining of sensitive skin. Studies by Heft et al. (15,16) demonstrate elevation in the sensory thresholds in the elderly compared to the younger age group by various stimuli in the face. Also, another study has shown significant decrease in the performance of sensory skin properties (structural and functional) in elderly skin (17). These studies are in accordance with the previously mentioned age differences in visible skin irritation responses. A small study on stinging with lactic acid, which is a common objective test for sensitive skin, revealed a tendency of increased sensitivity in women, but it has no correlation when comparing discomfort in different areas of the face in the individual test persons (18).

As discussed earlier, underneath and elsewhere in this book, a key challenge is to find suitable objective tests that embrace this population subjectively reporting suffering from sensitive skin. This of course also applies when investigating gender and age differences.

Self-Reported Gender- and Age-Related Sensitive Skin

Table 15.1 provides an overview of selected larger epidemiological studies of prevalence of self-reported sensitive skin worldwide. For further studies and analyses on this subject, please see Chapters 1 and 2.

One should keep in mind that various methodologies have been applied in the different studies, and therefore, have caution in interpreting and comparing data.

All studies showed higher prevalence of some grade of self-reported sensitive skin among women, most of which to a significant degree. Specific prevalence varied between studies from 15.9% to 82.6% in women and 8.6% to 64.4% in men.

TABLE 15.1

Prevalence of Self-Reported Sensitive Skin in Selected Larger Cohorts

Author and Reference	Country	Interview Mode	N	Percentage of Women of N (%)	Percentage of SS Prevalence in Women (%)	Percentage of SS Prevalence in Men (%)	Gender Difference in Prevalence
Misery et al. (19)	United States	Telephone interview	994	50.2	50.9	38.2	No difference
Farage (20)	United States	Written questionnaire	1039	84	69.0	64.4	No difference
Kamide et al. (21)	Japan	Telephone interview	1500	51.8	56.0	52.8	Significantly more in 20–29 y group compared to >50 y group
Xu et al. (22)	China	Face-to-face interview	9154	57.1	15.9	8.6	Significantly more in <25 y and 25–49 y compared to >50 y group
Taïeb et al. (23)	Brazil	Telephone interview	1022	NA	45.7	22.3	No difference
	Russia		1500	NA	50.1	25.4	Significantly younger with SS
Willis et al. (24)	United Kingdom	Written questionnaire	2316	88.9	51.4	38.2	NA
Misery et al. (25)	Eight European countries	Telephone interview	4506	NA	49.4	37.0	No difference
Guinot et al. (26)	France	Written questionnaire	8522	59.5	61	32	Significantly more younger with SS
Löffler et al. (27)	Germany	Written questionnaire	420	61.4	82.6	63.6	No difference

Note: *N*: number of participants; NA: not applicable; SS: sensitive skin; *y*: year.

A more varied picture appears with respect to age. About one-half of the studies report no difference. The rest report that significantly more young people than elderly complain of sensitive skin.

Potential Causes of Gender and Age Differences

Taking into consideration that it is well documented that more women than men suffer from self-declared sensitive skin and that there is tendencies toward more younger people than the elderly who experience this, surprisingly little research on gender- and age-related differences exist.

Age

As reported earlier, some studies indicate that the elderly exhibit a tendency to have higher sensation irritation thresholds (15–17), which was in accordance with the studies on visible skin irritants such as the tests with SLS (5–7). But if this was true, why do we only see a tendency of lower prevalence in elderly in half of the studies on self-reported sensitive skin? Xu et al.'s (22) and Guinot et al.'s (26) studies found significantly fewer persons with sensitive skin among the elderly compared to younger individuals in both genders (Table 15.1). They state that this finding might be linked to age-related experience and behavior and, therefore, a tendency to avoid environmental conditions and contact with certain triggering substances/products. Another possible explanation expressed by Xu et al. (22) is the fact that the elderly simply are not familiar with terms such as sensitive or skin susceptibility and, therefore, either do not express or experience suffering from it.

Gender

In general, more women than men report suffering from sensitive skin (Table 15.1). At this point, however, no evidence exists on the objective increase of skin susceptibility in women compared to men. Löffler's group is the only one known to directly investigate a full cohort with prevalence of self-reported sensitive skin and physical skin tests (27). They investigated 420 volunteers, who completed a questionnaire with self-estimation of enhanced skin susceptibility. Volunteers were also tested with TEWL, cutaneous blood flow, and skin hydration. The researchers furthermore patch-tested 152 volunteers with SLS on the forearm. There were significantly more women than men reporting enhanced skin susceptibility, but no correlation was found between self-estimated skin susceptibility and the bioengineering values. Other groups have, as mentioned earlier, investigated variation in skin characteristics between genders, but unfortunately, it is not directly linked to prevalence of sensitive skin in the same cohorts. For example, it is shown that women have significantly thinner epidermis compared to men (but, curiously, it had no correlation with age) (4). It can be questioned if the right objective tests are being applied. As seen elsewhere in this book, many new modalities of physical examinations of patients reporting suffering from sensitive skin are in the pipeline, hopefully providing us with further knowledge.

Some have expressed that fluctuations in hormone levels in women could help explain why the reported prevalence of sensitive skin in women is around double that of men in some parts of the world. Among others, Misery et al. (19) expressed this theory, because the fluctuation in sex hormone levels seem to alter skin reactivity as demonstrated in 42 atopic women who underwent skin prick test and blood samples for sex hormones during their menstrual cycle. Others have also investigated this area and proposed that hormonal differences between genders may produce a greater inflammatory response in women compared to men (28–30).

As mentioned in the discussion on reasons of age variation, behavior and cultural differences should also be discussed as factors of gender variations. Firstly, it is noteworthy, that in some parts of the world, for example, China, people report a remarkably low prevalence of sensitive skin. One explanation for this can be the lack of knowledge of the relatively new term *sensitive skin* in certain parts of the population (22). Secondly, it is possible that parts of the gender-specific prevalence in sensitive skin may be related to women's more frequent use of cleansers, cosmetics, and facial products, some of which may produce some irritation in some individuals. In addition, women may be more conscious than men of appearance and visual signs of irritation on the face and, therefore, more likely to perceive their facial skin as more sensitive (20). Thirdly and lastly, but in the same vein of behavior, as discussed by, for example, Löffler et al. (27), Farage and Maibach (28), and Farage (31), is the evident gender variation influenced by education and mass media's commercials. This could explain aspects such as lower prevalence in some countries/area due to lower exposure to modern commercials. This could also explain the tendency in other countries/areas such as some parts of the United States, Japan, and some European countries, where prevalence of self-reported sensitive skin between genders is almost equal. With increased marketing of products for sensitive skin in men, it might have become more culturally acceptable for men to define themselves as having sensitive skin.

REFERENCES

1. M. K. Robinson, Age and gender as influencing factors in skin sensitivity, in *Sensitive Skin Syndrome*, 1st ed., E. Berardesca, J. W. Fluhr, and H. I. Maibach, Eds. Boca Baton, FL: CRC Press, 2006, pp. 169–180.
2. M. K. Robinson, Population differences in skin structure and physiology and the susceptibility to irritant and allergic contact dermatitis: Implications for skin safety testing and risk assessment, *Contact Dermat.*, vol. 41, no. 2, pp. 65–79, 1999.
3. H. Sumino, S. Ichikawa, S. Kasama, T. Takahashi, H. Kumakura, Y. Takayama, T. Kanda, M. Murakami, and M. Kurabayashi, Effects of raloxifene and hormone replacement therapy on forearm skin elasticity in postmenopausal women, *Maturitas*, vol. 62, no. 1, pp. 53–57, 2009.
4. J. Sandby-Møller, T. Poulsen, and H. C. Wulf, Epidermal thickness at different body sites: Relationship to age, gender, pigmentation, blood content, skin type and smoking habits, *Acta Derm. Venereol.*, vol. 83, no. 6, pp. 410–413, 2003.
5. E. Lejman, T. Stoudemayer, G. Grove, and A. M. Kligman, Age differences in poison ivy dermatitis, *Contact Dermat.*, vol. 11, no. 3, pp. 163–167, 1984, September.
6. A. B. Cua, K. P. Wilhelm, and H. I. Maibach, Cutaneous sodium lauryl sulphate irritation potential: Age and regional variability, *Br. J. Dermatol.*, vol. 123, no. 5, pp. 607–613, 1990, November.
7. M. K. Robinson, Population differences in acute skin irritation responses: Race, sex, age, sensitive skin and repeat subject comparisons, *Contact Dermat.*, vol. 46, no. 2, pp. 86–93, 2002, February.
8. C. L. Goh, Prevalence of contact allergy by sex, race and age, *Contact Dermat.*, vol. 14, no. 4, pp. 237–240, 1986, April.
9. M. Schwartz, Eczematous sensitization in various age groups, *J. Allergy*, vol. 24, no. 2, pp. 143–148, 1953, March.
10. E. Young, H. van Weelden, and L. van Osch, Age and sex distribution of the incidence of contact sensitivity to standard allergens, *Contact Dermat.*, vol. 19, no. 4, pp. 307–308, 1988, October.
11. L. Kanerva, R. Jolanki, and J. Toikkanen, Frequencies of occupational allergic diseases and gender differences in Finland, *Int. Arch. Occup. Environ. Health*, vol. 66, no. 2, pp. 111–116, 1994.
12. W. P. Jordan and S. E. King, Delayed hypersensitivity in females: The development of allergic contact dermatitis in females during the comparison of two predictive patch tests, *Contact Dermat.*, vol. 3, no. 1, pp. 19–26, 1977, February.
13. J. L. Rees, P. S. Friedmann, and J. N. Matthews, Sex differences in susceptibility to development of contact hypersensitivity to dinitrochlorobenzene (DNCB), *Br. J. Dermatol.*, vol. 120, no. 3, pp. 371–374, 1989, March.
14. J. J. Leyden and A. M. Kligman, Allergic contact dermatitis: Sex differences, *Contact Dermat.*, vol. 3, no. 6, pp. 333–336, 1977, December.
15. M. W. Heft, B. Y. Cooper, K. K. O'Brien, E. Hemp, and R. O'Brien, Aging effects on the perception of noxious and non-noxious thermal stimuli applied to the face, *Aging (Albany, NY)*, vol. 8, no. 1, pp. 35–41, 1996, February.
16. M. W. Heft and M. E. Robinson, Age differences in orofacial sensory thresholds, *J. Dent. Res.*, vol. 89, no. 10, pp. 1102–1105, 2010, October.
17. R. I. Kelly, R. Pearse, R. H. Bull, J. L. Leveque, J. de Rigal, and P. S. Mortimer, The effects of aging on the cutaneous microvasculature, *J. Am. Acad. Dermatol.*, vol. 33, no. 5 Pt 1, pp. 749–756, 1995, November.

18. M. Marriott, E. Whittle, and D. A. Basketter, Facial variations in sensory responses, *Contact Dermat.*, vol. 49, no. 5, pp. 227–231, 2003.

19. L. Misery, V. Sibaud, C. Merial-Kieny, and C. Taïeb, Sensitive skin in the American population: Prevalence, clinical data, and role of the dermatologist, *Int. J. Dermatol.*, vol. 50, no. 8, pp. 961–967, 2011.

20. M. A. Farage, Does sensitive skin differ between men and women? *Cutan. Ocul. Toxicol.*, vol. 29, no. 3, pp. 153–163, 2010.

21. R. Kamide, L. Misery, N. Perez-Cullell, V. Sibaud, and C. Taïeb, Sensitive skin evaluation in the Japanese population, *J. Dermatol.*, vol. 40, no. 3, pp. 177–181, 2013, March.

22. F. Xu, S. Yan, M. Wu, F. Li, Q. Sun, W. Lai, X. Shen, N. Rahhali, C. Taïeb, and J. Xu, Self-declared sensitive skin in China: A community-based study in three top metropolises, *J. Eur. Acad. Dermatol. Venereol.*, vol. 27, no. 3, pp. 370–375, 2013, March.

23. C. Taïeb, M. Auges, V. Georgescu, N. Perez Cullell, and L. Miséry, Sensitive skin in Brazil and Russia: An epidemiological and comparative approach, *Eur. J. Dermatol.*, vol. 24, no. 3, pp. 372–376, 2014.

24. C. M. Willis, S. Shaw, O. De Lacharrière, M. Baverel, L. Reiche, R. Jourdain, P. Bastien, and J. D. Wilkinson, Sensitive skin: An epidemiological study, *Br. J. Dermatol.*, vol. 145, no. 2, pp. 258–263, 2001, August.

25. L. Misery, S. Boussetta, T. Nocera, N. Perez-Cullell, and C. Taïeb, Sensitive skin in Europe, *J. Eur. Acad. Dermatology Venereol.*, vol. 23, no. 4, pp. 376–381, 2009.

26. C. Guinot, D. Malvy, E. Mauger, K. Ezzedine, J. Latreille, L. Ambroisine, M. Tenenhaus et al., Self-reported skin sensitivity in a general adult population in France: Data of the SU.VI.MAX cohort, *J. Eur. Acad. Dermatology Venereol.*, vol. 20, no. 4, pp. 380–390, 2006.

27. H. Löffler, H. Dickel, O. Kuss, T. L. Diepgen, and I. Effendy, Characteristics of self-estimated enhanced skin susceptibility, *Acta Derm. Venereol.*, vol. 81, no. 5, pp. 343–346, 2001.

28. M. A. Farage and H. I. Maibach, Sensitive skin: Closing in on a physiological cause, *Contact Dermat.*, vol. 62, no. 3, pp. 137–149, 2010, March.

29. M. Lee, The sodium laurylsulphate model: An overview, *Cont. Dermatol.*, vol. 33, pp. 1–7, 1995.

30. M. A. Farage, Vulvar susceptibility to contact irritants and allergens: A review, *Arch. Gynecol. Obstet.*, vol. 272, no. 2, pp. 167–172, 2005.

31. M. A. Farage, How do perceptions of sensitive skin differ at different anatomical sites? An epidemiological study, *Clin. Exp. Dermatol.*, vol. 34, no. 8, pp. e521–530, 2009, December.

16

Sensitive Skin: Do We Observe an Impact on Quality of Life?

Laurent Misery and Charles Taïeb

Countless studies and publications describe the impact of various dermatoses on the quality of life of patients. Over the past 2 years, the quality of life was more or less specifically assessed 800 times in acne, 250 times in vitiligo, 1450 times in the AD, and nearly 1250 times in psoriasis (1)!

These skin diseases (and many others) share a number of characteristics to which the patient and their families are subjected, such as the high impact in terms of the daily life, psychiatric morbidity, and cost of healthcare. All these skin diseases share the common characteristic of being *visible* and consequently exclude patients from their social and/or family environment.

On the contrary, there are very few evaluations of the impact of sensitive skin on the quality of life of individuals who complain. We performed such a study (2).

Among the French population over the age of 15, the impact of sensitive skin on quality of life was studied through the use of two validated questionnaires: the SF-12 scale (for quality of life) and the Hamilton Anxiety and Depression scale (HAD; for depression).

In order to assess the quality of life, SF-12 is relevant and very frequently used. In fact, the SF-12v2® is a shorter version of the SF-36v2® Health Survey, but SF-12v2 uses just 12 questions to measure functional health and well-being from the patient's point of view.

Taking only 2–3 minutes to complete, the SF-12v2 is a practical, reliable, and valid measure of physical and mental health and is particularly useful in large population health surveys or for applications that combine a generic and disease-specific health survey. SF-12 is available in multiple languages who respect the linguistic and cultural steps of translations.

Two separate summary scores are obtained for each of the physical and mental domains by summing across all 12 items for each. Higher scores indicate higher levels of quality of life. Values that can be considered as normal in healthy conditions in the general population have been reported for many countries (around 50 in France).

A study was carried out by a polling organization in July 2004 (2). A sample was made up of 1001 individuals selected among a national representative sample of the French population over 15 years old. Subjects were interviewed by phone according to the quota method (gender, age, profession of head of family, town category, and region).

Questions on how they perceived their skin sensitivity and possible aggravating factors were asked. The quality of life was then assessed by using the SF-12.

When asked, "Do you have sensitive skin?" 20.7% answered, "very sensitive"; 38.2%, "sensitive"; 27.5%, "hardly sensitive"; 13.2%, "not sensitive"; and 0.5% gave no answer (Table 16.1).

The SF-12 questionnaire was administered to all men and women of the representative sample. The scores obtained for each dimension respectively in men and in women are described in Table 16.2. If the physical dimension (PCS) was not different according to gender ($P = .2$), a statistically significant difference for the mental dimension (MCS) was observed ($P = .0005$).

TABLE 16.1

Prevalence of Sensitive Skin According to Sex

	Men (%)	Women (%)	Global (%)	P Value χ^2
Very sensitive	12.53	28.43	20.7	
Rather sensitive	33.82	42.55	38.2	
Slightly sensitive	32.99	22.63	27.5	
Not sensitive	20.67	6.38	13.2	<.001

TABLE 16.2

Score of the Two Dimensions of the SF-12

	Men	Women	Global	P Value χ^2
PCS-12	50.2 ± 7.9	49.7 ± 8.6	49.9 ± 8.3	0.2806
MCS-12	47.9 ± 9.1	45.7 ± 9.8	46.8 ± 9.5	0.0005

There was no significant difference in mental and physical scores according to skin sensitivity. However, the mental scores were statistically different according to skin sensitivity, with some differences between men and women:

- Males: 45.6 for the sensitive skin group versus 49.7 for the not sensitive group ($P < .0001$)
- Females: 44.6 for the sensitive skin group versus 47.3 for the not sensitive group ($P = .0024$)

The fact that the MCS is altered, while the PCS is not, is not surprising! This result is usually found in all publications that evaluated the SF-12 in various dermatoses (3–7) because SF-12 is the general scale for the measurement of quality of life and not a specific scale for patients with disorders.

Comparisons of the mental scores according to the levels of perceived intensity of sensitive skin (very sensitive, rather sensitive, slightly sensitive, not sensitive) show that the MCS of quality of life is more altered when the intensity of the declared skin sensitivity is more severe (Tables 16.3 and 16.4).

Evaluation of depressive symptomatology using the HAD scale showed that there was no significant link between depressive symptomatology and skin sensitivity; in the group that answered, "sensitive

TABLE 16.3

Score of the Two Dimensions of the SF-12 as Expressed Sensitivity

	PCS-12 Men	PCS-12 Women	MCS-12 Men	MCS-12 Women
Sensitive	49.8 ± 8.4	49.5 ± 8.2	45.6 ± 9.9	44.6 ± 10.3
Not sensitive	50.6 ± 7.7	49.8 ± 9.1	49.7 ± 7.8	47.3 ± 8.7

TABLE 16.4

Score of the Two Dimensions of the SF-12 According to the Severity of Skin Sensitivity

	PCS-12 Male	PCS-12 Women	MCS-12 Male	MCS-12 Women
Very sensitive	48.0 ± 9.9	49.3 ± 8.9	43.6 ± 11.7	42.2 ± 11.9
Rather sensitive	50.9 ± 7.9	49.6 ± 7.9	46.1 ± 9.4	45.5 ± 9.6
Slightly sensitive	50.9 ± 7.1	50.4 ± 8.4	48.4 ± 7.9	46.9 ± 8.9
Not sensitive	50.2 ± 7.7	48.7 ± 10.1	51.3 ± 7.4	47.8 ± 84

skin," 4.3% of the subjects presented a certain depressive symptomatology against 4.8% in the group that answered, "not sensitive skin."

In conclusion, the MCS of quality of life, measured by the SF-12 scale, is altered in people who suffer from sensitive skin, and the higher the sensitivity, the more affected is the quality of life. These results are similar to those that are observed in skin diseases.

REFERENCES

1. *Science Direct*, http://www.sciencedirect.com/, 2015, May.
2. Misery L, Myon E, Martin N et al. Sensitive skin: Psychological effects and seasonal changes. *J Eur Acad Dermatol Venereol*. 2007; 21: 620–628.
3. Sibaud V, Dalenc F, Chevreau C et al. HFS-14, a specific quality of life scale developed for patients suffering from hand-foot syndrome. *Oncologist* 2011; 16: 1469–1478.
4. Boccara O, Méni C, Léauté-Labreze C et al. Haemangioma family burden: Creation of a specific questionnaire. *Acta Derm Venereol*. 2015; 95: 78–82.
5. Dufresne H, Hadj-Rabia S, Méni C, Sibaud V, Bodemer C, Taïeb C. Family burden in inherited ichthyosis: Creation of a specific questionnaire. *Orphanet J Rare Dis*. 2013; 8: 28.
6. Méni C, Bodemer C, Toulon A et al. Atopic dermatitis burden scale: Creation of a specific burden questionnaire for families. *J Eur Acad Dermatol Venereol*. 2013; 27: 1426–1432.
7. Taïeb A, Boralevi F, Seneschal J, Merhand S, Georgescu V, Taïeb C, Ezzedine K. The atopic dermatitis burden scale for adults: Development and validation of a new assessment tool (ABS-A). *Acta Derm Venereol*. 2015; 5: 700–705.

17

Perceived Sensitive Skin at Different Anatomical Sites

Miranda A. Farage

What Is Sensitive Skin?

The term *sensitive skin* is commonly used to describe a number of subjective, unpleasant sensations in response to a wide variety of external and internal stimuli (1). The specific sensations can vary from one individual to the next but are generally described as stinging, burning, pain, tingling sensations, or feelings of tightness or dryness. Objective signs of skin irritation, such as redness and swelling, seldom accompany the unpleasant sensations experienced by individuals with sensitive skin. In fact, many people who profess sensitive skin do not predictably experience visible signs of the sensations reported, whereas some who describe themselves as nonsensitive strongly react to tests of objective irritation (2). One possible explanation for the observed breakdown between sensory effects and objective signs is the fact that an objective sign such as erythema is the result of a complex, multistep physiological process. Underlying processes such as changes in blood flow, moisture content, and/or pH would be expected to occur before the appearance of visible external changes (3,4).

The global prevalence of sensitive skin has been largely explored throughout much of the world using epidemiological surveys. Table 17.1 summarizes the results of such surveys on sensitive skin not associated with a particular anatomical site. In European countries and the United States, the prevalence is over 50%. The literature indicates that self-assessed claims to skin sensitivity have steadily increased over time (5). In studies comparing sensitive skin between genders, a higher proportion of women claim to have sensitive skin compared to men. However, there is evidence that the gap between men and women may be closing (6). In South American and Asian countries, the prevalence of individuals claiming sensitive skin shows greater variation. In a recent study in Brazil, Taïeb et al. (7) found that over 80% of women and over 50% of men reported some degree of sensitive skin (Table 17.1), with the proportion reporting very or moderately sensitive skin at 45.9% for women (i.e., 16.67% and 29.22%) and 22.5% for men (i.e., 3.16% and 19.33%). In contrast, a study conducted in Mexico by Hernández-Blanco et al. (8) reported a prevalence of 36%. In Asia, the reported prevalences in Japan (9) and Russia (7) were comparable to some European countries, but two separate studies from China (10,11) indicate that a smaller proportion of the general population claim to have sensitive skin: 23% and 39.5%, respectively.

Differences in prevalence between countries regarding the perception of sensitive skin may be related to some of the underlying physiological causes and environmental triggers for sensitive skin that will be discussed in greater detail in the following sections, such as darker skin type and prevailing weather conditions. However, cultural influences likely account for some of this difference. In a study conducted among 9154 subjects from three urban areas in China (Beijing, Shanghai, and Guangzhou), Xu et al. (11) hypothesized that some of the participants, especially older individuals, were not familiar with sensitive skin, and therefore, the condition may have been underreported. This hypothesis was supported by the observations that (a) some individuals who did not claim to have sensitive skin responded that they experienced adverse sensory effects after using cosmetic products and (b) the reported prevalence was inversely proportional to the age group of the responders.

Cultural expectations also seem to play a role in the prevalence. Manufacturers of consumer products have increasingly marketed products targeted for sensitive skin. This may partially explain why the proportion of the population that claims to have sensitive skin appears to be increasing (10). The study

TABLE 17.1

Self-Declared Sensitive Skin Overall

Country	Year	Population	Number of Subjects	Any Sens.[a]	Degree of Self-Proclaimed Sensitivity (%)			References
					Very	Moderate	Slight	
Europe								
Europe (total)	2009[b]	General population by phone	4506 total	74.7	13	25.1	36.6	(7,12)
Belgium	2009[b]	General population by phone	500 total	60	10[c]	16[c]	4[c]	(7,12)
England	2001[b]	General population by mailed questionnaire (Y/N question)	2316 total	49.95[c]	NA	NA	NA	(13)
			2058 women	51.4	NA	NA	NA	
			258 men	38.2	NA	NA	NA	
France	March 2004	General population by questionnaire	1006 total	80.8	12	40.1	28.7	(14)
			women	85.5	14.9	44.4	26.2	
			men	74.8	8.7	35	31.1	
France	July 2004	General population by questionnaire	1001 total	86.7	21.1	38.2	27.4	(15)
			women	91.2	28.2	41.1	21.9	
			men	77.9	12.5	33.3	32.1	
France	2009[b]	General population by phone	1006 total	82	12.1[c]	39.9[c]	30[c]	(7,12)
Germany	1999	Dermatology patients with unrelated complaints	420 total	75.2	28.1	34.2	25.1	(16)
			258 women	82.6	19	34.9	28.7	
			162 men	63.5	15.4	21	27.1	
Germany	2009[b]	General population by phone	500 total	59	15.8[c]	20[c]	23.2[c]	(7,12)
Greece	2005	Female panelists	25 atopic women	100	44	36	20	(17)
			25 women with nonrelated complaints	64	0	16	48	
Greece	2009[b]	General population by phone	500 total	70	8.6	22.4[c]	29[c]	(7,12)
Italy	2004	General population	9154 total (88.5% women)	56.5	NA	NA	NA	(18)

(Continued)

TABLE 17.1 (CONTINUED)

Self-Declared Sensitive Skin Overall

Country	Year	Population	Number of Subjects	Any Sens.[a]	Degree of Self-Proclaimed Sensitivity (%)			References
					Very	Moderate	Slight	
Italy	2009[b]	General population by phone	500 total	90.6	17.4[c]	37.2[c]	36[c]	(7,12)
Portugal	2009[b]	General population by phone	500 total	86	16.2[c]	13.4[c]	56.4[c]	(7,12)
Spain	2009[b]	General population by phone	500 total	88	13[c]	20[c]	55[c]	(7,12)
Switzerland	2009[b]	General population by phone	500 total	59	13[c]	18[c]	28[c]	(7,12)
North America								
United States	2006	Female panelists (age: ≥50)	29 incontinent women	82.8	17.2	41.4	24.1	(19)
			42 age matched control	76.2	2.4	23.8	23.8	
United States	2007	General population by phone	994 total	NA	44.6 (very and sens)	NA	NA	(20)
			499 women	NA	50.9 (very and sens)	NA	NA	
			495 men	NA	38.2 (very and sens)	NA	NA	
United States	2009	General population in Cincinnati, Ohio	1039 total	68.4	4.9	23	40.5	(6)
			869 women	69	5.1	23.8	40.2	(21)
			163 men	64.4	4.3	19	41.1	(22)
United States (Mississippi)	2013[b]	General population in rural Mississippi	89 women	77.5	11.2	31.5	34.8	(23)
South America								
Brazil	2014[b]	General population by phone	1022 total					(7)
			women	80.4[c]	16.67	29.22	34.51	
			men	53.06[c]	3.16	19.33	30.57	
Mexico	2011–2012	Healthy volunteers	246 total	36	NA	NA	NA	(8)
			168 women	42.2	NA	NA	NA	
			78 men	23	NA	NA	NA	

(*Continued*)

TABLE 17.1 (CONTINUED)

Self-Declared Sensitive Skin Overall

Country	Year	Population	Number of Subjects	Any Sens.[a]	Very	Moderate	Slight	References
					Degree of Self-Proclaimed Sensitivity (%)			
Asia								
China	2009[b]	General population in China	408 women	23	2	5	16	(10)
China (urban dwellers)	2009	General population by questionnaire	9154 total	39.53	2.94	9.85	26.74	(11)
			5223 women	NA	15.93 (very and sens)		NA	
			3931 men	NA	8.62 (very and sens)		NA	
Japan	2011	General population by phone	1500 total		54.5 (very and rather)		NA	(9)
			777 women	95.6	7.5	48.5	39.6	
			723 men	93.5	9.5	43.3	40.7	
Russia	2014[b]	General population by phone	1500 total					(7)
			women	85.84[c]	13.02	37.04	35.78	
			men	66.9[c]	6.65	18.74	41.51	

Note: NA: not available.

[a] Any sensitivity, for example, very, moderate, or slight.

[b] If year of study is not given, the date corresponds to the year of publication.

[c] Percentages are not reported but interpreted from other data in publication.

conducted by Misery et al. (12) in eight European countries is consistent with a cultural component. In Portugal, Italy, and Spain, 80–90% of the subjects reported at least some skin sensitivity, while Germany, Belgium, and Switzerland reported just a little more than half (Table 17.1). Since the European population is essentially considered to be a genetically homogenous population, the authors attributed this unexpected finding to substantially more fashion and beauty-related advertising in specific European countries.

Differing cultural practices may produce widely different exposures to potential irritants and, therefore, to perceptions of sensitive skin. Women are more likely to use cosmetic products on the face and, therefore, more likely to experience unpleasant sensory effects as a result. Similarly, in most countries women are more frequently exposed to household cleaners and products compared to men and, as a result, have more opportunities to experience reactions to these products. Hygiene practices and the use of feminine products, such as douches, perfumes, medications, antifungal medications, and contraceptives, are a common cause of vulvar irritation in women (24). These practices can vary between different countries or between socioeconomic groups within countries (25). Based on the differing uses of these products, older women are more likely to report irritation due to incontinence products, whereas younger women are more likely to report irritation due to tampons (26). These findings are almost certainly based on culturally driven levels of exposure rather than on actual physiological differences.

There is no consensus on a classification for sensitive skin; however, several have been proposed (27). A number of these include consideration of objective signs of irritation, such as inflammation, or visible dermatological disorders. Since the etiology of sensitive skin and its association with frank skin inflammation or underlying dermatological disease is still not well understood, Misery (27) has proposed classifying sensitive skin according to severity, that is, *very sensitive*, *sensitive*, *slightly sensitive*, and *nonsensitive*.

Physiological and External Factors That Contribute to Sensitive Skin

The etiology of sensitive skin is unknown, but the disorder is believed to be related to a number of intrinsic physiological characteristics and other causes (Table 17.2), including alterations in skin barrier function, neurosensory function, and other host and external factors (3,28–30).

TABLE 17.2

Possible Contributing Factors to Sensitive Skin

Factor	References
Alterations in Barrier Function	
Thin SC	(31–34)
Decreased hydration of SC	(35–37)
Disruption of SC	(38)
Increased sweat glands	(32)
Increase neutral lipids and decreased sphingolipids	(39)
Decreased lipids	(40–44)
High-baseline TEWL	(45)
Neurosensory Function	
Increased epidermal innervations	(35,46)
Other Host Factors	
Fair skin	(13)
Susceptibility to blushing and/or flushing	(13)
Atopy and other skin conditions	(13,17,47)
Female sex	(13,16)
Hormonal status	(48)
External Factors	
Cultural expectations in technologically advanced countries	(16)

Barrier Function

Poor barrier function can result in abnormal penetration of potentially irritating substances and a decrease in the skin tolerance threshold (35). A number of early studies have suggested a link between sensitive skin and alterations in barrier function (49). Berardesca et al. (50) studied hyperreactors to nicotinate and concluded that they may have a thinner SC with a reduced corneocyte area resulting in a higher transcutaneous penetration of water-soluble chemicals. Seidenari et al. (40) concluded that alterations of baseline capacitance values indicates a tendency to barrier impairment and supported the view that skin hyperreactivity to water-soluble irritants is induced by the absorption of greater amounts of irritants. Corneosurfametry data were used by Goffin et al. (51) to demonstrate significant differences in SC reactivity between individuals with sensitive or nonsensitive skin. However, increased absorption is not the only explanation for sensitive skin. Cho et al. (52) evaluated individuals classified into sensitive skin and nonsensitive skin based on a LAST performed on the face. These investigators demonstrated no differences in TEWL as a measure of barrier function, but a significant difference in the mean quantity of SC ceramides, which were significantly lower in the sensitive skin group compared to the nonsensitive group. In a series of studies on individuals with sensitive skin, Roussaki-Schulze et al. (53) concluded that patients with sensitive skin had significantly lower levels of sebum and hydration than nonsensitive individuals. In addition, individuals with sensitive skin were more likely to develop alkali resistance and had significantly higher hyperreactivity of blood vessels in response to the application of methyl nicotinate.

Barrier function requires a well-organized, multilayered lipid structure between corneocytes (29). Further, the barrier properties of the SC are dependent on the precise lipid composition. Regions with higher neutral lipids and lower sphingolipids are associated with superior barrier properties (39,54). A weak barrier would not only facilitate the penetration of potentially irritating substances, but may also inadequately protect nerve endings resulting in hyperreactivity.

Neurosensory Function

The pain and other unpleasant sensations that are the hallmark of sensitive skin imply a likely relationship to neurosensory dysfunction, probably involving several neuromediators and sensory receptors. Possible mechanisms for neural system hyperreactivity include nerve fibers; endothelin receptors; burn, itch, and heat receptors; cold receptors; and neutrophins (55). Dermal nerve fibers extend throughout viable epidermis as free nerve endings, but the epidermal component of this network is still poorly characterized (46).

Besne et al. (56) evaluated epidermal innervation of biopsy samples from different anatomical sites; two facial sites (upper eyelid and preauricular area), the abdomen, and the mammary area. The innervation of the facial areas was significantly higher than the other anatomical sites. With increasing age, the dermal innervation of the facial sites decreased, while it increased in the mammary skin and was unchanged on the abdominal skin. These authors proposed that epidermal nerve density variation could explain the different sensitivity thresholds in various anatomical sites.

Skin sensations such as itching, pain, and warmth are mediated by unmyelinated C fibers (29,57). Kim et al. (58) evaluated C fiber measurements at 5 Hz electric current stimulation in a study on a small number of young adult male volunteers. The individuals prone to sensitive skin showed a tendency toward a decreased sensory perception threshold compared with the individuals who were not prone to sensitive skin.

Querleux et al. (59) used lactic acid to induce slight painful stimulation and a feeling of discomfort while monitoring brain activity using fMRI. The test was performed on nine subjects with self-declared sensitive skin and nine subjects with nonsensitive skin. During the study, the individuals with sensitive skin had a higher level of declared discomfort as a result of lactic acid application compared to the individuals with nonsensitive skin. Brain activity recording using the fMRI showed striking differences between the two groups. In the nonsensitive individuals, activity was concentrated in the left primary sensorimotor area, contralateral to the side of application of the lactic acid. By contrast, in the sensitive skin group, the discomfort-related activity was found in the sensorimotor cortex in both hemispheres. In addition, in the sensitive group only, specific discomfort-related activity was observed in the bilateral peri-insular regions classically considered as secondary the somatosensory area. This study indicated that subjects with sensitive skin have a specific CNS response during a LAST and suggests that the excitability of sensitive nerves in the facial epidermis lead to brain activation very similar to those observed in the pain process.

Other Contributing Causes

Individuals with fair skin are more likely to have skin sensitivity. Willis et al. (13) found that individuals susceptible to blushing were more likely to have sensitive skin, as were individuals with atopy or other skin conditions such as rosacea and acne. A similar observation was reported by Kamide et al. (9) based on a survey conducted among 1500 individuals in Japan. Sensitive skin was more likely to be declared by individuals who flush easily and are susceptible to sunburn. In contrast, Jourdain et al. (60) conducted a survey among 811 women in the San Francisco area in 1998 and found no significant differences between the incidence of sensitive skin among ethnic groups (i.e., African Americans, Asians, Euro-Americans, and Hispanics).

There appears to be an association between perceived sensitive skin and AD. In a study conducted in 2005 in a dermatology clinic in Greece, Farage et al. (17) surveyed 25 women diagnosed with AD and 25 women with unrelated complaints. All patients in the group with AD described their skin as sensitive to some degree, with 80% claiming their skin was either very or moderately sensitive (44% and 36%, respectively). The remaining 20% described their skin as slightly sensitive. By contrast, 64% of the individuals in the control group described their skin as sensitive to some degree, with none of the patients claiming to have very sensitive skin, and only 16% of the subjects claim that their skin was moderately sensitive. The association between the clinical diagnosis of AD and self-declared sensitive skin was statistically significant ($P < .0001$). Misery et al. (12) conducted a study in eight European countries and reported that a history of childhood AD was more frequent among individuals with sensitive or very sensitive skin compared to individuals with slight or nonsensitive skin. In contrast, in a 2001 publication, Willis et al. (13) found no association between the incidence of self-perceived sensitive skin when atopic subjects were compared to nonatopics (49% and 51%, respectively).

Gender plays a role in the perception of sensitive skin. Generally, the proportion of women who claim sensitive skin is cited as 50–70%; and the proportion of men, 30–60% (21). In a study conducted among 420 volunteer subjects (162 men and 258 women), Loffler et al. (16) reported a higher proportion of women claiming some degree of skin sensitivity (moderate, strong, or severe) compared to men (82.6% and 63.6%, respectively). In a study conducted in the United Kingdom among 3300 women and 500 men, Willis et al. (13) reported an incidence of perceived sensitive skin of 51.4% among women and 38.2% among men.

Misery et al. (15) conducted a study to compare perceptions of sensitive skin in summer versus winter. A higher percentage of women claimed to have very sensitive skin in both seasons, and a higher percentage of men declared that their skin was slightly or nonsensitive. In a study conducted in eight countries in Europe, investigators reported that a higher proportion of women declared sensitive skin compared to men (49.4% and 37%, respectively; $P < .05$) (16). In studies reported by Farage (21), there was no significant difference between genders when all degrees of general skin sensitivity were considered. However, women consistently reported a higher proportion of very and moderately sensitive skin. Men reported a higher proportion of slightly sensitive skin.

The gender difference in the perception of sensitive skin may be due to a variety of factors. Men's and women's skin differs in a number of physiological parameters, including skin thickness, hormone metabolism, hair growth, sweat rate, sebum production, surface pH, fat, and collagen content (28). Women tend to be exposed to a wider variety of cosmetics and household products, creating more opportunities to experience the sensations associated with sensitive skin. Further, perhaps it has been more culturally acceptable for women to claim sensitivity compared to men, although with the growth in the popularity of men's products formulated for sensitive skin, this may cease to be the case in the modern consumer world.

Interestingly, skin barrier function and reactivity to some irritants exhibit a cyclical variability in women that demonstrates hormonal influences in sensitive skin (61). Harvell et al. (62) investigated water barrier function on the back and forearm and found that the TEWL value was significantly higher on the day of minimal estrogen/progesterone secretion compared to the day of maximal estrogen secretion. This suggests that the skin barrier function is less complete on the days just prior to the onset of the menses compared to the days just prior to ovulation. In women, the forearm skin exhibited stronger reactions to SLS on day 1 than during days 9–11 of the menstrual cycle, while no difference was detected in a male control group evaluated during the same time period (63).

A number of test methods have been developed to objectively identify individuals with sensitive skin. A few examples are listed in Table 17.3. Some of these methods evaluate sensory responses such as stinging in response to the application of lactic acid (64) or capsaicin (55) or irritant reactions to materials such as SLS (65). However, there is a great deal of interpersonal variability in individual responses to specific irritants (3,54,66), even among chemicals with similar modes of action (67). Reactivity to one chemical is not necessarily predictive of reactivity to other materials (68). Biometric measures of possible underlying physical effects show promise, such as TEWL to assess barrier function, cross-polarized light and/ or temperature differences to evaluate underlying blood flow, or measurement of cytokines. However, to date, no single objective test exists to identify individuals with hyperreactive or sensitive skin.

Triggering Factors of Sensitive Skin

Questionnaire-based surveys have identified a variety of external stimuli as triggers of sensitive skin. Reactions to weather, climate, and environmental conditions are commonly associated with sensitive skin. In a 2008 publication by Saint-Martory et al. (69), environmental triggering factors for sensitive skin at various body sites included cold (66% of sensitive skin group), sun exposure (51%), wind (42%), heat (28%), and pollution (18%). In a study of 994 individuals in the United States, Misery et al. (16) reported that the percentage of subjects experiencing cutaneous reactivity to all climatic and environmental factors, such as dry air, cold, wind, heat, and pollution, was significantly higher in the sensitive skin group compared to that in the nonsensitive skin group. In our studies conducted in the United States, we found a similar result (6,22,23). Perceived irritation to each of the weather conditions listed in the survey (i.e., cold, hot, dry, and humid) was associated with sensitive skin to a significant degree. Similar data were reported by Kamide et al. (9) in a study conducted in Japan. In individuals with sensitive skin, weather and climate conditions were identified as potential triggers by large portions of the sensitive skin group (dry air, 70.5%; cold climate, 53.2%; temperature shifts, 46.9%; air-conditioning, 40.0%; and pollution, 39.3%).

Weather and climate triggers for sensitive skin are dependent on the local conditions. In a recent survey among the general populations of Brazil and Russia, Taïeb et al. (7) found a difference in the most frequently identified environmental triggering factors for sensitive skin. In Russia, the most frequently named factors among the very or rather sensitive individuals were wind (59%), cold (56%), water (54%), temperature shifts (51%), and pollution (47%). In Brazil, where climatic conditions are more homogeneous, sensitivity to cold was less pronounced. The most frequently cited triggers were warm climate (37%), temperature shifts (30%), and pollution (28%), with cold cited by a smaller proportion of subjects (26%).

Misery et al. (14,15) conducted a study during two seasonal periods in France. These investigators reported a higher percentage of the general population claiming sensitive skin in July (86.7% reporting some degree of sensitivity) compared to March (80.8%), leading the authors to conclude that sensitive skin appears more frequently in summer than in winter. In addition, the severity of sensitive skin was worse, as reflected by the number of individuals claiming their skin was very sensitive (21.1% versus 12%, respectively). Cold is a very common triggering factor for sensitive skin. In addition, cooler, dryer weather has been demonstrated to result in higher TEWL values in facial skin which would reflect poorer skin barrier function (70). In light of these observations, it is a bit unexpected that the prevalence of sensitive skin would be higher in the summer (14,15). However, other triggering factors in the summer months, such as sun exposure, air-conditioning, frequent temperature changes, and greater air pollution, may play a role in increasing the perception of sensitive skin (15).

Another commonly cited trigger for sensitive skin is stress or emotions. In our investigation among 1039 individuals in the United States (22), stress was identified as a cause of skin irritation by 63% of

TABLE 17.3

Examples of Test Methodologies Used to Identify Individuals with Sensitive Skin

Methodology	Sensory Effect Evaluated	Physical Effect Evaluated	Relevant Irritants	Advantages	Disadvantages	References
Lactic acid	Stinging	None	Cosmetics, other personal preparations meant to be left on	Highly sensitive and specific	Does not predict sensitivity to other irritants	(64)
Capsaicin	Stinging	None	Cosmetics, other personal preparations meant to be left on	Sensitive, detection threshold well correlated (inversely) to perception of sensitive skin	Does not predict sensitivity to other irritants	(55)
SLS	Burning	Erythema	Industrial exposures, cleaning products	Cheap, quick, reliable assessment of individual susceptibility to specific irritant	Sensitivity to one irritant not predictive of general sensitivity, relationship to sensitive skin in question	(45)
TEWL	None	Barrier function	Any potential irritant	Noninvasive, objective, quantitative	Requires specialized equipment	(40,65)
Cross-polarized light	None	Subclinical erythema	Any potential irritant	Permits detection of physical changes not apparent by standard visual scoring, noninvasive	Requires specialized equipment	(71)
Thermoscan	None	Temperature increases resulting from inflammatory processes related to skin injury	Any potential irritant	Noninvasive, objective, quantitative	Requires specialized equipment	(72)
Sebutape	None	Measurement of cytokines produced by injured skin	Any potential irritant	Noninvasive, objective, quantitative, potentially very sensitive	Requires training, specialized equipment; utility for sensitive skin still unassessed	(73)

Source: Farage, M. A., and Maibach, H. I., *Contact Dermat*, 62, 137–149, 2010. With permission.

the sensitive skin group and 24% of the nonsensitive group. In a study conducted in Italy among 2101 individuals (18), emotions were cited as one of the main triggers for irritation by a large proportion of the sensitive skin group (52% of women and 27.9% of men). In a study in France conducted to evaluate the prevalence of sensitive skin at specific body sites, Saint-Martory et al. (69) reported that 61% of sensitive skin subjects identified stress as a triggering factor, a frequency second only to cold (66%). Animal models have demonstrated that stress can activate dermal mast cells and skin nerves (1). Further, individuals with reactive skin (as determined by electric current perception) have been demonstrated to have a higher density of mast cells (74).

Sensitive skin is often associated with cosmetics and other consumer products (22). Among women with sensitive skin, 60% indicated a response to cosmetics (21). Only 14% of women without sensitive skin claimed such a response. In a 2001 study conducted in England, Willis et al. (13) reported that 80.11% of the sensitive skin group have experienced an adverse reaction to a cosmetic product compared to 32.61% of the nonsensitive group.

In both men and women, many household and personal hygiene products have been identified as potential triggering factors for skin irritation among individuals with sensitive skin, including laundry detergents, hand and body soaps, deodorants, and sunscreens (21). In their study on 400 women in France, Saint-Martory et al. (69) reported that soaps and cosmetics were identified as potential triggers by 42% and 28%, respectively, of sensitive skin responders.

Women seem more susceptible to adverse effects from products. In a study among 1093 individuals in Ohio, we reported that a higher percentage of women claim to have adverse reactions to facial products such as moisturizers, lotions, astringents, and cleansers (21). However, for both men and women, there was a significant difference between those with sensitive skin and those with nonsensitive skin.

One observation that may be of particular importance to sensitive skin at sites other than the face is the reaction to rough fabrics. For both men and women, this seems to be a frequent triggering factor for sensitive skin. In our US study, 69% of men with sensitive skin and 71% of women indicated rough fabric causes some degree of irritation (21). For the nonsensitive group, the proportion of men and women were 33% and 45%, respectively. Friction from clothes was identified as a trigger by 28% of responders in a study in France among 400 women (69).

There has not been a great deal of investigative work to correlate specific triggering factors for sensitive skin with specific anatomical sites; however, it is apparent that different triggers are important based on the potential exposures for those sites. Facial skin is somewhat unique since it is exposed to all types of weather and environmental conditions and to many cosmetics and personal care products. Other areas of the body may have more limited exposure to weather conditions, but greater exposure to fabrics in clothing. The genital area is exposed to specific potential triggers such as incontinent products (19).

Sensitive Skin at Different Anatomical Sites

It is becoming increasingly clear that individuals can have very different perceptions about the degree of skin sensitivity at different anatomical sites. Table 17.4 provides a brief overview of studies specifically inquiring about the perception of sensitive skin at particular anatomical sites. (Further details on individual studies are discussed in subsequent sections of this chapter.)

Structural differences in the skin can contribute to differences in barrier function and, therefore, differences in skin sensitivity between anatomical regions. The SC density tremendously varies by anatomical site. As reviewed by Tagami (75), genital skin demonstrated the thinnest SC, followed by the face, neck, scalp, trunk, and extremities. Location-related differences in percutaneous absorption have also been identified. Feldmann and Maibach (76) monitored the excretion of topically applied C14-hydrocortisone from a number of body sites and compared the rate of material applied to the volar surface of the forearm. These investigators found a large variation in the absorption and subsequent excretion, from trace amounts when the material was applied to the plantar foot arch (0.14 times that of the volar surface of the forearm) to extremely high amounts when the material was applied to the scrotum (42 times that of the forearm). The areas of the forehead and jaw angle demonstrated absorption that was 6 times and 13 times that of the forearm, respectively. Similar studies with additional materials

TABLE 17.4

Overview of Self-Proclaimed Sensitive Skin at Specific Anatomical Sites

Anatomical Site	Any Sensitivity[a] (%)	Country	References
Face	34	England	(13)
	49–85	France	(69,77,78)
	52–86	United States	(6,19,23,60)
	20	China	(10)
Scalp	23.5	England	(13)
	29–70	France	(69,79,80)
Genital skin	44–68[b]	United States	(6,19,23)
	6	China	(10)
Other Body Sites			
Hands	58	France	(69)
Feet	34	France	(69)
Neck	27	France	(69)
Torso	23	France	(69)
Back	21	France	(69)
Body	60–75	United States	(6,23)
Body	9	China	(10)

[a] Further details on individual studies are contained in subsequent tables.
[b] Among incontinent women, prevalence was 86%.

(benzoic acid, benzoic acid sodium salt, caffeine, and acetyl salicylic acid) were conducted by Rougier et al. (81). Results showed that permeability considerably varied depending on the anatomical location and the physicochemical nature of the substance. Generally, the forehead was more permeable than the postauricular area, followed by the abdomen and the arm. The presence of skin appendages such as hair follicles and sweat ducts result in incomplete SC barrier function (75) and provide a pathway for the penetration of substances through the skin.

Measurements of TEWL tend to be parallel to both the thickness of the SC and the percutaneous permeation. In vivo TEWL measurements demonstrate high variation depending on body site (75). The TEWL measured on facial skin is >10 g/m^2/h, about twice that of the forearm, upper arm, trunk, and lower extremities (i.e., around 5 g/m^2/h). On the scalp and axilla, TEWL measurements of around 7 g/m^2/h have been reported. The female vulva, which has an SC layer that is the thinnest of measured body sites, demonstrated TEWL measurements of up to 25 g/m^2/h.

As corneocytes mature, they begin to more firmly attach to the intercellular lipids that compose the cornified envelope. Thus, larger, flattened, mature corneocytes result in superior barrier function compared to areas with rounder, smaller, less mature epidermal cells. The SC of areas of high epidermal cell proliferation, such as the face and scalp, tend to demonstrate corneocytes smaller in size than areas of slower proliferation, such as the trunk or extremities (75). Similarly, these corneocytes are less mature and, therefore, less firmly attached.

Variability in perceived sensitivity is likely related, at least in part, to structural differences. This is especially apparent in investigations in which the same group of individuals was asked about perceived sensitivity at more than one anatomical site. In a study conducted in 2006, 1039 men and women completed a survey questionnaire related to their perceptions of sensitive skin. Within this group, 77.3% reported perceived sensitivity of the face, compared with 60.7% for the body, and 56.2% specifically with regard to genital skin (6). The prevalence of sensitive skin of the genital area differed significantly based on gender (women reported 58.1% and men reported 44.2%; $P = .03$) (6), ethnicity (Caucasian men versus women reported 37.3% and 57%, respectively; $P < .0001$; African American men versus women, 65% and 66.7%, respectively; $P = .84$) (21), and age (increasing from 53% in the <30 years age group to 66% in the >50 years age group; $P = 0.012$) (6). In contrast, the perception of sensitive skin of the face and body did not differ between these demographic subgroups. Saint-Martory et al. (69) reported on a survey questionnaire study conducted in 2004–2005 among 400 individuals in France (69). The face was most often reported as the site of sensitivity (85% of responders). However, other anatomical sites were also reported as sensitive: the hands (58%), scalp (36%), feet (34%), neck (27%), torso (23%), and back (21%), in order of frequency.

Face

The face is a common area of concern for skin sensitivity. Stinging sensations, particularly, are readily elicited on facial skin (82), and the face is readily accessible for both visual (83) and biophysical assessments (40). Further, facial skin is highly innervated, has an abundant blood circulation, and is metabolically active (75). The nasolabial fold has been reported to be the most sensitive region (68) of the facial area, followed by themalar eminence (68), chin, forehead, and upper lip (69). Factors contributing to facial sensitivity are likely the number of products used on the face (particularly in women), a thinner barrier in facial skin, and an abundance of nerve endings (84).

In Western industrialized countries, the percentage of individuals who perceived sensitive facial skin appears to be increasing. As shown in Table 17.5, a study conducted in England prior to 2001 (13) reported that the percentage of participants who responded positively to a yes/no question about perceived sensitive skin of the face was 34%. A 1998 study conducted in France (64,78) reported that 49% of participants perceived sensitive skin of the face. Both investigators found that a greater proportion of women had this perception compared to men. A study in France (conducted in 2004–2005) reported that 85% of women in the survey perceived that they had sensitive skin (69). In a study conducted in 1998 in the United States, Jourdain et al. (60) reported that a total of 52% of women perceived their facial skin to be very or moderately sensitive. Studies conducted since 2006 in the United States report the proportion of subjects who perceived their facial skin as sensitive to some degree as 68–86% (6,19,21,23).

In China, the proportion of women who perceive their facial skin as sensitive is much lower (20%) (10). The only other reported study in China (summarized in Table 17.1) did not ask, specifically, if participants had sensitive facial skin (11). However, the questionnaire asked about specific symptoms of the face and irritation after cosmetic usage. About 5% of the participants who reported burning or pruritus after using cosmetics and 9.4% of the participants who reported prickling did not claim to have sensitive skin. Approximately 28% of the participants who experienced irritation on the face often or sometimes did not report sensitive skin. The differences between China and the western, industrialized countries could be in part related to cultural differences. As discussed earlier, cultural influences likely account for some of this difference. A lack of familiarity with the term *sensitive skin* may result in underreporting.

Scalp

Based on three studies conducted in France, sensitive scalp is reported by about a third of the population (Table 17.6). Willis et al. (13) reported that about a quarter of the participants in a study in England perceived that they had sensitive scalp. In the 2004–2005 survey study conducted by Saint-Martory et al. (69) among 400 women, 36% claimed to have sensitive scalp. Misery et al. (79) reported on two survey studies conducted in France. In a 2008 study among 1011 subjects, 14.5% reported suffering from very sensitive scalp and 29.4% from moderately sensitive scalp. Women suffered more frequently from a sensitive scalp compared to men (47.4% of men and 40.8% of women; $P < .05$). Cold and emotions were identified as triggers (79). In a subsequent study conducted in France, in 2009, involving 2117 individuals, 682 (32.2%) declared they had a sensitive scalp (29.1% of men and 35.6% of women) (80). There was no association between sensitive scalp and a particular scalp disease, such as hair loss, dandruff, seborrheic dermatitis, psoriasis, and allergy (79,80). However, the frequency of all scalp diseases increased in parallel with the perceived severity of the scalp sensitivity (80). The proportion of people declaring sensitive scalp increased with age (80). Itching was the most commonly reported symptom (59%), with prickling (33%), tightness (16%), pain (13%), and burning (11%) also reported (80).

TABLE 17.5

Self-Declared Sensitive Skin of the Face

Country	Year	Population	Number of Subjects	Any Sens.[a]	Degree of Self-Proclaimed Sensitivity (%)			References
					Very	**Moderate**	**Slight**	
Europe								
England	2001[b]	General population by mailed questionnaire	2316 total	34[c]	NA	NA	NA	(13)
			2058 women	34.6	NA	NA	NA	
			258 men	29.1	NA	NA	NA	
France	1998	General population (35–60 years of age) by questionnaire	8522 total	49[c]			NA	(7,77)
			5074 women	61	NA	NA	NA	
			3448 men	32	NA	NA	NA	
France	2004–2005	Hospital outpatients and healthy volunteers	400 women	85	30.5	NA	NA	(69)
North America								
United States	1998	General population in San Francisco	811 women		31[c]	21[c]	NA	(60)
United States	2006	Female panelists (age: ≥50)	29 incontinent women	86.2	10.3	41.4	34.5	(19)
			42 age matched control	82.9	4.9	31.7	46.3	
United States	2009	General population in Cincinnati, Ohio	1039 total	77.3	10.7	23.7	42.9	(6)
			869 women	78.6	11.2	25.3	42.1	(21)
			163 men	68.1	8.6	15.3	44.2	(22)
United States (Mississippi)	2013[b]	General population in rural Mississippi	89 women	79.8	21.3	30.5	28	(23)
Asia								
China	2009[b]	General population in China	408 women	20	3	5	12	(10)

Note: NA: not available.

[a] Any sensitivity, for example, very, moderate, or slight.

[b] If year of study is not given, the date corresponds to the year of publication.

[c] Percentages are not reported but interpreted from other data in publication.

Vulva and Genitalia

The vulvar epithelium exhibits marked regional differences in structure (66). The cutaneous epithelium of the mons pubis and labia majora exhibits a keratinized, stratified, squamous structure. The degree of keratinization and thickness of the epidermis decreases toward the labia minora, and the inner third of the labia minora is a nonkeratinized mucosal tissue.

Although the labia majora is composed of keratinized epithelium comparable to exposed skin, it is more hydrated and, therefore, more permeable to some materials (61) and more susceptible to friction effects. The nonkeratinized vulvar skin of the labia minora exhibits increased permeability related to the absence of keratin and loosely packed, less structured lipid barrier (24,66). In addition, the thinner, inner epithelia represent a shorter distance for penetration of substances (66). Differences in susceptibility to irritation seem to be dependent on the relative permeability of the irritant in the skin of the vulva. For example, vulvar skin is significantly more reactive than forearm skin to benzalkonium chloride and maleic acid (85), but less reactive than the forearm to SLS (28,66). When both venous

TABLE 17.6

Self-Declared Sensitive Scalp

Country	Year	Population	Number of Subjects	Any Sens.[a]	Very	Moderate	Slight	Reference
					Degree of Self-Proclaimed Sensitivity (%)			
England	2001[b]	General population by mailed questionnaire	2316 total	23.5[c]	NA	NA	NA	(13)
			2058 women	23.25	NA	NA	NA	
			258 men	25.38	NA	NA	NA	
France	2004–2005	Hospital outpatients and healthy volunteers	400 women	36	NA	NA	11.9	(69)
France	2008[b]	General population in France	1011 total	69.8	14.5	29.4	25.9	(79)
			women	NA	47.4[c] (very and moderate)		NA	
			men	NA	40.8[c] (very and moderate)		NA	
France	2009	General population in France	2117 total	32.22	8.8[c]	16.4[c]	6.9[c]	(80)
			women	35.56	NA	NA	NA	
			men	29.1	NA	NA	NA	

Note: NA: not available.
[a] Any sensitivity, for example, very, moderate, or slight.
[b] If year of study is not given, the date corresponds to the year of publication.
[c] Percentages are not reported but interpreted from other data in publication.

blood and menses were evaluated for irritant potential, the vulva was less responsive to both than was the upper arm (86,87) suggesting that the labia majora is adapted to be less sensitive to menses-induced skin irritation (87).

Several studies using the identical questionnaire have been conducted in the United States (Cincinnati, Ohio, and rural Mississippi) and China (Table 17.7). The proportion of subjects in the United States who perceive that they have sensitive genital skin is 44–58% (6,21,23). In contrast, the proportion of subjects with this same perception in China is only 6% (10).

Unlike perceived sensitive skin at some other anatomical sites, sensitive genital skin is related to gender and ethnicity. In the study conducted among 1039 subjects in a metropolitan area in Ohio, there was a significant difference in the perception of sensitive genital between women and men (58.1% and 44.2%, respectively; $P = .030$) (6,88). Further, this same study showed that a higher proportion of African Americans described themselves as having sensitive genital skin compared to Caucasians (66.4% and 54.2%, respectively; $P = .012$) (88). Among different age groups (i.e., <30, 31–39, 40–40, and >50), sensitive skin of the genital area was more likely to be declared by subjects aged 50 and older than the subjects in the other age groups ($P = .012$). Of the three specific anatomical sites included in the questionnaire (i.e., face, body, and genital skin), the skin of the genital area was the only site where the perception of sensitive skin was influenced by gender, ethnicity, and age.

A separate study evaluated perceptions of sensitive skin in women with urinary incontinence compared to a group of age-matched controls (19). Surprisingly, a lower percentage of incontinent subjects described their genital skin as very or moderately sensitive compared to control subjects. The explanation for this surprising result is unclear. It is possible that incontinent individuals may attribute adverse sensory effects or irritation to their incontinent status, rather than to the notion that they have sensitive skin of the genital area (88). In this study, the triggering factor most strongly associated with sensitive genital skin was rough fabrics.

TABLE 17.7

Self-Declared Sensitive Genital Skin

Country	Year	Population	Number of Subjects	Any Sens.[a]	Degree of Self-Proclaimed Sensitivity (%)			References
					Very	Moderate	Slight	
United States	2006	Female panelists (age: ≥50)	29 incontinent women	86.2	6.9	27.6	51.7	(19)
			42 age matched control	68.3	12.2	14.6	41.5	
United States	2009	General population in Cincinnati,	1039 total	56.3	8.5	13.6	43.7	(6,21,22)
			869 women	58.1	9.4	14.5	34.2	
			163 men	44.2	3.7	8	32.5	
United States (Mississippi)	2013[b]	General population in rural Mississippi	89 women	57.3	3.4	20.2	33.7	(23)
China	2009[b]	General population in China	408 women	6	1	1	4	(10)

[a] Any sensitivity: For example, very, moderate, or slight.
[b] If year of study is not given, the date corresponds to the year of publication.

Other Body Sites

Survey data relating specifically to sensitive skin of other body sites is summarized in Table 17.8. As mentioned earlier, Saint-Martory et al. (69) conducted a survey in 2004–2005 among 400 individuals in the general population in France. The face was most often reported as the site of sensitivity (85% of responders, as shown in Table 17.4). However, other anatomical sites were also reported as sensitive: the hands (58%), scalp (36%), feet (34%), neck (27%), torso (23%), and back (21%), in order of frequency.

In a study conducted in the United States (urban area of Cincinnati, Ohio), the proportion of the subjects claiming to have sensitive body skin was 60.7%, with a similar proportion of women and men (60.2% and 62%, respectively) (6,21,22). A higher proportion of women claimed some degree of sensitive body skin in the study conducted in rural Mississippi (i.e., 74.2%) (23). Mississippi and Ohio have dramatically different climates. Mississippi experiences mild winters and long summers with high temperatures and humidity; Cincinnati, Ohio, has cold winters and milder summers. Dramatically different cultural factors may also influence southern women as compared to those farther north.

As with other body sites the prevalence of self-declared sensitive body skin was much lower in China than in other geographical sites, suggesting at least some cultural component (10). Only 9% of the surveyed population claimed some degree of sensitivity of the skin on the body.

Conclusion

Sensitive skin is a real phenomenon, and it is clear that specific individuals have heightened sensory responses to different kinds of external irritants and other stimuli. We are beginning to understand some of the physiological basis for this condition. However, a thorough understanding of the underlying physiological causes remains elusive. Difficulties in progress are magnified by the variability of this condition based on geography, culture, season, and even anatomical site. A lack of correlation between sensory symptoms and objective signs presents a serious challenge in developing reliable diagnostic tests. It is

TABLE 17.8

Self-Declared Sensitive Skin at Other Body Sites

Country	Year	Population	Number of Subjects	Body Site	Any Sens.[a]	Degree of Self-Proclaimed Sensitivity (%)			References
						Very	**Moderate**	**Slight**	
France	2004–2005	Hospital outpatients and healthy volunteers	400 women	Hands	58	20.1	NA	NA	(69)
				Feet	34	11.3	NA	NA	
				Neck	27	8.7	NA	NA	
				Torso	23	5.9	NA	NA	
				Back	21	5.2	NA	NA	
United States	2009	General population in Cincinnati, Ohio	1039 total	Body	60.7	1.8	18.3	4.06	(6,21,22)
			869 women	Body	60.2	1.8	18.6	39.7	
			163 men	Body	62	1.8	16	44.2	
United States (Mississippi)	2013[b]	General population in rural Mississippi	89 women	Body	74.2	9	31.5	33.7	(23)
United States	2006	Female panelists (age: ≥50)	29 incontinent women	Body	69	3.4	31	34.5	(19)
			42 age matched control	Body	65.9	2.4	22	41.5	
China	2009[b]	General population in China	408 women	Body	9	1	2	6	(10)

Note: NA: not available.

[a] Any sensitivity: For example, very, moderate, or slight.

[b] If year of study is not given, the date corresponds to the year of publication.

becoming increasingly clear that the phenomenon of sensitive skin is the product of multiple etiologies with multiple components. Our challenge is that we must continue to incorporate these new understandings as we chip away at a more complete understanding of sensitive skin.

REFERENCES

1. Berardesca E, Farage MA, Maibach H. Sensitive skin: An overview. *Int J Cosmet Sci.* 2013;35:2–8.
2. Farage MA, Maibach HI. Sensitive skin: New findings yield new insights. In: Baran R, Maibach HI, editors. *Textbook of Cosmetic Dermatology.* New York: Informa Healthcare; 2010. pp. 73–83.
3. Farage MA, Maibach HI. Sensitive skin: Closing in on a physiological cause. *Contact Dermat.* 2010;62:137–149.
4. Farage MA. Are we reaching the limits or our ability to detect skin effects with our current testing and measuring methods for consumer products? *Contact Dermat.* 2005;52:297–303.
5. Escalas-Taberner J, Gonzalez-Guerra E, Guerra-Tapia A. Sensitive skin: A complex syndrome. *Actas Dermosifiliogr.* 2011;102:563–571.
6. Farage MA. How do perceptions of sensitive skin differ at different anatomical sites? An epidemiological study. *Clin Exp Dermatol.* 2009;34:e521–e530.
7. Taïeb C, Auges M, Georgescu V, Perez Cullell N et al. Sensitive skin in Brazil and Russia: An epidemiological and comparative approach. *Eur J Dermatol.* 2014;24:372–376.
8. Hernández-Blanco D, Castanedo-Cázares JP, Ehnis-Pérez A, Jasso-Ávila I et al. Prevalence of sensitive skin and its biophysical response in a Mexican population. *World J Dermatol.* 2013;2:1–7.
9. Kamide R, Misery L, Perez-Cullell N, Sibaud V et al. Sensitive skin evaluation in the Japanese population. *J Dermatol.* 2013;40:177–181.

10. Farage MA, Mandl CP, Berardesca E, Maibach HI. Sensitive skin in China. *J Cosmet Dermatol Sci Appl.* 2012;2:184–195.
11. Xu F, Yan S, Wu M, Li F et al. Self-declared sensitive skin in China: A community-based study in three top metropolises. *J Eur Acad Dermatol Venereol.* 2013;27:370–375.
12. Misery L, Boussetta S, Nocera T, Perez-Cullell N et al. Sensitive skin in Europe. *J Eur Acad Dermatol Venereol.* 2009;23:376–381.
13. Willis CM, Shaw S, De Lacharriere O, Baverel M et al. Sensitive skin: An epidemiological study. *Br J Dermatol.* 2001;145:258–263.
14. Misery L, Myon E, Martin N, Verriere F et al. Sensitive skin in France: An epidemiological approach. *Ann Dermatol Venereol.* 2005;132:425–429.
15. Misery L, Myon E, Martin N, Consoli S et al. Sensitive skin: Psychological effects and seasonal changes. *J Eur Acad Dermatol Venereol.* 2007;21:620–628.
16. Loffler H, Dickel H, Kuss O, Diepgen TL et al. Characteristics of self-estimated enhanced skin susceptibility. *Acta Derm Venereol.* 2001;81:343–346.
17. Farage MA, Bowtell P, Katsarou A. Self-diagnosed sensitive skin in women with clinically diagnosed atopic dermatitis. *Clin Med Dermatol.* 2008;2:21–28.
18. Sparavigna A, Di Pietro A, Setaro M. "Healthy skin": Significance and results of an Italian study on healthy population with particular regard to "sensitive" skin. *Int J Cosmet Sci.* 2005;27:327–331.
19. Farage MA. Perceptions of sensitive skin: Women with urinary incontinence. *Arch Gynecol Obstet.* 2009;280:49–57.
20. Misery L, Sibaud V, Merial-Kieny C, Taïeb C. Sensitive skin in the American population: Prevalence, clinical data, and role of the dermatologist. *Int J Dermatol.* 2011;50:961–967.
21. Farage MA. Does sensitive skin differ between men and women? *Cutan Ocul Toxicol.* 2010;29:153–163.
22. Farage MA. Perceptions of sensitive skin: Changes in perceived severity and associations with environmental causes. *Contact Dermat.* 2008;59:226–232.
23. Farage MA, Miller KW, Wippel AM, Berardesca E et al. Sensitive skin in the United States: Survey of regional differences. *Family Med Medical Sci Res.* 2013;2:1–8.
24. Farage MA. Vulvar susceptibility to contact irritants and allergens: A review. *Arch Gynecol Obstet.* 2005;272:167–172.
25. Farage MA, Lennon L. Products for vulvar hygiene. In: Farage MA, Maibach HI, editors. *The Vulva: Anatomy, Physiology and Pathology,* first edition. New York: Informa Healthcare; 2006. pp. 217–233.
26. Farage MA. Perceptions of sensitive skin with age. In: Farage MA, Miller KW, Maibach HI, editors. *Textbook of Aging Skin.* Berlin Heidelberg: Springer-Verlag; 2010. pp. 1027–1046.
27. Misery L. Sensitive skin. *Expert Rev Dermatol.* 2013;8:631–637.
28. Farage MA, Robinson MK. Sensitive skin: Intrinsic and extrinsic contributors. In: Loden M, Maibach HI, editors. Treatment of Dry Skin Syndrome. Berlin: Springer-Verlag; 2012. pp. 95–109.
29. Inamadar AC, Palit A. Sensitive skin: An overview. Indian J Dermatol Venereol Leprol. 2013;79:9–16.
30. Farage MA, Maibach HI. Sensitive skin: New findings yield new insights (submitted). Textbook on Cosmetic Dermatology, fifth edition. 2015.
31. Robinson MK. Racial differences in acute and cumulative skin irritation responses between Caucasian and Asian populations. *Contact Dermat.* 2000;42:134–143.
32. Aramaki J, Kawana S, Effendy I, Happle R et al. Differences of skin irritation between Japanese and European women. *Br J Dermatol.* 2002;146:1052–1056.
33. Freeman RG, Cockerell EG, Armstrong J, Knox JM. Sunlight as a factor influencing the thickness of epidermis. *J Invest Dermatol.* 1962;39:295–298.
34. Thomson ML. Relative efficiency of pigment and horny layer thickness in protecting the skin of Europeans and Africans against solar ultraviolet radiation. *J Physiol.* 1955;127:236–246.
35. Pons-Guiraud A. Sensitive skin: A complex and multifactorial syndrome. *J Cosmet Dermatol.* 2004;3:145–148.
36. Corcuff P, Lotte C, Rougier A, Maibach HI. Racial differences in corneocytes: A comparison between black, white and oriental skin. *Acta Derm Venereol.* 1991;71:146–148.
37. Berardesca E, Maibach HI. Racial differences in sodium lauryl sulphate induced cutaneous irritation: Black and white. *Contact Dermat.* 1988;18:65–70.
38. Farage MA, Stadler A. Risk factors for recurrent vulvovaginal candidiasis. *Am J Obstet Gynecol.* 2005;192:981–2; author reply 982.

39. Lampe MA, Burlingame AL, Whitney J, Williams ML et al. Human stratum corneum lipids: Characterization and regional variations. *J Lipid Res*. 1983;24:120–130.

40. Seidenari S, Francomano M, Mantovani L. Baseline biophysical parameters in subjects with sensitive skin. *Contact Dermat*. 1998;38:311–315.

41. Reinertson RP, Wheatley VR. Studies on the chemical composition of human epidermal lipids. *J Invest Dermatol*. 1959;32:49–59.

42. Brod J. Characterization and physiological role of epidermal lipids. *Int J Dermatol*. 1991;30:84–90.

43. Elias PM, Menon GK. Structural and lipid biochemical correlates of the epidermal permeability barrier. *Adv Lipid Res*. 1991;24:1–26.

44. Swartzendruber DC, Wertz PW, Kitko DJ, Madison KC et al. Molecular models of the intercellular lipid lamellae in mammalian stratum corneum. *J Invest Dermatol*. 1989;92:251–257.

45. Lee CH, Maibach HI. The sodium lauryl sulfate model: An overview. *Contact Dermat*. 1995;33:1–7.

46. Marriott M, Whittle E, Basketter DA. Facial variations in sensory responses. *Contact Dermat*. 2003;49:227–231.

47. Farage MA. Self-reported immunological and familial links in individuals who perceive they have sensitive skin. *Br J Dermatol*. 2008;159(1):237–238.

48. Britz MB, Maibach HI, Anjo DM. Human percutaneous penetration of hydrocortisone: The vulva. *Arch Dermatol Res*. 1980;267:313–316.

49. Farage MA, Berardesca E, Maibach HI. Sensitive skin: A valid syndrome of multiple origins. In: Wilhelm K-P, Zhai H, Maibach HI, editors. *Marzulli and Maibach's Dermatotoxicology*, eighth edition. London: Informa Healthcare, Inc; 2012. pp. 238–247.

50. Berardesca E, Cespa M, Farinelli N, Rabbiosi G et al. In vivo transcutaneous penetration of nicotinates and sensitive skin. *Contact Dermat*. 1991;25:35–38.

51. Goffin V, Pierard-Franchimont C, Pierard GE. Sensitive skin and stratum corneum reactivity to household cleaning products. *Contact Dermat*. 1996;34:81–85.

52. Cho HJ, Chung BY, Lee HB, Kim HO et al. Quantitative study of stratum corneum ceramides contents in patients with sensitive skin. *J Dermatol*. 2012;39:295–300.

53. Roussaki-Schulze AV, Zafiriou E, Nikoulis D, Klimi E et al. Objective biophysical findings in patients with sensitive skin. *Drugs Exp Clin Res*. 2005;31 Suppl:17–24.

54. Cua AB, Wilhelm KP, Maibach HI. Cutaneous sodium lauryl sulphate irritation potential: Age and regional variability. *Br J Dermatol*. 1990;123:607–613.

55. Stander S, Schneider SW, Weishaupt C, Luger TA et al. Putative neuronal mechanisms of sensitive skin. *Exp Dermatol*. 2009;18:417–423.

56. Besne I, Descombes C, Breton L. Effect of age and anatomical site on density of sensory innervation in human epidermis. *Arch Dermatol*. 2002;138:1445–1450.

57. Green BG. Measurement of sensory irritation of the skin. *Am J Contact Dermat*. 2000;11:170–180.

58. Kim SJ, Lim SU, Won YH, An SS et al. The perception threshold measurement can be a useful tool for evaluation of sensitive skin. *Int J Cosmet Sci*. 2008;30:333–337.

59. Querleux B, Dauchot K, Jourdain R, Bastien P et al. Neural basis of sensitive skin: An fMRI study. *Skin Res Technol*. 2008;14:454–461.

60. Jourdain R, de Lacharriere O, Bastien P, Maibach HI. Ethnic variations in self-perceived sensitive skin: Epidemiological survey. *Contact Dermat*. 2002;46:162–169.

61. Farage MA, Maibach HI. Tissue structure and physiology of the vulva. In: Farage MA, Maibach HI, editors. *The Vulva: Anatomy, Physiology and Pathology*, first edition. New York: Informa Healthcare; 2006. pp. 9–26.

62. Harvell J, Hussona-Saeed I, Maibach HI. Changes in transepidermal water loss and cutaneous blood flow during the menstrual cycle. *Contact Dermat*. 1992;27:294–301.

63. Agner T, Damm P, Skouby SO. Menstrual cycle and skin reactivity. *J Am Acad Dermatol*. 1991;24:566–570.

64. Kligman A. Human models for characterizing "sensitive skin." *Cosmet Dermatol*. 2001;14:15–19.

65. Pinto P, Rosado C, Parreirao C, Rodrigues LM. Is there any barrier impairment in sensitive skin?: A quantitative analysis of sensitive skin by mathematical modeling of transepidermal water loss desorption curves. *Skin Res Technol*. 2011;17:181–185.

66. Farage MA, Maibach HI. The vulvar epithelium differs from the skin: Implications for cutaneous testing to address topical vulvar exposures. *Contact Dermat*. 2004;51:201–209.

67. Farage MA, Katsarou A, Maibach HI. Sensory, clinical and physiological factors in sensitive skin: A review. *Contact Dermat.* 2006;55:1–14.

68. Marriott M, Holmes J, Peters L, Cooper K et al. The complex problem of sensitive skin. *Contact Dermat.* 2005;53:93–99.

69. Saint-Martory C, Roguedas-Contios AM, Sibaud V, Degouy A et al. Sensitive skin is not limited to the face. *Br J Dermatol.* 2008;158:130–133.

70. Tan YM, Wang XM, Yuan C, Tang YW et al. Skin sensitivity and intolerance in Shanghai: Cumulative influence of different meteorological parameters. *Cutan Ocul Toxicol.* 20141–7.

71. Farage MA. Enhancement of visual scoring of skin irritant reactions using cross-polarized light and parallel-polarized light. *Contact Dermat.* 2008;58:147–155.

72. Farage MA, Wang B, Miller KW. Surface skin temperature in tests for irritant dermatitis. In: Berardesca E, Maibach H, Wilhelm K, editors. *Non Invasive Diagnostic Techniques in Clinical Dermatology.* Berlin: Springer; 2013. pp. 383–394.

73. Perkins MA, Osterhues MA, Farage MA, Robinson MK. A noninvasive method to assess skin irritation and compromised skin conditions using simple tape adsorption of molecular markers of inflammation. *Skin Res Technol.* 2001;7:227–237.

74. Quatresooz P, Pierard-Franchimont C, Pierard GE. Vulnerability of reactive skin to electric current perception—A pilot study implicating mast cells and the lymphatic microvasculature. *J Cosmet Dermatol.* 2009;8:186–189.

75. Tagami H. Location-related differences in structure and function of the stratum corneum with special emphasis on those of the facial skin. *Int J Cosmet Sci.* 2008;30:413–434.

76. Feldmann RJ, Maibach HI. Regional variation in percutaneous penetration of 14C cortisol in man. *J Invest Dermatol.* 1967;48:181–183.

77. Morizot F, Guinot C, Lopez S, Le Fur I et al. Sensitive skin: Analysis of symptoms, perceived causes and possible mechanisms. *Cosmet Toilet.* 2000;115:83–89.

78. Guinot C, Malvy D, Mauger E, Ezzedine K et al. Self-reported skin sensitivity in a general adult population in France: Data of the SU.VI.MAX cohort. *J Eur Acad Dermatol Venereol.* 2006;20:380–390.

79. Misery L, Sibaud V, Ambronati M, Macy G et al. Sensitive scalp: Does this condition exist? An epidemiological study. *Contact Dermat.* 2008;58:234–238.

80. Misery L, Rahhali N, Ambonati M, Black D et al. Evaluation of sensitive scalp severity and symptomatology by using a new score. *J Eur Acad Dermatol Venereol.* 2011;25:1295–1298.

81. Rougier A, Lotte C, Maibach HI. In vivo percutaneous penetration of some organic compounds related to anatomic site in humans: Predictive assessment by the stripping method. *J Pharm Sci.* 1987;76:451–454.

82. Farage MA, Bowtell P, Katsarou Z. The relationship among objectively assessed vulvar erythema, skin sensitivity, genital sensitivity, and self-reported facial skin redness. *J Appl Res.* 2006;6:272–281.

83. Vie K, Pons-Guiraud A, Dupuy P, Maibach H. Tolerance profile of a sterile moisturizer and moisturizing cleanser in irritated and sensitive skin. A*m J Contact Dermat.* 2000;11:161–164.

84. Chew A, Maibach H. Sensitive skin. In: Loden M, Miabach H, editors. *Dry Skin and Moisturizers: Chemistry and Function.* Boca Raton, FL: CRC Press; 2000. pp. 429–440.

85. Britz MB, Maibach HI. Human cutaneous vulvar reactivity to irritants. *Contact Dermat.* 1979;5:375–377.

86. Farage MA, Hood WH, Hillard P. The menstrual cycle, the composition of menses, and the effect of menses on skin. In: Farage MA, Maibach HI, editors. *The Vulva: Anatomy, Physiology and Pathology,* first edition. New York: Informa Healthcare; 2006. pp. 151–165.

87. Farage MA, Warren R, Wang-Weigand S. The vulva is relatively insensitive to menses-induced irritation. *Cutan Ocul Toxicol.* 2005;24:243–246.

88. Farage MA. Perceptions of sensitive skin of the genital area. In: Surber C, Elsner P, Farage MA, editors. *Topical Applications and the Mucosa.* Basel: Karger; 2011. pp. 142–154.

18

Sensitive Skin and Noneczematous Dermatoses

Ian McDonald, Helen Rea, and Martin Steinhoff

Introduction

Sensitive skin is a clinical syndrome defined by the self-reported facial presence of different sensory perceptions, including tightness, stinging, burning, tingling, pain, and/or pruritus (1). It is also known as *reactive* or *overreactive skin* or *intolerant* or *irritable skin*, and symptoms may occur in response to multiple factors including physical (UV, heat, cold, wind), chemical (cosmetics, soaps, water, pollutants) psychological (stress), or hormonal (menstrual cycle). In surveys, approximately 50% of women and 40% of men may report having sensitive skin (2). Complaints of sensitive skin most frequently relate to the face. Indeed, products that are tolerated on other sites can cause irritation on the face with the eyelids being especially sensitive. A study showed that 70% of patients reporting reactive facial skin also exhibited involvement of extrafacial sites, such as the hands, scalp, feet, neck, torso, or back (3). Genital involvement is also likely to be underestimated in prevalence with 56% of people in one study reporting having had sensitive genital skin (4).

The etiology of sensitive skin is thought to be multifactorial. Pathophysiologically, it is thought to result from interactions in the sensory nervous system, TRP ion channels including TRPV1 (localized on small to medium diameter sensory nerve endings [C fibers]), Merkel cells, and keratinocytes, skin cells including keratinocytes and blood vessels resulting in neurogenic inflammation. Atopic predisposition, other dermatoses, and a disrupted skin barrier function are additional predisposing factors. Other contributing factors are environmental triggers (e.g., UV irradiation), lifestyle (e.g., irritating makeup), and endogenous factors (e.g., hormonal changes, pH changes). In fact, the key role of sensory nerve endings has been highlighted (5) showing a decrease of intraepidermal nerve fiber density in patients with sensitive skin and, in particular, a decrease in the peptidergic C fiber density. However, as to whether a decrease in immunostaining clearly represents diminished nerve fiber numbers is controversial. To date, the treatment of sensitive skin is mainly to avoid certain irritants and to protect keratinocytes and epidermal barrier function (6,7). Most results suggest that the prevention and treatment of sensitive skin may be aided by protecting the survival of intraepidermal nerve fibers and by promoting their development. Thus, sensitive skin appears to be a more complex condition than a *cosmetic* syndrome. Although the pathophysiology of sensitive skin remains unclear (8), the underlying mechanism is not allergic and not in keeping with irritant-toxic eczema, which has a classical histology, time kinetic, and epidermal component.

Diagnosis

Sensitive skin remains a clinical diagnosis made on the grounds of typical symptoms and clinical features reported by patients. Tests that may help to establish the diagnosis include the stinging test, heat sensitivity test, and capsaicin test. However, because skin sensitivity occurs in response to a variety of factors either of nonallergic or more rarely allergic origin, accurate history-taking remains the most reliable diagnostic method (6).

Sensitive skin may occur in individuals with a variety of dermatoses, both eczematous and noneczematous. This chapter will concentrate on noneczematous dermatoses associated with symptoms of skin sensitivity. These include rosacea, perioral dermatitis (PD), and seborrhoeic dermatitis (SD). We will also briefly discuss noneczematous occupational dermatoses including irritant and allergic contact dermatitis, dry skin, and cutaneous dysthesias.

Rosacea

Rosacea is a common, chronic, and recurrent inflammatory skin disease that may be associated with ocular involvement. It primarily affects people of northern and western European descent and is often referred to as the *curse of the Celts* (9). Rosacea is associated with significant psychological morbidity and impaired health-related quality of life (10). Indeed, a survey performed by the National Rosacea Society involving over 500 people reported 42% of patients with rosacea feeling sad or depressed by the appearance of their skin.

The disease is characterized by a variety of primary and secondary features. Primary features include flushing (transient erythema) persistent erythema, teleangiectasia, papules, and pustules. Secondary features include symptoms of burning, stinging, and tightness of the skin. Secondary morphological features also include plaques, dry appearance, edema, or phymatous skin changes (10). Four distinct subtypes of rosacea have been recognized by the National Rosacea Society Expert Committee. These include erythematotelangiectatic rosacea (ETR), papulopustular, phymatous, and ocular rosacea. Subtype 1, ETR, is defined by the presence of flushing and central facial erythema. Additional possible features are edema, stinging, and burning sensations, as well as roughness or scaling. Subtype 2, papulopustular rosacea, is defined by persistent erythema and transient papules or pustules. Subtype 3, phymatous rosacea, presents with thickening skin, irregular surface nodularities, and enlargement. Areas affected by phymatous rosacea are the chin, forehead, cheeks, ears, and nose, with nasal involvement or rhinophyma being the most common phenotype. Ocular rosacea, finally, is defined as subtype 4 (11).

The exact pathogenesis of rosacea is poorly understood (12). Dysregulation of the innate and adaptive immune system with prolonged cytokine and chemokine release, overgrowth of commensal skin organisms, demodex infestation, and aberrant neurovascular signaling may all have a role in promoting the clinical features of rosacea (13). In response to environmental exogenous trigger factors (temperature changes, microbes, mites, spicy food) or endogenous trigger factors (exercise with subsequent vasodilation, ethanol, microbiota imbalance), toll-like receptors and other pattern recognition receptors induce the release of antimicrobial peptides, such as cathelicidin (LL-37), or proteases (e.g., kallikreins like KLK-5), matrix metalloproteinases (MMPs), reactive oxygen species, nitric oxides, cytokines, and chemokines, which initiate and perpetuate inflammation (14,15). The dermal structure is modified by these effectors through vascular changes (prolonged vasodilation, plasma extravasation, and, later, also angiogenesis) which also leads to extracellular matrix (especially collagen) degeneration, probably induced by MMPs. Infiltrated macrophages and mast cells, as well as T cells, produce more effector molecules, resulting in chronic inflammation (16). See Figure 18.1.

Current treatments for rosacea target many of these pathological processes partly, although with limited efficacy. One licensed treatment for the management of ETR is brimonidine 0.33% topical gel, which is an alpha-2 adrenergic agonist that acts on vascular smooth muscle cells (17). It is a symptomatic treatment specifically developed and indicated for the persistent facial erythema of rosacea (18). Topical ivermectin, which is an antiparasitic and anti-inflammatory agent, is also now fully licensed for the treatment of papulopustular rosacea. It reduces the number of inflammatory lesions and also erythema. Other approved medications include topical azelaic acid, topical metronidazole, and slow-release doxycycline. Off-label therapies include laser therapy or medications such as alpha1 antagonists, beta-adrenergic antagonists, sodium sulfacetamide, sulfur, clindamycin, and systemic low-dose isotretinoin, for example.

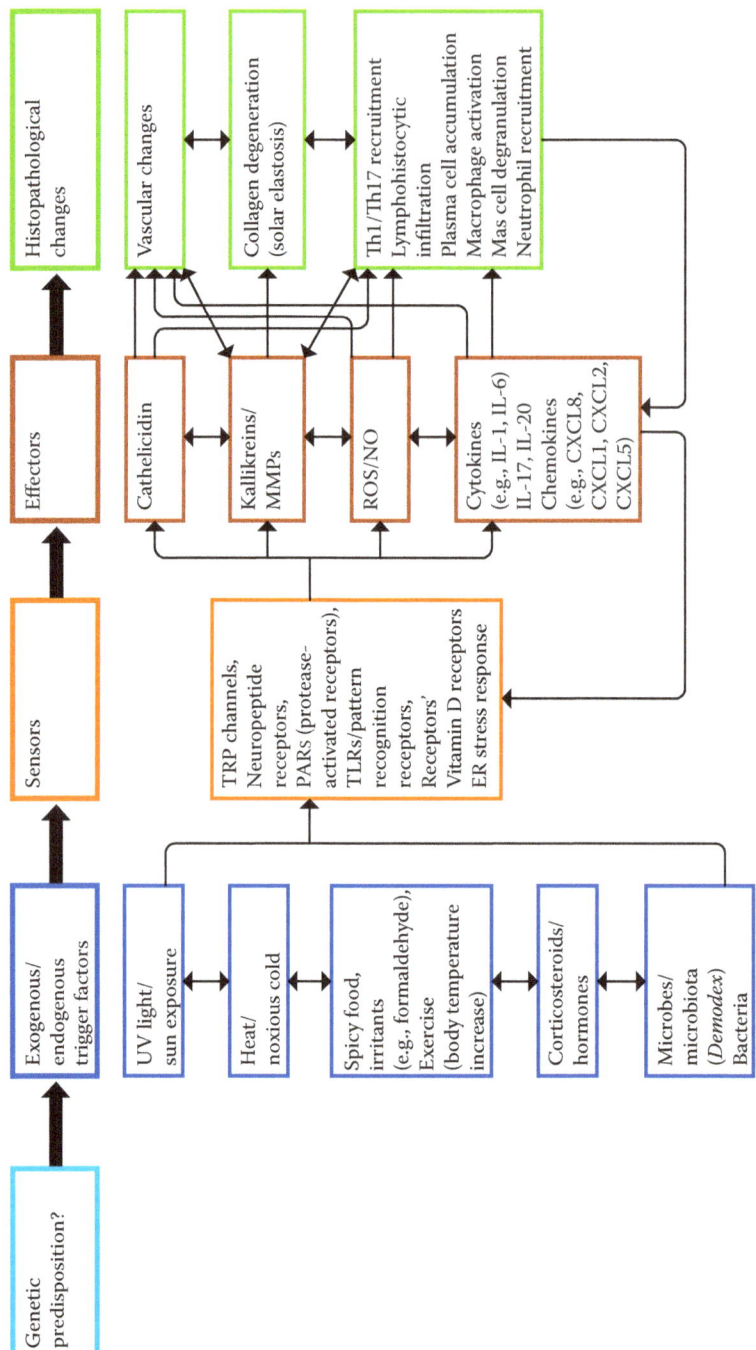

FIGURE 18.1 Possible mechanisms and pathways in the pathogenesis of rosacea.

Perioral Dermatitis

PD is a common, chronic inflammatory, papulopustular/vesicular dermatitis with morphological and histological similarities to rosacea. It was first described in 1957 as a cyclical, light-sensitive seborrhoeid affecting the perioral area in young women (19). The term *perioral dermatitis* was later introduced by Mihan and Ayres in 1964 after describing the condition in 21 patients (20). PD is associated with symptoms of skin sensitivity including burning and stinging and has a significant impact on patient quality of life (21). Like many patients with skin sensitivity, affected individuals also describe intolerance of sunlight, heat, and wind in addition to various cosmetics that tend to exacerbate their symptoms (22).

It has a spectrum of clinical manifestations lending itself to many synonyms including periorofacial dermatitis, rosacea-like dermatitis, chronic papulopustular facial dermatitis, facial Afro-Caribbean childhood eruption, lupus-like PD, and granulomatous perioral/periorofacial dermatitis.

PD predominantly affects young to middle-aged women who account for approximately 90% of cases (23). It is now however becoming increasingly common in men and can also occur in children and adolescents. In childhood and infancy, it has a slight female predominance and can present as early as 6 months with a peak incidence in those younger than 5 years of age (24).

The morphological features of PD consist of small (1–2 mm) grouped, superficial, erythematous papules, papulovesicles, or papulopustules in a predominantly perioral distribution. This distinctive pattern in the perioral area and nasolabial folds helps distinguish PD from rosacea, which is mainly centrofacial in presentation. The lesions of PD can also affect the periorbital area and lateral portion on the lower eyelids. Papules may be superimposed on thin confluent erythematous plaques resembling a nonspecific dermatitis, and the sparing of vermillion border is a characteristic clinical finding in many patients.

Although the pathogenesis and etiology of PD is still unclear, several factors and causes have been postulated. The overuse of emollients on affected skin areas is thought to be a relevant contributing factor, while topical steroids, although initially improving symptoms, can result in significant rebound after cessation of use. Indeed, systemic and inhaled corticosteroids can also lead to the development of PD (25,26). Infective agents are also thought to play a role in the pathogenesis of PD. Fusiform spirilla bacteria, demodex folliculorum, and candida, for example, have all been cultured from lesions of patients with PD. Whether their presence is causative or consequential of the environment is yet to be established. A hormonal link has also suggested given its temporal association with menses, pregnancy, and the oral contraceptive pill (27).

Histopathologically, the papules of PD have a granulomatous component similar to that of rosacea. Early papules demonstrate an eczematous picture, while later, more chronic lesions reveal diffused hypertrophy of connective tissue and hyperplasia of sebaceous follicles.

Although there is no accepted, standard treatment regime for PD at the time of writing, initial measures should include appropriate skin care advice. As a first step, discontinuation of potential causative and exacerbating agents such as cosmetics, emollients, and topical corticosteroids is advised. Patients are advised to wash their face with warm water only and to use liquid or gel sunscreens if required. Although some authors suggest a *watch-and-wait approach*, this can be unacceptable for many patients. Topical treatments include antibiotics such as metronidazole, erythromycin, or clindamycin, which have been found to be moderately effective in the treatment of PD (28). Topical calcineurin inhibitors (pimecrolimus, tacrolimus) have also demonstrated efficacy, particularly in the setting of steroid-induced PD. However, caution is advised given the occasional reports of granulomatous eruptions after using these preparations (29,30). More recently, Praziquantel 3% ointment was shown to improve symptoms of PD and quality of life in adult patients treated daily for 4 weeks (31). Systemic treatment includes the use of oral antibiotics for a period of 4–6 weeks. Commonly used agents include oxytetracycline, doxycycline, and erythromycin (particularly in the pediatric population where tetracycline-induced teeth staining is a concern). The option of oral isotretinoin is reserved for patients failing to respond to oral antibiotics. It is prescribed at doses between 0.05 and 0.1 mg/kg, lower than that used in acne vulgaris (31).

Although sharing many clinical features with rosacea including symptoms of skin sensitivity, the natural history of PD thankfully bears less resemblance. Following appropriate treatment and clearance, subsequent relapses are uncommon.

Seborrhoeic Dermatitis

SD is a common, chronic, and recurrent inflammatory skin disease characterized by the presence of thin erythematous scaly plaques and patches with ill-defined borders. It mainly affects sebum-rich areas of the body such as the scalp, face, upper chest, and back and may be associated with symptoms of sensitive skin such as pruritus (32). SD is common, affecting approximately 11% of the general population and up to 70% of infants in the first 3 months of life (33). Among adults, the peak incidence is in the third and fourth decades of life and is often associated with a substantially negative impact on quality of life (34). The severity of SD is highly variable and occurs more frequently in certain medical conditions including Parkinson's disease, familial amyloidosis, and trisomy 21. Abrupt onset and severe recalcitrant SD may also be the result of underlying human immunodeficiency virus infection where it is the most common dermatoses (occurring in 31% of patients including those on antiretrovirals). It can occur in the setting of immunosuppressant medication (renal transplant patients) and with certain psychotropic medications. Patients also report emotional stress and fatigue as exacerbating factors (35).

The diagnosis of SD is a clinical one characterized by the presence of itchy erythematous patches with greasy scales. Commonly affected sites include the scalp, anterior hairline, eyebrows, glabella region of the forehead, nasolabial folds, ears, central chest (petaloid appearance), and genital region. Scalp involvement typically results in fine scale/dandruff that may be associated with signs of inflammation such as erythema, or indeed, local or generalized scaling may appear in isolation.

Although the exact pathogenesis of SD is not completely understood, it is thought to be dependent upon three factors: sebum, microbial metabolism (specifically, Malassezia yeasts), and individual susceptibility (36–39). There appears to be a strong association with yeast colonization particularly of the genus *Malassezia* spp (40). This is evidenced by the clinical improvement observed in patients treated with antifungal medication and a reduction in *Malassezia* spp. seen. Sebum lipid degradation and subsequent production of modified unsaturated short-chain fatty acids by *Malassezia* spp. means they are more capable of penetrating skin and inducing inflammation. Applications of genetic and proteomic techniques have also resulted in a greater understanding of the mechanisms involved in SD and dandruff. It now appears likely that yeast genes are switched on to produce different irritants or metabolites on both dandruff and SD-affected skin. The *Malassezia* species, *M. globosa* and *M. restricta*, are most commonly associated with these conditions. The production of oleic acid and other inflammatory molecules by these species can induce scaling and immunostimulation as oleic acid is a ligand for aryl hydrocarbon receptors involved in contact sensitization (39).

Several treatment options exist for the management of SD. These include topical antifungals and anti-inflammatories, keratolytics, and tar products.

Topical antifungals, particularly the azoles (ketoconazole), are established and effective treatment for SD (41). They can also be used intermittently to maintain remission and in combination with topical anti-inflammatories such as topical steroids or calcineurin inhibitors. The latter is used to effectively control the inflammatory component of SD although tacrolimus also has demonstrated potent fungicidal activity against Malassezia in vitro. Other nonprescription antifungal treatments include selenium sulfide which is present in many over-the-counter (OTC) shampoos and has demonstrated efficacy as a twice-weekly treatment regime. Tea tree oil and zinc pyrithione present in antidandruff shampoos are also commonly used by patients as OTC alternatives.

Occupational Dermatoses

Overview

Occupational skin diseases (OSDs) are the second most common occupational diseases worldwide (42). Occupational contact dermatitis (OCD) is the most frequent OSD, and comprises irritant contact dermatitis (ICD), allergic contact dermatitis (ACD), and physical and contact uritarial dermatoses. There are many endogenous and exogenous factors which affect the development of OCD, including age, atopic skin diathesis, sex, ethnicity, certain occupations, and environmental factors.

One of the most important contributing causes is skin barrier dysfunction. The skin provides a first-line defense from environmental assaults and provides physical, chemical, and biological protection. Skin barrier disturbance plays an important role in skin diseases such as ICD, ACD, ichthyosis, and AD. Genetic factors, such as filaggrin gene (FLG) mutations, and extrinsic factors, such as skin irritants interfering with SC structure and composition, may lead to abnormalities in skin barrier function and increased vulnerability to skin diseases. FLG encodes the cornified envelope protein filaggrin, which plays a key role in skin barrier function. FLG mutation is implicated in the development of OCD (43).

Occupations with the highest propensity to OCD include healthcare workers, hairdressers, and construction workers. There are often multiple contributing causes to OCD, as workers are exposed to both irritants and allergens. ICD often precedes and facilitates the development of ACD, with impairment of the skin barrier contributing to the concurrence of ICD and ACD in many workers with OCD.

Irritant Contact Dermatitis

The term *sensitive skin* most commonly refers to a form of ICD. This is defined as an inflammatory response of the skin to an externally applied agent or factor without requiring prior sensitization, that is, it is not due to allergy. Examples of such agents/factors include skin irritants, of which wet work is the most important. *Wet work* is defined as unprotected exposure to humid environments/water; high frequencies of hand washing procedures or prolonged glove occlusion (44). Although some chemicals can cause skin irritation in most people if exposed, it is usually a combination of several mild irritant agents accumulating in ICD.

Irritating body fluids such as sweat, urine, and feces, environmental factors such as heat, cold, low humidity, and UV light and mechanical factors, for example, friction, pressure, and vibration may all contribute to the development of ICD. However, host factors also influence susceptibility, and these include age, sex, skin site, and history of eczema. Ten clinical types of ICD have been recognized, of which eight present with clinically perceivable changes in the skin. Two forms of ICD show no clinical changes, and these are therefore worth mentioning in more depth.

1. Subjective/sensory irritation, also known as *sensorineural irritation*: Subjective/sensory irritation is characterized by sensory discomfort such as itching, stinging, tingling, or burning, but in the absence of any clinical or histological evidence of inflammation. Involvement of nerves and blood vessels contribute to the development of the symptoms. Lactic acid and propylene glycol in cosmetic agents are common causes of this. It is generally of acute onset. Avoiding the irritant or using personal protective equipment such as gloves and the frequent use of generous amounts of moisturizer usually results in a good outcome.

2. Nonerythematous irritation, also called *suberythematous irritation*: Nonerythematous irritation differs from subjective irritation in that there are changes of inflammation seen on skin biopsy. It often develops slowly, and discomfort is experienced with multiple chemicals. Cocamidopropyl betaine and coconut diethanolamide are common causes of this and are often ingredients in cosmetics. The outcome with this form of ICD is variable.

There have been a number of advances in the understanding of ICD. While there is still no routine test and ICD is often a diagnosis of exclusion, some interesting new areas of research include the role of TNF-a gene polymorphism and use of confocal microscopy (45). The definitive treatment of ICD is the identification and removal of any potential causal agents.

Allergic Contact Dermatitis

ACD is a skin reaction following the development of a type IV hypersensitivity reaction to an externally applied agent. It is less common than irritant contact dermatitis. It typically develops increasing intensity with time. Approximately 3000 chemicals are well documented as specific causes of ACD. Compounds must be less than 500 d for efficient penetration through the SC barrier. The main difference between the rash caused by ACD and the one caused by ICD is that the first one tends to be confined to the area where the trigger touched the skin, whereas in the second case, the rash is more likely to be more widespread on the skin. The definitive treatment of allergic contact dermatitis is the identification and removal of any potential causal agents; otherwise, the patient is at increased risk for chronic or recurrent dermatitis.

Other Noneczematous Dermatoses

Dry skin (xerosis), from any cause, is irritable and sensitive. Skin may be dry for a variety of reasons including genetic, that is, ichthyosis; environmental, that is, low humidity; or indeed from excessive washing (46,47). General health issues such as thyroid disease or certain medications may also contribute to the problem. Dry skin tends to be itchy, especially if overheated (environmental or endogenous). Patients are advised to use regular emollients to improve skin barrier function and relieve symptoms of pruritus. Emollients act by filling spaces around desquamating but attached skin cells, sealing moisture into the skin through the production of an occlusive barrier (48). The net effect is softening of the skin. Ingredients in emollients include mineral oils (e.g., liquid paraffin, petrolatum), waxes (e.g., lanolin, beeswax, and carnauba), long-chain esters, fatty acids, and mono-, di-, and triglycerides.

Cutaneous Dysthesias

Many cutaneous dysthesias are associated with predominant symptoms of burning, stinging, and itch/pruritus. They typically exist within well defined areas in the absence of primary cutaneous signs. Although the exact pathomechanism in all dysthesias is not entirely clear, some are thought to result from specific nerve root pathology. They include scalp dysthesias *buring scalp syndrome*, anogenital dysthesa *burning scrotum/vulva syndrome*, brachioradial pruritus, meralgia parasthetica, notalgia parasthetica, and trigeminal tropic syndrome. Management of dysthesias begins by aiming to identify underlying causes (nerve root impingement). Treatment strategies depend on the subtype involved and include topical corticosteroids, capsaicin, some antidepressants (amitriptyline, venlafaxine), gabapentin, carbamazepine, and lamotrigine among others.

Conclusion

Sensitive skin is an important clinical entity characterized by symptoms of stinging, burning, tightness, itch, and pain. It can exacerbate the impact of already distressing skin disorders with significant impairment on patient quality of life. It exists as a common symptom in many inflammatory and noneczematous dermatoses as discussed within this chapter. Given the heterogenous morphology and pathophysiology of these skin diseases, it may be that a common, but as yet undefined, mechanistic pathway exists to produce many of these ubiquitous and characteristic symptoms.

REFERENCES

1. Misery L, Loser K, Ständer S. Sensitive skin. A review article. *J Eur Acad Dermatol Venereol.* 2016, February;30 Suppl 1:2–8.
2. Fluhr JW et al. Skin irritation and sensitization: Mechanisms and new approaches for risk assessment. *D Skin Pharmacol Physiol.* 2008;21:124–135.
3. Saint-Martory C et al. Sensitive skin is not limited to the face. *Br. J. Dermatol.* 2008;158(1):130–133.
4. Farage MA. How do perceptions of sensitive skin differ at different anatomical sites? An epidemiological study. *Clin. Exp. Dermatol.* 2009;34:e521–e530.
5. Buhe et al. Pathophysiological study of sensitive skin: Investigative report. *Acta Derm Venereol.* 2016, March;96(3):314–318.
6. Misery L. Sensitive skin. *Expert Rev Dermatol.* 2013;8:631–637.
7. Berardesca E, Farage M, Maibach H. Sensitive skin: An overview. *Int J Cosmet Sci.* 2013;35:2–8.
8. Ständer S, Schneider SW, Weishaupt C, Luger TA, Misery L. Putative neuronal mechanisms of sensitive skin. *Exp. Dermatol.* 2009;18(5):417–423.

9. University College Dublin Charles Institute. Update on rosacea. *1st International Symposium, March, 2014, Dublin.*

10. Wilkin J et al. Standard classification of rosacea: Report of the National Rosacea Society Expert Committee on the classification and staging of rosacea. *J Am Acad Dermatol.* 2002;46:584–587.

11. Gerber P, Buhren B, Steinhoff M, Homey B. Rosacea: The cytokine and chemokine network. *J Investig Dermatol Symp Proc.* 2011, December;15(1):40–477.

12. Steinhoff M et al. Clinical, cellular, and molecular aspects in the pathophysiology of rosacea. *J Investig Dermatol Proc.* 2011;15:2–11.

13. Two AM, Wu W, Gallo RL, Hata TR. Rosacea: Part I. Introduction, categorization, histology, pathogenesis, and risk factors. *J Am Acad Dermatol.* 2015;72:749–758.

14. Buhl T et al. Molecular and morphological characterization of inflammatory infiltrate in rosacea reveals activation of Th1/Th17 pathways. *J Invest Dermatol.* 2015, September;135(9):2198–2208.

15. Sulk M et al. Distribution and expression of non-neuronal transient receptor potential (TRPV) ion channels in rosacea. *J Invest Dermatol.* 2012, April;132(4):1253–1262.

16. Steinhoff M, Schmelz M, Schauber J. Facial erythema of rosacea—Aetiology, different pathophysiologies and treatment options: A review article. *J Acta Derm Venereol.* 2016, June;96(5):579–586.

17. Fowler J Jr et al. Efficacy and safety of once-daily topical brimonidine tartrate gel 0.5% for the treatment of moderate to severe facial erythema of rosacea: Results of two randomized, double-blind, and vehicle-controlled pivotal studies. *Drugs Dermatol.* 2013, June;12(6):650–656.

18. Fowler J et al. Once-daily topical brimonidine tartrate gel 0.5% is a novel treatment for moderate to severe facial erythema of rosacea: Results of two multicentre, randomized and vehicle-controlled studies. *Br J Dermatol.* 2012, March;166(3):633–641.

19. Frumess GM, Lewis HM, Light-sensitive seborrheid. *AMA Arch Derm.* 1957, February;75(2):245–248.

20. Mihan R, Ayres S Jr. Perioral dermatitis. *Arch Dermatol.* 1964, June;89:803–805.

21. Fritsch P, Pichler E, Linser I. Perioral dermatitis. *Hautarzt.* 1989, August;40(8):475–479.

22. Ljubojević S, Lipozencić J, Turcić P. Perioral dermatitis. *Acta Dermatovenerol Croat.* 2008;16(2):96–100.

23. Nguyen V, Eichenfield LF. Periorificial dermatitis in children and adolescents. *J Am Acad Dermatol.* 2006, November;55(5):781–5.

24. Dirschka T, Weber K, Tronnier H. Topical cosmetics and perioral dermatitis. *J Dtsch Dermatol Ges.* 2004, March;2(3):194–199.

25. Hengge UR, Ruzicka T, Schwartz RA, Cork MJ. Adverse effects of topical glucocorticosteroids. *J Am Acad Dermatol.* 2006, January;54(1):1–15.

26. Tempark T, Shwayder TA. Perioral dermatitis: A review of the condition with special attention to treatment options. *Am J Clin Dermatol.* 2014, April;15(2):101–113.

27. Veien NK et al. Topical metronidazole in the treatment of perioral dermatitis. *J Am Acad Dermatol.* 1991, February;24(2 Pt 1):258–260.

28. Schwarz T et al. A randomized, double-blind, vehicle-controlled study of 1% pimecrolimus cream in adult patients with perioral dermatitis. *J Am Acad Dermatol.* 2008, July;59(1):34–40.

29. Lipozencic J, Ljubojevic S. Perioral dermatitis. *Clin Dermatol.* 2011, March–April;29(2):157–161.

30. Bribeche MR, Fedotov VP, Jillella A. Topical praziquantel as a new treatment for perioral dermatitis: Results of a randomized vehicle-controlled pilot study. *Clin Exp Dermatol.* 2014, June;39(4):448–453.

31. Lipozenčić J, Hadžavdić SL. Perioral dermatitis. *Clin Dermatol.* 2014, January–February;32(1):125–130.

32. Berk T, Scheinfeld N. Seborrheic dermatitis. P T. 2010, June;35(6):348–352.

33. Bikowski J. Facial seborrheic dermatitis: A report on current status and therapeutic horizons. *J Drugs Dermatol.* 2009, February;8(2):125–133.

34. Reider N, Fritsch PO. Seborrheic dermatitis. In: Bolognia JL, Jorizzo JL, Schaffer JV, editors. *Dermatology*, third ed. Philadelphia, PA: Elsevier; 2012.

35. Peyrí J, Lleonart M, Grupo español del Estudio SEBDERM. Clinical and therapeutic profile and quality of life of patients with seborrheic dermatitis. *Actas Dermosifiliogr.* 2007, September; 98(7):476–482.

36. Buhl T, Sulk M, Nowak P et al. Molecular and morphological characterization of inflammatory infiltrate in rosacea reveals activation of Th1/Th17 pathways. *J Invest Dermatol.* 2015, September;135(9):2198–2208.

37. Tajima M, Sugita T, Nishikawa A, Tsuboi R. Molecular analysis of Malassezia microflora in seborrheic dermatitis patients: Comparison with other diseases and healthy subjects. *J Invest Dermatol.* 2008;128(2):345–351.

38. Dawson TL. Malassezia globosa and restricta: Breakthrough understanding of the etiology and treatment of dandruff and seborrheic dermatitis through whole-genome analysis. *J Investig Dermatol Symp Proc.* 2007, December;12(2):15–19.

39. Hay RJ. Malassezia, dandruff and seborrhoeic dermatitis: An overview. *Br J Dermatol.* 2011, October;165 Suppl 2:2–8.

40. Gupta AK et al. Identification and typing of *Malassezia* species by amplified fragment length polymorphism and sequence analyses of the internal transcribed spacer and large-subunit regions of ribosomal DNA. *J Clin Microbiol.* 2004;42(9):4253–4260.

41. Okokon EO, Verbeek JH, Ruotsalainen JH, Ojo OA, Bakhoya VN. Topical antifungals for seborrhoeic dermatitis. *Cochrane Database Syst Rev.* 2015, May;2(5):CD008138.

42. Kasemsarn P, Bosco J, Nixon RL. The role of the skin barrier in occupational skin diseases. *Curr Probl Dermatol.* 2016;49:135–143.

43. Visser MJ et al. Impact of atopic dermatitis and loss-of-function mutations in the filaggrin gene on the development of occupational irritant contact dermatitis. *Br J Dermatol.* 2013, February; 168(2):326–332.

44. Fartasch M. Wet work and barrier function. *Curr Probl Dermatol.* 2016;49:144–151.

45. Slodownik D, Lee A, Nixon R. Irritant contact dermatitis: A review. *Australas. J. Dermatol.* 2008;49:1–11.

46. Norman RA. Xerosis and pruritus in the elderly: Recognition and management. *Dermatol Ther.* 2003;16: 254–259.

47. Lodén M. Role of topical emollients and moisturizers in the treatment of dry skin barrier disorders. *Am J Clin Dermatol.* 2003;4:771–788.

48. Van der Linden et al. Health-related quality of life in patients with cutaneous rosacea: A systematic review. *Acta Derm Venereol.* 2015, April;95(4):395–400.

19

Sensitive Skin and Eczematous Dermatoses

Arun C. Inamadar and Aparna Palit

Introduction

Sensitive skin is defined as a "skin less tolerant to frequent and prolonged use of cosmetics and toiletries and is self diagnosed, unaccompanied by any evident physical signs of irritation" (1). Currently, sensitive skin is a commonly encountered entity among cosmetic consumers and professionals. *Sensitive skin subjects* have been described as "people complaining of severe sensations of discomfort such as burning, stinging or itching after application of cosmetics or toiletries, such as sunscreens and soaps without any clinical stigmata like scaling, induration and/or erythema that would be expected in known inflammatory or allergic processes" (2).

Eczematous dermatoses are common dermatological disorders. The most common type of eczematous dermatitis is atopic dermatitis (AD). Other common eczematous dermatoses are allergic contact dermatitis (ACD), irritant contact dermatitis (ICD), and seborrheic dermatitis (SD). Principles of treatment of eczematous dermatoses include general skin care, patient education about avoidance of irritants, skin hydration, and the use of topical corticosteroids as and when necessary (3).

The eczematous skin of allergic contact dermatitis is more susceptible to various environmental influences, for example, chemical or mechanical irritation, climatic conditions, and skin care products. On the other side, irritated skin might imply a risk for enhanced sensitization.

The interrelation between eczematous dermatoses and sensitive skin is complex and can be discussed from various perspectives. It appears that individuals with a contact allergy/eczematous dermatitis do have higher skin sensitivity. For example, the eczematous skin of ACD is more susceptible to various environmental influences, such as chemical or mechanical irritation, climatic conditions, and skin care products. However, the mechanism is rather complex.

In this chapter, an attempt has been made to differentiate these two different but often confused conditions. In addition, the pathomechanism, clinical features, diagnosis, and management of these conditions have been discussed (4).

Pathophysiology

The etiology of sensitive skin is poorly understood. There is a decrease in the *tolerance threshold* of the skin without any immune or allergic mechanism (5). The condition is generally attributed to heightened neurosensory input and/or jeopardized skin barrier (6).

Figure 19.1 depicts the pathomechanism involved in sensitive skin.

The pathophysiological mechanism of the most common form of contact dermatitis (CD), the ICD, is as follows (7): There is inflammation arising due to release of proinflammatory cytokines derived mainly from the keratinocytes, usually in response to chemical stimuli, resulting in direct recruitment and activation of T lymphocytes. The main pathophysiological changes are skin barrier disruption, epidermal cellular changes, and cytokine release.

Individuals with a history of AD are prone to develop ICD of the hands. Polymorphisms in the *FLG* gene, which result in loss of filaggrin production, may alter the skin barrier and are a predisposing factor for AD. *FLG* null alleles are associated with increased susceptibility to chronic ICD (8). ACD results

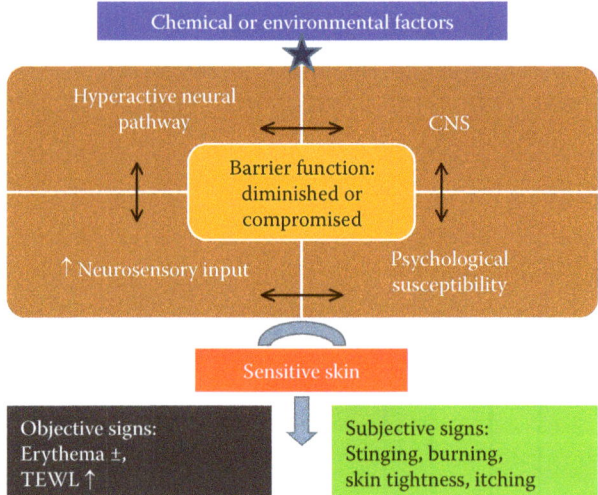

FIGURE 19.1   Pathomechanism of sensitive skin.

from a T cell-mediated, delayed type of hypersensitivity reaction elicited by the contact of the skin with the offending chemical in individuals who have been previously sensitized to the same chemical.

AD and ACD are both common skin diseases having an immune pathogenesis (9). AD is a common skin condition, characterized by a complex, heterogeneous pathogenesis, including skin barrier dysfunctions and significant pruritus. Recently, the skin barrier dysfunction induced by the *FLG* mutation has been demonstrated in AD. The barrier dysfunction shifts Th1 to Th2 response. Th2 cells produce IL-31, which provokes pruritus, and Th2 cytokines decrease filaggrin expressions by keratinocytes. These findings suggest that the evolution of a Th2 response lead to pruritus and barrier dysfunctions in patients with AD (10,11).

There is some similarity between sensitive skin and AD. It is likely that the same factors that play a role in the development of sensitive skin are also operative in AD. The most common and an important factor is skin-barrier dysfunction. There may also be differences among neural thresholds. Some patients have an abnormal response to mediators such as histamine. In some, exposure to histamine generates a significant wheal, whereas in others, there is only an insignificant response or none at all. This differing response can be due to their diverse neural threshold.

Atopic Diathesis and Sensitive Skin

It was thought that patients with AD were unable or less likely to develop contact dermatitis. In various studies, patients with AD stimulated with strong allergens failed to develop sensitization at rates similar to patients without AD. However, recent literature evidence from the United States and Europe has shown that patients with AD have similar if not higher rates of positive patch test results to common contact allergens, than in patients without AD (12).

There are studies supporting the link between sensitive skin and an atopic diathesis (13). It was first suggested by Thiers that features of atopic diathesis could explain sensitive skin syndrome (SSS) (14).

In a survey from the United Kingdom, only 49% of persons with sensitive skin had atopic diathesis concurrently. Hence, all cases with sensitive skin cannot be attributed to underlying atopic diathesis (15).

Clinical Features

The most practical, functional clinical description of sensitive skin is the one that reacts to cosmetic products. That is the hallmark feature of sensitive skin. It is mainly diagnosed by the subjective perceptions of the patient or from patient observation.

The usual complaints with which the patients approach the dermatologists are "I applied that moisturizer and it irritated me so much" or "I cannot find a sunscreen that feels good" or "Everything I apply to my skin burns and stings," and so on. These are the clues toward the diagnosis of sensitive skin. Demonstrable clinical signs are rare or none in these patients. Only identifiable clinical features may be less hydrated and less supple skin (1). Subjective, sensorial signs, such as stinging, burning, and itching sensations on an apparently normal-looking skin are the clinching points for the diagnosis of sensitive skin (16). The face is the main target of cosmetic use and, hence, the main body part affected. However, *sensitive skin* may as well involve other locations, such as the hands or scalp (5). In contrast, all the eczematous dermatoses have specific clinical signs and symptoms, specific distribution or body site predilection, and well-defined diagnostic criteria.

People with sensitive skin may identify and mention various aggravating factors for their condition; these include environmental factors such as cold, wind, sun, heat, humid weather, pollution, and exposure to water during showers and in swimming pools (17). Such triggering factors may be part of various eczematous disorders, such as AD, and may even be misdiagnosed as rosacea.

Diagnosis

The diagnosis of sensitive skin is challenging, as there is no consensual definition and way of objective assessment of the condition. The diagnosis mostly relies upon the way subjects report about their feeling of sensations; assessment can also be undertaken by using a questionnaire, prepared by the clinician based upon the existing knowledge on sensitive skin. A provocative test lactic acid stinging test (LAST) can be performed with patients' consent in order to reproduce the symptoms, which can be considered as indirect evidence of the condition (16). A thorough clinical examination to eliminate obvious as well as more subtle contact eczemas, AD, etc., is mandatory in all patients with sensitive skin (2).

In vivo and *in vitro* tests for evaluation of sensitive skin are mentioned in Table 19.1. Hematological investigations such as absolute eosinophil count and serum immunoglobulin E level help in the diagnosis of AD. Patch tests and photopatch tests are diagnostic of CD and photocontact dermatitis (18). Some *in vivo* tests similar to patch tests are in use for the detection of sensitive skin. One of these is the *repeat insult patch test*, where the product to be tested is applied on the patient's skin multiple times per week and evaluated for irritation or sensitization. Another such test is the *chamber scarification test*, where an area of skin is scratched to cause little damage, and then the product is applied to evaluate the reaction.

The main pathogenesis of sensitive skin is impaired barrier function. Physiological changes associated with sensitive skin can be detected when the patient is minimally symptomatic. Noninvasive biophysical instruments can be used for such objective detection of sensitive skin. Such techniques are detection of transepidermal water loss (TEWL), corneometry, skin capacitance, and estimation of skin hydration and skin pH. These tests should be undertaken either at baseline or after a provocative test to identify the biophysical variations linked to sensitive skin (6).

TABLE 19.1

In Vivo Tests for Evaluation of Sensitive Skin (6)

In Vivo Test	Method/Evaluation
Patch test	Performed with raw ingredients or finished products.
Repeat insult patch test	Ten patches are applied to the same site at 48–72 hour intervals for 3–4 week periods; after 2 weeks of rest, test site is rechallenged and graded.
Chamber scarification test	Volar aspect of the forearm is scarified, and the test product is applied under a Finn chamber repetitively for 3 days and evaluated up to 1 week after patch removal.
Cumulative irritancy test	Patch test is applied to the same test site for 10–21 days and evaluated for irritant reaction.

Source: Draelos, ZD, *Am J Contact Dermat*, 8, 67–78, 1997.

Management

Management of sensitive skin due to cosmetics involves simple procedures with a step-by-step elimination, avoidance, and introduction of cosmetics (1). The skin should be prepared and strengthened with barrier repair creams. Good moisturizers should be applied to dry skin and, moreover, to dampen the skin immediately after bathing to improve hydration and enhance the skin barrier. Water-based products are better avoided as these may result in dryness. Water-based products also generally contain more preservatives, which may be the source of irritants or allergens.

Harsh cleansers and soaps should be avoided, and synthetic detergents should be used sparingly when needed. The natural *acid mantle* can be preserved by using products that are at least pH neutral, ideally a little bit acidic, by avoiding alkaline soaps and moisturizing the skin to strengthen the barrier. If the acid mantle turns alkaline due to use of harsh cleansers or creams, the barrier is damaged very quickly and it promotes Staphylococcal growth (19).

Even in AD, it is important to moisturize the skin effectively to correct or repair the associated barrier dysfunction. The same principles of managing disrupted barrier apply in both AD and sensitive skin. Whereas other eczematous dermatoses are managed by the standard disease-specific protocols/guidelines designed and updated for these disorders regularly.

REFERENCES

1. Inamadar AC, Palit A. Sensitive skin: An overview. *Indian J Dermatol Venereol Leprol* 2013; 79:9–16.
2. Lev-Tov H, Maibach HI. The sensitive skin syndrome. *Indian J Dermatol* 2012; 57:419–423.
3. Zug KA, McKay M. Eczematous dermatitis: A practical review. *Am Fam Physician* 1996; 54:1243–1250.
4. Loffler H. Contact allergy and sensitive skin. In: Berardesca E, Maibach HL, Fluhr JW, Eds. *Sensitive Skin Syndromes*. New York: CRC Press; 2006. pp. 225–230.
5. Saint-Martory C, Roguedas-Contios AM, Sibaud V, Degouy A, Schmitt AM, Misery L. Sensitive skin is not limited to the face. *Br J Dermatol* 2008; 158:130–133.
6. Draelos ZD. Sensitive skin: Perceptions, evaluation and treatment. *Am J Contact Dermat* 1997; 8:67–78.
7. Ale IS, Maibach HI. Irritant contact dermatitis. *Rev Environ Health* 2014; 29:195–206.
8. de Jongh CM, Khrenova L, Verberk MM, Calkoen F, van Dijk FJ, Voss H et al. Loss-of-function polymorphisms in the filaggrin gene are associated with an increased susceptibility to chronic irritant contact dermatitis: A case-control study. *Br J Dermatol* 2008; 159:621–627.
9. Thyssen JP, McFadden JP, Kimber I. The multiple factors affecting the association between atopic dermatitis and contact sensitization. *Allergy* 2014; 69:28–36.
10. Yokozeki H. The research for atopic dermatitis: Up to date. *Nihon Rinsho* 2014; 72:1503–1509 [Article in Japanese].
11. Kabashima K. New concept of the pathogenesis of atopic dermatitis: Interplay among the barrier, allergy, and pruritus as a trinity. *J Dermatol Sci* 2013; 70:3–11.
12. Aquino M, Fonacier L. The role of contact dermatitis in patients with atopic dermatitis. *Allergy Clin Immunol Pract* 2014; 2:382–387.
13. Kamide R, Misery L, Perez-Cullell N, Sibaud V, Taïeb C. Sensitive skin evaluation in the Japanese population. *J Dermatol* 2013; 40:177–181.
14. Thiers H. Peau sensible. In: Thiers H, editor. Les Cosmétiques. second ed. Paris: Masson; 1986. pp. 266–268.
15. Willis CM, Shaw S, de Lacharrière O et al. Sensitive skin: An epidemiological study. *Br J Dermatol* 2001; 145:258–263.
16. Jourdain R, Amaral F, Inamadar AC, Godse K. Sensitive skin. In: Srinivas C, Verschoore M, Eds. *Basic Science for Modern Cosmetic Dermatology*. New Delhi: Jaypee Brothers Medical Publishers; 2015. pp. 127–137.
17. Farage M. Perceptions of sensitive skin: Changes in perceived severity and associations with environmental causes. *Contact Dermat.* 2008; 59:226–232.
18. Ali SM, Yosipovitch G. Skin pH: From basic science to basic skin care. *Acta Derm Venereol* 2013; 93:261–267.
19. Ale IS, Maibach HA. Diagnostic approach in allergic and irritant contact dermatitis. *Expert Rev Clin Immunol* 2010; 6:291–310.

Section V

Environmental Factors and Everyday Products

20

Influence of Air Pollution on Skin

Sparsha Saxena and Golara Honari

Introduction

Skin as the first line of contact between our body and the external surrounding has a critical role in protecting us against environmental exposures such as UV radiation, microbial agents, and ambient pollution. Numerous studies have examined effects of sun exposure, specifically UV A and B radiations on skin. Sensitive skin syndrome (SSS), also referred to as *hyperreactive skin*, is a common condition in which affected individuals are suffering from unpleasant sensations of itching, burning, and stinging with minimal environmental stimulation. Multiple factors are involved in the pathophysiology of SSS, such as impaired barrier function, chronic inflammation, impaired or increased sensation, and hyper-reactive neurosensory responses to even subtle stimuli. Symptoms are often manifested as affected individuals are topically exposed to various environmental products, including cosmetics (1). For cosmetics alone, Jourdain et al. (2) found that 78% of consumers report intolerance to certain cosmetic toiletries. This intolerance includes, but is not limited to, prickling, burning, redness, or tingling sensations (3,4). While negative impacts of pollution on respiratory and cardiovascular and cutaneous systems have been shown, much needs to be learned (5,6). This chapter provides an overview of common air pollutants other than UV radiation and how they can affect skin.

Air Pollutant Overview

Contamination of air by any chemical, physical, or biological compound that affects natural characteristics of air is known as *air pollution*. Pollutants are organic and inorganic compounds that can be derived from natural sources or created by human activities (anthropogenic pollution). Both indoor and outdoor (ambient) air pollution are important environmental hazards that can potentially affect skin. Important pollutants other than UV radiations include gaseous pollutants, persistent organic pollutant, particulate matters (PMs), heavy metals, and mobile source air toxics.

Gaseous pollutants mostly consist of sulfur dioxide, carbon monoxide, nitrogen oxides, ground level ozone, and volatile organic compounds (VOCs) (7). Ozone is made of three oxygen atoms (O_3) and can be found in the upper atmosphere of earth, as well as at ground level (tropospheric ozone). Unlike atmospheric ozone, also known as *good ozone*, which provides a protective shield against the sun's hazardous UV radiation, the ground level ozone can adversely affect life on earth. Ground level ozone, or so-called bad ozone, is a by-product of chemical reactions between nitrogen oxides and VOCs in the presence of UV rays. Ozone is a main component of photochemical smog and is known to pose oxidative stress on skin (8).

Persistent organic pollutants (POPs) are anthropogenic compounds that are resistant to natural degradation in the environment. POPs are mainly formulated for industrial or agricultural use or are unwanted by-products of certain chemical and combustion reactions, and due to their persistence, they can pose a global concern. Well-known POPs include dichlorodiphenyltrichloroethane, polychlorinated biphenyls, and dioxins. Dioxins are long known to cause chloracne and are known as aryl hydrocarbon receptor ligands that can affect FLG expression and epidermal barrier protein regulation (9,10).

TABLE 20.1

Overview of Pollutants

Pollutant	Indoor or Outdoor	Sources
Combustion related	Indoor	Burning of wood, charcoal, agricultural residues, and dung
Biologicals	Indoor	Microbial cells such as bacteria and viruses, fungal spores, protozoans, algae, and pollen (11)
Radons	Indoor/outdoor	Dust particles in air
Lead	Outdoor	Motor vehicles and industrial sources
Polycyclic aromatic hydrocarbons	Outdoor	Exhaust
Particle matter	Outdoor	Traffic, soot, construction byproducts, dust
VOCs	Outdoor	Solvents, thinners, degreasers, cleaners, lubricants, and liquid fuels
Oxides (carbon monoxide and nitrogen oxides and sulfur dioxides)	Outdoor	Power generation is responsible for nitrogen oxide emission
Ozone (ground level)	Outdoor	Smog

Mobile source air toxics include any pollutants that are emitted from motor vehicle and nonroad engines. Examples of mobile source air toxics include lead, benzene, 1,3-butadiene, formaldehyde, acetaldehyde, acrolein, polycyclic organic matters, naphthalene, and diesel PM. Exposure to traffic-related air pollutants can affect multiple organs including the skin (12–14).

The US Environmental Protection Agency (EPA) sets six principal pollutants as National Ambient Air Quality Standards, which are referred to as *criteria* pollutants and are routinely monitored in ambient air. They include the following (15):

- Ozone (ground-level ozone)
- PMs (including particles <2.5 μm found in smoke and particles between 2.5 and 10 μm found near road ways)
- Carbon monoxide
- Nitrogen oxide
- Sulfur dioxide
- Lead

Indoor pollution has many sources including combustion products such as coal, wood, gas, cigarette smoke, certain furniture or carpets, building materials, household cleaning products, central air conditions, insecticides, and outdoor sources such as radon and outdoor air pollution (5,15,16).

See Table 20.1.

Skin and Pollution

Air pollution can potentially affect skin via different mechanisms including oxidative stress and induction of inflammation and by changing normal skin microbiome.

Oxidative stress is involved in pathogenesis of multiple skin disorders including inflammatory and neoplastic skin disorders (17). A number of gaseous pollutants, UV radiation, and ground level ozone can create oxidative stress in skin (18).

There is substantial evidence on the role of oxidative stress in cutaneous carcinogenesis as well as its effects on inflammation and aging (8,17,19,20). Oxidative stress was the subject of investigation by Thiele in the late 1990s, who showed on a series of studies on hairless mice that exposure to ozone causes lipid peroxidation in SC and depletes skin's natural antioxidants such as vitamins E and C and adversely affects the barrier function of the epidermis, making it potentially susceptible to inflammation. Other investigators have also shown oxidative stress and free radical formation due to ozone exposure (18,21–26).

McCarthy et al. (27) in a study exposing normal human epidermal keratinocytes (NHEK) to ozone (at levels comparable to levels of ambient ozone in cities), observed an increase in levels of hydrogen peroxide and IL-1 alpha indicating the presence of oxidative stress and induction of a proinflammatory response as well as evidence of increased DNA breaks.

He at al. (28) showed that exposure to ozone using exposure chambers on human skin led to more than a twofold increase in lipid hydroperoxides in the superficial SC and 70% decrease in vitamin E, but it did not increase some of the enzymes involved in epidermal desquamation (28). Subjects in this study were exposed to ozone at 0.8 ppm for 2 hours, which is higher than the 0.075 ppm limit by EPA (15). It is of note that the ozone level as high as 0.68 ppm was recorded in Los Angeles in 1955 (29). Authors suggested that ozone in realistic environmental levels can pose a moderate oxidative stress, but these effects may be much less than the toxic effects showed in in vitro studies.

Inflammatory reactions mediated via various inflammatory cytokines are associated with pollution. Increased inflammatory cytokines such as IL-1 beta was observed with in vitro exposure of human keratinocytes to diesel exhaust particles (30). The induction of nuclear factor kappa B, which is a transcription factor largely known to have proinflammatory effects via the expression of proinflammatory cytokines, chemokines, and adhesion molecules, has been associated with exposure to diesel exhaust dust in mouse epidermal cell lines (31). Another important pathway that pollution can potentially affect skin is through the aryl hydrocarbon receptor (AhR). AhR is a multifunctional ligand-dependent cytosolic transcription factor, initially discovered as a cytosolic receptor and transcription factor for polycyclic aromatic hydrocarbons, such as 2,3,7,8-tetrachlorodibenzo-*p*-dioxin (9,32–34). AhR is a ligand with an affinity for a wide range of low-molecular weight chemicals including dioxins, coal tar, tryptophan photoproducts, and flavonoids. After ligation, cytoplasmic AhR translocates to the nucleus via heterodimerization with AhR nuclear translocator and mediates multiple physiological and pathological cascades in the cell. AhR-dependent signal transduction pathways produce diverse biological and toxicological effects following activation with endogenous or xenobiotic ligands (35). For example, dioxin-activated AhR ligand induces the activation of various transcription factors including cytochrome P4501A1 (CYP1A1). While it exhibits a physiological role in detoxification of these compounds, the activation of CYP1A1 enzyme actually leads to the generation of ROS and causes oxidative stress (9). Interestingly, the activation of AhR with another set of ligands such as coal tar, ketoconazole, and other chemicals mediates antioxidant signaling via nuclear factor-erythroid 2-related factor-2 (9,36,37). Increased expression of FLG has been observed with both oxidative and antioxidative ligand activation of AhR (9). While the role of AhR in skin hemostasis, cellular proliferation, epidermal barrier protein metabolism, melanogenesis, and inflammation has been the subject of extensive research; its physiological and toxicological effects still need to be better elucidated (9,35,38). Nonetheless, pollutants such as dioxins and ozone are shown to be among the oxidative ligand activators of AhR and can adversely affect the cutaneous biology (8).

Barrier function can also be affected with ambient air pollution. Pan et al. (39) in a recent study, showed that PMs in ambient air (using some heavy metals and polycyclic aromatic hydrocarbons) can increase TEWL, mildly damage tight junctions, increase annexin A2 (which can indicate barrier dysfunction) and consequently increase the absorption of topically applied substances such as tretinoin. Suggested barrier dysfunction due to pollution needs to be further investigated in human skin with exposure to ambient pollution at realistic concentrations.

See Table 20.2.

TABLE 20.2

Studies on Impact of Pollution on Skin

Study	Purpose	Design	Results
Kramer et al. (13)	To investigate whether exposure to TAP affects symptoms of eczema and respiratory allergies in less populated, small-town areas	Observational study following 3390 newborns from small-town areas through annual questionnaires; 77% of families continued to participate until age 6. Symptoms were correlated with TAP measurements.	Prevalence of eczema was significantly higher in areas with higher measured TAP.
Afaq et al. (8)	To determine effects of ozone exposure on family of CYP isoforms, which are involved in biotranformation of environmental pollutants	NHEKs were exposed to ozone. Protein and messenger ribonucleic acid (RNA) expression of AhR (a ligand-activated transcription factor which regulates CYP gene expression) was measured as well as marker for CYP.	Exposure to ozone led to the activation of AhR, which mediated increased expression of CYP isoforms in NHEKs.
Vierkotter et al. (40)	To assess the relationship between airborne particle pollution and extrinsic skin aging	Traffic-related pollution was determined by measurements of ambient PM at place of residence in 400 Caucasian women. Skin aging was clinically assessed by means of the SCINEXA.	Ambient pollution was significantly associated with extrinsic aging, particularly with increased pigment spots (and less with wrinkling).
Choi et al. (41)	To examine effect of dust particles from Asian dust particles on expression of CYP isoforms in NHEKs	NHEKs were exposed to Asian dust particles and expression of CYP proteins in RNA was measured by PCR analysis.	Asian dust storm particles significantly upregulated AhR activation, proinflammatory IL-6 and IL8, and expression of CYP proteins in NHEKs.
McCarthy et al. (27)	To assess effects of ozone on NHEK	NHEKs were exposed to ozone equivalent to ambient air and subsequently keratinocyte levels of mitochondrial sirtuin, SIRT3, hydrogen peroxide, ATP and IL-1 alpha, and other parameters were measured.	Increase levels of hydrogen peroxide and IL-1 alpha were observed pointing to oxidative stress and a proinflammatory response. Also, an increase in comet tail as an indicator of increased DNA breaks was observed.
Kim et al. (42)	To assess clinical effects of outdoor air pollution on AD	Observational study conducted with 22 patients with AD; followed for 18 months. Individuals recorded results in a symptom diary, in addition to their frequency of bathing and application of lotion. Daily concentration of pollutants near their residence was correlated with the scoring AD index.	Findings revealed that outdoor pollution aggravates AD.
Kim et al. (43)	To evaluate the impact of indoor air quality on AD	Changes in AD in 425 children was assessed using EASI and IGA at base line and 7 months later, while during that period, measures to improve indoor air quality were implemented.	Indoor air pollution reduction caused statistically significant decrease in AD and eczema.

(Continued)

TABLE 20.2 (CONTINUED)

Studies on Impact of Pollution on Skin

Study	Purpose	Design	Results
Jin et al. (44)	Gene expression signatures of normal human keratinocytes (NHKs) when exposed to inflammatory cytokines	Whole genome microarray analysis of NHKs after exposure to T-helper cytokines (INF gamma, IL-4, IL17, and IL-22) as well as acute phase proinflammatory cytokines (IL-1beta, IL-6, and TNF alpha) as well as SLS and UVB radiation.	IL-24 was found among the genes that were expressed in NHKs exposed to inflammatory cytokines, SLS, and UVB, suggesting a role for environmental irritants and UVB and epidermal inflammation.
Lefebvre et al. (45)	To test impact of outdoor pollution on skin of individuals living in large urban areas compared to individuals living far from urban pollution, by assessing biochemical and biophysical measures	Biochemical and physical measures including skin PH, sebum production, corneodesmosin, ATP, oxidized proteins, and erythema were compared between 96 volunteers exposed to high levels of urban pollution and 93 volunteers from a smaller city with lower levels of urban pollution.	Higher levels of oxidized proteins and lower levels of squalene and vitamin E were noted in individuals living in polluted urban areas.

Note: CYP: cytochrome P450; EASI: eczema area and severity index; IGA: investigator's global assessment; INF: interferon; PCR: polymerase chain reaction; SCINEXA: score of intrinsic and extrinsic skin aging; SIRT3: mitochondrial sirtuin 3; TAP: traffic-related air pollution.

Conclusion

Multiple factors are involved in the pathophysiology of sensitive skin such as impaired barrier function, chronic inflammation, impaired or increased sensation, and hyperreactive neurosensory responses to even subtle stimuli (please refer to Chapter 5 for detailed discussion). While studies on direct effects of pollution on individuals with sensitive skin are lacking, environmental pollution has been associated with the induction of oxidative stress, cutaneous inflammation, and potential impairment of cutaneous barrier function. It is plausible that individuals with sensitive skin may be more prone to developing symptoms with exposure to pollution, but further investigation is needed.

REFERENCES

1. Marriott, M. et al. The complex problem of sensitive skin. *Contact Dermat.* 53, 93–99 (2005).
2. Jourdain, R., de Lacharriere, O., Bastien, P., and Maibach, H. I. Ethnic variations in self-perceived sensitive skin: Epidemiological survey. *Contact Dermat.* 46, 162–169 (2002).
3. Loffler, H., Dickel, H., Kuss, O., Diepgen, T. L., and Effendy, I. Characteristics of self-estimated enhanced skin susceptibility. *Acta Derm. Venereol.* 81, 343–346 (2001).
4. Farage, M. A., and Maibach, H. I. Sensitive skin: Closing in on a physiological cause. *Contact Dermat.* 62, 137–149 (2010).
5. Raaschou-Nielsen, O. et al. Air pollution and lung cancer incidence in 17 European cohorts: Prospective analyses from the European Study of Cohorts for Air Pollution Effects (ESCAPE). *Lancet Oncol.* 14, 813–822 (2013).
6. Ezzati, M., and Kammen, D. Indoor air pollution from biomass combustion and acute respiratory infections in Kenya: An exposure-response study. *Lancet* 358, 619–624 (2001).
7. Sarnat, J. A., Schwartz, J., Catalano, P. J., and Suh, H. H. Gaseous pollutants in particulate matter epidemiology: Confounders or surrogates? *Environ. Health Perspect.* 109, 1053–1061 (2001).
8. Afaq, F. et al. Aryl hydrocarbon receptor is an ozone sensor in human skin. *J. Invest. Dermatol.* 129, 2396–2403 (2009).

9. Furue, M. et al. Gene regulation of filaggrin and other skin barrier proteins via aryl hydrocarbon receptor. *J. Dermatol. Sci.* 80, 83–88 (2015).

10. US Environmental Protection Agency. Risk assessment. US Environmental Protection Agency, Arlington, VA. Available at http://www.epa.gov/risk/expobox/chemicalclass/other-pop.htm, accessed September 4, 2015.

11. Chen, B. H., Hong, C. J., Pandey, M. R., and Smith, K. R. Indoor air pollution in developing countries. *World Health Stat. Q.* 43, 127–138 (1990).

12. US Environmental Protection Agency. Mobile source pollution and related health effects. US Environmental Protection Agency, Arlington, VA. Available at http://www.epa.gov/otaq/toxics.htm, accessed September 4, 2015.

13. Kramer, U. et al. Eczema, respiratory allergies, and traffic-related air pollution in birth cohorts from small-town areas. *J. Dermatol. Sci.* 56, 99–105 (2009).

14. Morgenstern, V. et al. Atopic diseases, allergic sensitization, and exposure to traffic-related air pollution in children. *Am. J. Respir. Crit. Care Med.* 177, 1331–1337 (2008).

15. US Environmental Protection Agency. NAAQS table. US Environmental Protection Agency, Arlington, VA. Available at https://www.epa.gov/criteria-air-pollutants/naaqs-table, accessed September 4, 2015.

16. Roberts, W. E. Pollution as a risk factor for the development of melasma and other skin disorders of facial hyperpigmentation—Is there a case to be made? *J. Drugs Dermatol.* 14, 337–341 (2015).

17. Briganti, S., and Picardo, M. Antioxidant activity, lipid peroxidation and skin diseases: What's new. *J. Eur. Acad. Dermatol. Venereol.* 17, 663–669 (2003).

18. Pryor, W. A. Mechanisms of radical formation from reactions of ozone with target molecules in the lung. *Free Radic. Biol. Med.* 17, 451–465 (1994).

19. Thiele, J. J., Dreher, F., Maibach, H. I., and Packer, L. Impact of ultraviolet radiation and ozone on the transepidermal water loss as a function of skin temperature in hairless mice. *Skin Pharmacol. Appl. Skin Physiol.* 16, 283–290 (2003).

20. Bickers, D. R., and Athar, M. Oxidative stress in the pathogenesis of skin disease. *J. Invest. Dermatol.* 126, 2565–2575 (2006).

21. Thiele, J. J., Hsieh, S. N., Briviba, K., and Sies, H. Protein oxidation in human stratum corneum: Susceptibility of keratins to oxidation in vitro and presence of a keratin oxidation gradient in vivo. *J. Invest. Dermatol.* 113, 335–339 (1999).

22. Thiele, J. J., Traber, M. G., Polefka, T. G., Cross, C. E., and Packer, L. Ozone-exposure depletes vitamin E and induces lipid peroxidation in murine stratum corneum. *J. Invest. Dermatol.* 108, 753–757 (1997).

23. Thiele, J. J. et al. Ozone depletes tocopherols and tocotrienols topically applied to murine skin. *FEBS Lett.* 401, 167–170 (1997).

24. Thiele, J. J., Traber, M. G., Tsang, K., Cross, C. E., and Packer, L. In vivo exposure to ozone depletes vitamins C and E and induces lipid peroxidation in epidermal layers of murine skin. *Free Radic. Biol. Med.* 23, 385–391 (1997).

25. Weber, C. et al. Efficacy of topically applied tocopherols and tocotrienols in protection of murine skin from oxidative damage induced by UV-irradiation. *Free Radic. Biol. Med.* 22, 761–769 (1997).

26. Cotovio, J., Onno, L., Justine, P., Lamure, S., and Catroux, P. Generation of oxidative stress in human cutaneous models following in vitro ozone exposure. *Toxicol. In Vitro.* 15, 357–362 (2001).

27. McCarthy, J. T. et al. Effects of ozone in normal human epidermal keratinocytes. *Exp. Dermatol.* 22, 360–361 (2013).

28. He, Q. C. et al. Effects of environmentally realistic levels of ozone on stratum corneum function. *Int. J. Cosmet. Sci.* 28, 349–357 (2006).

29. Murdoch, J. C., Rahmatian, M., and Thayer, M. A. An analysis of improvements in urban air quality: Implications from the South Coast Air Basin. Available at http://iwlearn.net/publications/misc/caspianev_urbanair.pdf, accessed September 8, 2015 (2005).

30. Ushio, H., Nohara, K., and Fujimaki, H. Effect of environmental pollutants on the production of pro-inflammatory cytokines by normal human dermal keratinocytes. *Toxicol. Lett.* 105, 17–24 (1999).

31. Ma, C., Wang, J., and Luo, J. Activation of nuclear factor kappa B by diesel exhaust particles in mouse epidermal cells through phosphatidylinositol 3–kinase/Akt signaling pathway. *Biochem. Pharmacol.* 67, 1975–1983 (2004).

32. Poland, A., and Knutson, J. C. 2,3,7,8–Tetrachlorodibenzo-p-dioxin and related halogenated aromatic hydrocarbons: Examination of the mechanism of toxicity. *Annu. Rev. Pharmacol. Toxicol.* 22, 517–554 (1982).
33. Hahn, M. E. Aryl hydrocarbon receptors: Diversity and evolution. *Chem. Biol. Interact.* 141, 131–160 (2002).
34. Mimura, J., and Fujii-Kuriyama, Y. Functional role of AhR in the expression of toxic effects by TCDD. *Biochim. Biophys. Acta* 1619, 263–268 (2003).
35. Denison, M. S., Soshilov, A. A., He, G., DeGroot, D. E., and Zhao, B. Exactly the same but different: Promiscuity and diversity in the molecular mechanisms of action of the aryl hydrocarbon (dioxin) receptor. *Toxicol. Sci.* 124, 1–22 (2011).
36. van den Bogaard, E. H. et al. Coal tar induces AHR-dependent skin barrier repair in atopic dermatitis. *J. Clin. Invest.* 123, 917–927 (2013).
37. Tsuji, G. et al. Identification of ketoconazole as an AhR-Nrf2 activator in cultured human keratinocytes: The basis of its anti-inflammatory effect. *J. Invest. Dermatol.* 132, 59–68 (2012).
38. Luecke, S. et al. The aryl hydrocarbon receptor (AHR), a novel regulator of human melanogenesis. *Pigment Cell. Melanoma Res.* 23, 828–833 (2010).
39. Pan, T. L. et al. The impact of urban particulate pollution on skin barrier function and the subsequent drug absorption. *J. Dermatol. Sci.* 78, 51–60 (2015).
40. Vierkotter, A. et al. Airborne particle exposure and extrinsic skin aging. *J. Invest. Dermatol.* 130, 2719–2726 (2010).
41. Choi, H. et al. Asian dust storm particles induce a broad toxicological transcriptional program in human epidermal keratinocytes. *Toxicol. Lett.* 200, 92–99 (2011).
42. Kim, J. et al. Symptoms of atopic dermatitis are influenced by outdoor air pollution. *J. Allergy Clin. Immunol.* 132, 495–8.e1 (2013).
43. Kim, H. O. et al. Improvement of atopic dermatitis severity after reducing indoor air pollutants. *Ann. Dermatol.* 25, 292–297 (2013).
44. Jin, S. H., Choi, D., Chun, Y. J., and Noh, M. Keratinocyte-derived IL-24 plays a role in the positive feedback regulation of epidermal inflammation in response to environmental and endogenous toxic stressors. *Toxicol. Appl. Pharmacol.* 280, 199–206 (2014).
45. Lefebvre, M. A. et al. Evaluation of the impact of urban pollution on the quality of skin: A multicentre study in Mexico. *Int. J. Cosmet. Sci.* 37, 329–338 (2015).

21

Sensitive Skin, Skin Care Products, and Cosmetics

Enzo Berardesca

Skin care and cosmetics used in subjects affected by sensitive skin should be carefully selected in order to have a good compliance and possibly promote skin health. Indeed, sensitive skin has been classified primarily as a local reaction after the application of a cosmetic product (1).

Cleansers

Appropriate skin care includes cleansing, moisturizing, and application UV protection to maintain healthy skin. UV protection consists of sun avoidance, UV-protective clothing, and sunscreens (2). Therefore, effective cleansers for eczema and sensitive skin should provide effective cleansing without compromising the barrier integrity, and cosmetic or therapeutic moisturizers should be indicated as an important adjunct to alleviate dryness of the skin and restore skin barrier function (3).

Washing twice daily with a classic alkaline soap (pH 10.2) reduces the thickness of the SC cell layers, with associated attrition of intercellular lipids causing dryness, desquamation, and barrier damage (4). In diseased skin such as in sensitive or atopic skin, special cleansing agents are recommended consisting of non-soap-based surfactants, synthetic detergents (syndets) with an acidic or neutral pH, and lipid-free cleansing lotions. New formulations also include cleansers restoring intercellular lipids by delivering ceramides or similar lipids after washing (5). In a study of skin irritation of six cleansing agents designed for sensitive skin, 60 patients used a bar and a lipid-free liquid cleanser in a paired-comparison design. Among the users of the bar soaps, 41% of the patients discontinued because of facial erythema. However, there were no discontinuations among patients using the nonsoap cleansing lotion, which was also rated as causing the least irritation (6). Lipid-free cleansing lotions contain fatty alcohols and are designed for sensitive or dry skin; lotion formulations can be removed without water (7). Lipid-free cleansers also contain emollients and/or humectants to cleanse while protecting the skin from moisture loss. The pH of a cleanser is also important; neutral or acid pH cleansers (about 5.5), close to the normal pH of the epidermis, are recommended. It has been suggested that alkaline cleansing agents contribute to the dehydration of the SC and dry skin and should be avoided (8,9). Furthermore, the preventing loss of SC hydration can help in improving barrier performance.

Water alone is not recommended for cleansing. Barrier function is not improved by using water alone without soap because water is a uniphase element and is not immediately absorbed into the skin (3).

Moisturizers

Therapeutic moisturizers are important in the management of the treatment, as they improve skin hydration, reduce susceptibility to irritation, and restore integrity of the SC. There are three types of moisturizers: humectants (urea, propylenglicol, dexpanthenol, lactic acid), which have a water-binding capacity; emollients (petrolatum, lanolin, oils), which have an occlusive film that retains water; and physiological or structural lipids (ceramides or fatty acids), which fill the intercellular lipid layer. An effective moisturizer would include humectants, for hydration, and structural lipids, for replenishing the skin (10). However, most of the randomized controlled studies in this area refer to moisturizers designed to be used for atopic patients; nevertheless, due to the similarity in barrier function and the clinical overlap between AD and sensitive skin, most of the results of these studies are also applicable to sensitive skin. In a study of 580 consecutive patients affected by irritant dermatitis or AD, a combined lipid mixture containing ceramides was useful in relieving dry skin and improving barrier function with or without concurrent steroid treatment (11). Similarly, in an uncontrolled trial of 24 children with AD, the patients were treated with a barrier-repair emollient containing ceramides twice daily for 12 weeks while continuing prior topical treatment. Almost all (*n* = 22) patients showed significant improvement within 3 weeks (12).

The benefits of long-term use of moisturizers include changes in skin barrier function (13). A study on the effects of a urea-containing moisturizer on the barrier properties of atopic skin found that the moisturizer improved the water barrier function (as reflected by TEWL) and significantly reduced skin susceptibility to SLS (14).

Sunscreens

Since sensitive skin is occurring mainly on the face, UV exposure should be avoided. Besides skin damage induced by UV (photoaging), it is well established that photoexposure can trigger the onset of sensitive skin-related dermatoses such as rosacea (15). Therefore, the use of topical sunscreen is recommended. This could be included in a moisturizing day cream or lotion in winter, with SPF of up to 20; in summer; or when in outdoor activities; SPF 50 is needed with repeated application every 2–3 hours or after swimming or beach activities. Protective clothing may be extremely useful in order to avoid repeated application of chemicals on the skin.

Other general recommendations for use of cosmetics in sensitive skin are shown below

- Use cosmetics and makeup that are easy to remove with water or mild detergents.
- Prefer light makeup and not too much occlusive.
- Prefer makeup with sunscreen included.
- Prefer cosmetics tested for nickel and other heavy metals.
- Avoid cosmetics with preservatives and fragrances.
- Choose cosmetics with simple formulations, possibly with less than 10 ingredients.
- In case of very sensitive skin, test your cosmetic prior to regular use for a few days on the forearm.

REFERENCES

1. Kligman AM, Sadiq I, Zhen Y et al. Experimental studies on the nature of sensitive skin. *Skin Res Technol* 2006; 12(4): 217–22.
2. Burr S, Penzer R. Promoting skin health. *Nurs Stand* 2005 May 18–24;19(36):57–65.
3. Cheong WK. Gentle cleansing and moisturizing for patients with atopic dermatitis and sensitive skin. *Am J Clin Dermatol* 2009; 10 Suppl 1: 13–7.
4. White MI, Jenkinson DM, Lloyd DH. The effect of washing on the thickness of the stratum corneum in normal and atopic individuals. *Br J Dermatol* 1987; 116(4): 525–30.
5. Solodkin G, Chaudhari U, Subramanyan K et al. Benefits of mild cleansing: Synthetic surfactant based (syndet) bars for patients with atopic dermatitis. *Cutis* 2006; 77(5): 317–24.
6. Mills OH, Berger RS, Baker MD. A controlled comparison of skin cleansers in photoaged skin. *J Geriatr Dermatol* 1993; 1: 173–9.
7. Bikowski J. The use of cleansers as therapeutic concomitants in various dermatologic disorders. *Cutis* 2001 December; 68(5 Suppl): 12–9.
8. Ananthapadmanabhan KP, Lips A, Vincent C et al. pH-induced alterations in stratum corneum properties. *Int J Cosmet Sci* 2003 June; 25(3): 103–12.
9. Fluhr JW, Kao J, Jain M, Ahn SK, Feingold KR, Elias PM. Generation of free fatty acids from phospholipids regulates stratum corneum acidification and integrity. *J Invest Dermatol* 2001 July; 117(1): 44–51.

10. Loden M. The clinical benefit of moisturizers. *J Eur Acad Dermatol Venereol* 2005 November; 19(6): 672–88.
11. Berardesca E, Barbareschi M, Veraldi S, Pimpinelli N. Evaluation of efficacy of a skin lipid mixture in patients with irritant contact dermatitis, allergic contact dermatitis or atopic dermatitis: A multicenter study. *Contact Dermat* 2001; 45(5): 280–25.
12. Chamlin SL, Kao J, Frieden IJ et al. Ceramide-dominant barrier repair lipids alleviate childhood atopic dermatitis: Changes in barrier function provide a sensitive indicator of disease activity. *J Am Acad Dermatol* 2002 August; 47(2): 198–208.
13. Buraczewska I, Berne B, Lindberg M, Torma H, Loden M. Changes in skin barrier function following long-term treatment with moisturizers, a randomized controlled trial. *Br J Dermatol* 2007 March; 156(3): 492–8.
14. Loden M, Andersson AC, Lindberg M. Improvement in skin barrier function in patients with atopic dermatitis after treatment with a moisturizing cream (Canoderm). *Br J Dermatol* 1999 February; 140(2): 264–7.
15. Berardesca E, Iorizzo M, Abril E, Guglielmini G, Caserini M, Palmieri R, Pierard GE. Clinical and instrumental assessment of the effects of a new product based on hydroxypropyl chitosan and potassium azeloyl diglycinate in the management of rosacea. *J Cosmetic Dermatol* 2012; 11(1): 37–41.

22

Fabrics and Sensitive Skin

Gérald E. Piérard and Howard Maibach

Introduction

For lay people and scientists as well, the field of reactive (sensitive) skin remains in part controversial and complex to perceive (1–4). Everyone glibly provides his/her own definition for this condition. It corresponds to a set of subjective perceptions to extrinsic structures and compounds, without clearly causing an overt allergic or irritant dermatitis. It corresponds to a reactive susceptibility to xenobiotics showing obvious cultural and ethnic differences (5–7). Fabrics are occasionally involved in such a process, in particular, their fibers, dyes, pigments, finish chemicals, and various molecular residues collected during manufacturing, laundering, and cleaning (8,9). Some microorganisms bound to fabrics as well as antimicrobials associated with textiles (10–12) are occasionally involved in the chemically induced reactive skin condition.

Reactive skin to fabrics is rooted to at least two distinct definitions. On the one hand, the discomfort associated with reactive skin, in its restricted sense, corresponds to manifestations of a genuine exaggerated neural sensitivity and skin sensory irritation (SSI) to mechanical stimulations (13,14). This condition commonly remains invisible at the regular clinical inspection. On the other hand, a broader concept admits a variety of discrete biophysical changes and clinical signs in the skin including erythema, dryness, and xerosis (14,15). Indeed, this latter definition clearly encompasses some facets in common with allergic and irritant contact dermatitis, as well as the exacerbation of some other incipient dermatoses such as sudamina or AD. Anyway, reactive skin likely represents a multifactorial process leading to skin discomfort. In fact, skin readily experiences either reduced tolerance or heightened response to some external stress involving specific physical factors and/or chemical xenobiotics. The initial perception of the adverse discomfort is immediate or delayed after the offending contact. It corresponds to the neuro-sensory phenomenon of SSI including one or a series of feelings including tightness, pruritus, prickling, stinging, and tingling sensations. Over time in mild cases, subjective and subclinical symptoms bring about discrete visible effects, including erythema as well as rough and dry-looking skin. At that stage, the terms *irritant* or *allergic contact dermatitis* are possibly more relevant and should be distinctly evoked. In short, there is no scientific consensus, and identifying truly reactive skin is a challenging task. The precise pathomechanisms involved in reactive skin are largely unknown. This condition must be differentiated from symptoms or neurotic concerns, hypochondria, disturbed body image, chronic fatigue syndrome, and multiple chemical sensitive syndromes.

In short, sensitive skin is difficult to define and is a subject rife with controversy. This condition is the expression of sensory irritation in the absence of objective clinical signs, and it corresponds to exaggerated reactions to cosmetics, wool, cleansing products, and other compounds. It often worsens after exposure to a dry and cold environment. However, extending such a concept to environmentally induced dermatoses is probably not so productive since it introduces overlaps between allergic dermatitis, ICD, and various other dermatoses (16).

This review focuses on the invisible sensory irritation to fabrics. Interactions between cleansing products and human SC are complex and not fully understood. A series of clinical and noninvasive biometrological assessments possibly document specific aspects linked to sensory irritation (Table 22.1). This review encompasses measurements of TEWL, skin capacitance mapping, and squamometry. Fabric

TABLE 22.1

Noninvasive Experimental Methods Exploring Sensitive Skin

Mechanism	Method	References
Fabric feel	Subjective tactile sensory comfort	17
Geoclimate effect	Dew point determination	18,19
Mechanical irritation	Behind-the-knee test	20,21
SC barrier	TEWL	22
	Electrometric assessment	4,23
	Skin capacitance mapping	24
Corneocyte chemical reactivity	Squamometry	25
	Corneosurfametry	4,26,27
	Corneoxenometry	4,27,28

property data of interest are (a) low-stress mechanical properties, such as bending, shear, and tensile deformation, and (b) fabric surface data such as smoothness/evenness, roughness, and friction coefficient.

Fabric Feel

The fabric sensory comfort is a complex psychological process. Tactile or sensory comfort is thought to be directly unrelated with any particular nerve ending. When the fabric is held, handled, touches lightly, moves over, or is packed tightly to the skin, the individual describes how the skin feels and responds to fabrics (17). The same stimulus possibly elicits quite different responses from different individuals. Descriptors of the sensory attributes of tactile or sensory comfort such as soft, harsh, smooth, rough, sticky, damp, prickly, clammy, cool, warm, heavy, comfortable, or uncomfortable are used for describing the feelings. The intensity of the sensations defines the fabric feel ranges from soft to uncomfortable.

Two distinct situations are contrasted when assessing (a) perceived sensory attributes, including softness, smoothness, prickliness, and (b) other characteristics evaluating the fabric tactile comfort. Both test evaluations are possibly performed either by handling the fabrics or after wearing the fabrics on other parts of the body. In fact, the feel of a textile contact is frequently different on the palms from that on elsewhere. Indeed, the nature and density of neural receptors in the skin differ according to the body site. In addition, other skin structures are likely involved in abnormal sensory responses to contact with cleaned, laundered, or softened fabrics (9). This might suggest that a causative mechanism is associated with the chemicals involved in fabric processing. Changes in surface friction in part result from treating fabric with enzymes and softeners. The SC reactivity to cleaning agents for textiles is impaired in some subjects claiming SSI (13,14). Basically, two distinct chemical mechanisms, acting either singly or in combination, are involved in this process. On the one hand, surfactant interactions with regular corneocytes are unusual in their intensity, releasing a variety of mediators including cytokines, prostaglandins, and leukotrienes (15). In turn, these biomolecules boost the release of neuromediators from distinct cells leading to specific nerve ending stimulation (29). On the other hand, any impaired SC barrier function to surfactants possibly allows some xenobiotics to directly stimulate sensory nerve endings. Some chemicals are indeed released near the nerve endings. According to such hypothesis, SSI might be induced by subtle changes in the SC structure including a thinner layer with or without alteration of the corneocyte structure (30) and desquamation rate (31). Similarly, a reduced corneocyte size was suggested to enhance the penetration of water-soluble xenobiotics. Still another possibility involves an individual lowered threshold for skin nerve stimulation. Indeed, free nerve endings and specialized nerve corpuscles are under the influence of both excitation stimuli and antagonist signs (29,30,32). When the latter activity is lowered, it has been postulated that the efferent neurosensorial input is amplified and perceived as an SSI manifestation. As a result, lifestyle including psychological stress and emotions possibly influences the reactive skin condition.

Some subjects with SSI feel discomfort including itching and stinging when wearing garments. Unlike the majority of mild cleansers, some more aggressive cleaning agents including household cleaning products and laundering products possibly induce skin tightness, after about 5–10 minutes (14). Such unpleasant perception is ascribed to the physical attack of the upper SC by rapid water evaporation from the skin surface. In fact, harsh surfactants create an immediate corneocyte overhydration and swelling, followed by rapid water evaporation leading to an SC moisture level below the presurfactant treatment level (24). The overhydration process followed by the abated hydration level is responsible for a higher rate in skin surface water evaporation. Thus, a differential stress is created inside the upper SC. Such a condition is in part linked to epidermal lipid removal combined with surfactant binding to SC proteins and subsequent changes in the overall electrical charges at the skin surface.

In any case of surfactant-induced SSI, regional variability in the intensity of response is commonly present on different body sites (33). Moreover, the complex molecular composition of the cleansing products influences each individual skin surface overreactivity. In distinct individuals, these features are commonly restricted to limited sets of compounds. In addition, the SSI status is influenced by age, gender, and ethnicity, as well as by specific environmental and seasonal geoclimatic conditions (34). In particular, the negative geoclimatic influence manifests itself when the environmental dew point modifications in winter alter the SC physiology (18,19,35,36). The influence of the environmental dew point possibly participates to the variability in time of any reactive skin perception (18).

Similar to the decline in irritation reactivity with age, SSI to surfactants appears less frequent in older adults. In general, fair skin is believed to be more susceptible to SSI than darker skin. However, the situation is probably more complex when interpreting the heterogeneity in the mottled subclinical melanoderma (MSM) (37,38). This condition is likely due to the chronic effect of UV light exposure (38,39). The complaints about SSI appear to be more frequent when the extent in MSM pattern is enlarged (4).

Mechanical Skin Irritation

Fabrics are rubbed on the skin, sometime on preconditioned (inflamed) skin (17,20,21,40,41). The effects of gently rubbing semioccluded swatches of cotton terrycloth fabric are tested on the skin. Most mechanical irritation tests require panelists to wear laundered garments each day for several days. Alternatively, laundered fabric is worn in close proximity to the skin at a limited test site, such as in the diaper test and the axilla, the back of the knee, and the wrist ban wear test. The continuous friction through normal movement results in mechanical irritation. Of note, similar tests are used for assessing the skin effects associated with wearing fabrics washed with commercial laundry detergents with or without softeners. These procedures combine the potential for the mechanical and chemical irritations.

Chemical Skin Allergy and Irritation

For fabrics that remain in prolonged contact with the skin, two considerations are important with regard to their chemical composition: (a) the inherent irritation potential of the material and (b) a potential immune reaction promoting allergic reactions (4–61).

Bioengineering and Textile Skin Impact

Transepidermal Water Loss

In some individuals, SSI susceptibility appears correlated with an increased baseline TEWL. Accordingly, skin hyperreactivity to water-soluble shampoos is supposedly related to the increased SC permeating to such xenobiotics. Whether this condition is genuine or part of a self-exacerbating loop, once irritation is already initiated, the SC damaged is unsettled. The skin barrier function is also possibly tested by the determination of the passive sustainable test (62).

Placing fabric over the skin surface without any downward or lateral movement of the fabric relative to the skin possibly cause changes in the skin. One of the primary signs is hydration of the SC, because (a) the fabric usually acts as a barrier to the loss of TEWL at the skin surface or (b) the fabric is a source of water contributing to the SC hydration. The primary change, an increase in the SC hydration, commonly leads to other events such as increased susceptibility to microbial growth, abrasive damage, absorption of chemicals, and altered pH with inflammation of the skin as a final outcome or manifestation.

Two main types of assessments determine the effect of fabric on moisture in or on the skin. The first type involves the use of instruments measuring the water content of the SC or measuring the rate of evaporative water loss as an indication of the SC water content. Hydration due to fabric covering the skin is the difference between measurements taken after covering the skin with fabric and those taken on uncovered skin. The second type involves the use of rating scales by which subjects indicate skin wetness procedures.

Skin Capacitance Mapping

Skin susceptibility to SSI appears associated with decreased SC electric capacitance (24). The skin capacitance mapping procedure (Moisture Map MM10, CK technology) is a convenient way for assessing such changes. Such SSI nonoptical aspect is commonly present after SC preconditioning, and it does not always represent an initial step leading to reactive skin. By contrast, measuring the passive sustainable SC hydration and the SC water-holding capacity following the surfactant challenge is supposedly a tool discriminating some SSI and non-SSI skins (18).

Squamometry

Stripping the skin and sampling corneocytes using self-adhesive clear disks (Corneofix®, C+K electronic) and staining the harvested material with a toluidine blue-basic fuchsin dye represent the initial steps of the squamometry test (23). The squamometry index corresponds to the Chroma C* value of the sampling as assessed by reflectance colorimetry. This test is available for different purposes. When it deals specifically with the interaction of surfactants with SC, the method is called *squamometry S* (25). Indeed, after a preconditioning challenge with surfactants, the squamometry index increases. People with SSI to surfactants commonly show increased reactivity. This finding is possibly related to the presence of so-called immature corneocytes in the SC (26).

Ex Vivo Corneosurfametry

The ex vivo corneosurfametry and corneoxenometry bioassays (27,28) deal with surfactant SSI and other xenobiotic SSI assessments. Human SC harvested using cyanoacrylate skin surface strippings (CSSS; collected using the 3S Biokit [C+K technology, Visé, Belgium]) is the test substrate (27,28). Diluted or neat formulations are sprayed over the CSSS. The material is kept for 2 hours at room temperature in a moisturized environment. CSSS samples are then thoroughly rinsed using tap water, air-dried, and stained for 3 minutes with toluidine blue-basic fuchsin in 30% alcoholic solution. Their color is measured using reflectance colorimetry in the L*a*b* system (Chroma Meter® CR400 Minolta, Osaka, Japan), and the L* and Chroma C* values are recorded. The difference between L* and Chroma C* represents the so-called colorimetric index of mildness (CIM). This procedure increases the sensibility and repeatability of the test. Its value increases with the intensity of interaction between corneocytes and surfactants. For a given surfactant-based product, the CIM value is commonly increased in subjects complaining of sensitive skin to surfactants (27,28). In other types of reactive skin unrelated to surfactant, SSI does not show similar corneosurfametry characteristics. The advantage of corneosurfametry over in vivo tests relies on the avoidance of any discomfort and other hazards for human volunteers.

The reactivity of the superficial stratum disjunctum at the S-squamometry test appears different from that of the midpart of the SC as evaluated by corneosurfametry (4).

Conclusion

The individual perception of reactive skin by each subject involved in the process is impossible to be objectively controlled. The subjectivity of the complainant and of the test assessor is wide, and a number of seemingly objective assessments remain inconclusive. The sensory irritation is indeed an incipient manifestation of an allergic or an irritative reaction. Textile dermatitis is an example of a dual biological event.

REFERENCES

1. Slodownik D., Williams J., Lee A., and Piérard G. E. 2007. Controversies regarding the sensitive skin syndrome. *Expert Opinion: Dermatology* 2:579–84.
2. Farage M. A. and Maibach H. I. 2010. Sensitive skin: Closing in on a physiological cause. *Contact Dermatitis* 62:137–49.
3. Vanoosthuyze K., Zupkosky P. J., and Buckley K. 2013. Survey of practicing dermatologists on the prevalence of sensitive skin in men. *International Journal of Cosmetic Science* 35:388–93.
4. Piérard G. E., Hermanns-Lê T., Piérard-Franchimont C., Courtois J., and Piérard S. L. 2014. Analytical search of sensory irritation to shampoos in reactive scalp. *Labome Material and Methods* 4:1097.
5. Goffin V., Piérard-Franchimont C., and Piérard G. E. 1996. Sensitive skin and stratum corneum reactivity to household cleaning products. *Contact Dermatitis* 34:81–5.
6. Jourdain R., de Lacharriere O., Bastien P., and Maibach H. I. 2002. Ethnic variations in self-perceived sensitive skin: Epidemiological survey. *Contact Dermatitis* 46:162–9.
7. Robinson M. K. 2002. Population differences in acute skin irritation responses. Race, sex, age, sensitive skin and repeat subject comparisons. *Contact Dermatitis* 46:86–93.
8. Hatch K. L., Markee N. L., and Maibach H. I. 1992. Skin response to fabric, a review of studies and assessment methods. *Cloth Textitle Research Journal* 10:54.
9. Piérard G. E., Arrese J. E., Rodriguez C., and Daskaleros P. A. 1994. Effects of softened and unsoftened fabrics on sensitive skin. *Contact Dermatitis* 30:286–91.
10. Gauger A. 2006. Silver-coated textiles in the therapy of atopic eczema. *Current Problems in Dermatology* 33:152–64.
11. Teufel L., Schuster K. C., Merschak P., Bechtold T., and Redl B. 2008. Development of a fast and reliable method for the assessment of microbial colonization and growth on textiles by DNA quantification. *Journal of Molecular Microbiology and Biotechnology* 14:193–200.
12. Tavaria F. K., Soares J. C., Reis I. L., Paulo M. H., Malcata F. X., and Pintado M. E. 2012. Chitosan: Antimicrobial action upon staphylococci after impregnation onto cotton fabric. *Journal of Applied Microbiology* 112:1034–41.
13. Marriott M., Holmes J., Peters L., Cooper K., Rowson M., and Basketter D. A. 2005. The complex problem of sensitive skin. *Contact Dermatitis* 53:93–9.
14. Piérard-Franchimont C. and Piérard G. E. 2005. Spotlight on sensory irritation and its treatment. *Revue Médicale de Liege* 60:796–8.
15. Berardesca E., Farage M., and Maibach H. 2013. Sensitive skin: An overview. *International Journal of Cosmetic Science* 35:2–8.
16. Carter R., 3rd, Garcia A. M., and Souhan B. E. 2011. Patients presenting with miliaria while wearing flame resistant clothing in high ambient temperatures: A case series. *Journal of Medical Case Reports* 5:474.
17. Love W. E. and Nedorost S. T. 2009. Fabric preferences of atopic dermatitis patients. *Dermatitis: Contact, Atopic, Occupational, Drug* 20:29–33.
18. Paquet F., Piérard-Franchimont C., Fumal I., Goffin V., Paye M., and Piérard G. E. 1998. Sensitive skin at menopause; dew point and electrometric properties of the stratum corneum. *Maturitas* 28:221–7.
19. Devillers C., Piérard G. E., Quatresooz P., and Piérard S. 2010. Environmental dew point and skin and lip weathering. *Journal of the European Academy of Dermatology and Venereology* 24:513–7.
20. Farage M. A., Gilpin D. A., Enane N. A., and Baldwin S. 2001. Development of a new test for mechanical irritation: Behind the knee as a test site. *Skin Research and Technology* 7:193–203.

21. Farage M. A. 2006. The behind-the-knee test: An efficient model for evaluating mechanical and chemical irritation. *Skin Research and Technology* 12:73–82.

22. Raj N., Voegeli R., Rawlings A. V. et al. 2017. A fundamental investigation into aspects of the physiology and biochemistry of the stratum corneum in subjects with sensitive skin. *Int J Cosmet Sci.* 39:2–10.

23. Uhoda E., Paye M., and Piérard G. E. 2003. Comparative clinical and electrometric assessments of the impact of surfactants on forearm skin. *Exogenous Dermatology* 2:64–9.

24. Uhoda E., Lévêque J. L., and Piérard G. E. 2005. Silicon image sensor technology for in vivo detection of surfactant-induced corneocyte swelling and drying. *Dermatology* 210:184–8.

25. Piérard-Franchimont C., Henry F., and Piérard G. E. 2000. The SACD method and the XLRS squamometry tests revisited. *International Journal of Cosmetic Science* 22:437–46.

26. Piérard G. E., Goffin V., and Piérard-Franchimont C. 1994. Squamometry and corneosurfametry in rating interactions of cleansing products with strautm corneum. *Journal of the Society of Cosmetic Chemists* 45:269–77.

27. Piérard G. E., Piérard-Franchimont C., Hermanns-Lê T., and Paquet P. 2014. Recent advances in toxicological testing of the stratum corneum. *The British Journal of Dermatology* 171 Suppl 3:34–7.

28. Piérard G. E., Piérard-Franchimont C., Paquet P., Hermanns-Lê T., Radermacher J., and Delvenne P. 2014. Cyanoacrylate skin surface stripping and the 3S-Biokit advent in tropical dermatology: A look from Liege. *TheScientificWorldJournal* 2014:462634.

29. Boulais N. and Misery L. 2008. The epidermis: A sensory tissue. *European Journal of Dermatology* 18:119–27.

30. Hirao T., Denda M., and Takahashi M. 2001. Identification of immature cornified envelopes in the barrier-impaired epidermis by characterization of their hydrophobicity and antigenicities of the components. *Experimental Dermatology* 10:35–44.

31. Piérard G. E., Goffin V., Hermanns-Lê T., and Piérard-Franchimont C. 2000. Corneocyte desquamation. *International Journal of Molecular Medicine* 6:217–21.

32. Stander S., Schneider S. W., Weishaupt C., Luger T. A., and Misery L. 2009. Putative neuronal mechanisms of sensitive skin. *Experimental Dermatology* 18:417–23.

33. Farage M. A. 2009. How do perceptions of sensitive skin differ at different anatomical sites? An epidemiological study. *Clinical and Experimental Dermatology* 34:e521–30.

34. Farage M. A. 2011. Perceptions of sensitive skin of the genital area. *Current Problems in Dermatology* 40:142–54.

35. Piérard-Franchimont C. and Piérard G. E. 2002. Beyond a glimpse at seasonal dry skin: A review. *Exogenous Dermatology* 1:3–6.

36. Delvenne M., Piérard-Franchimont C., Seidel L., Albert A., and Piérard G. E. 2013. The weather-beaten dorsal hand clinical rating, shadow casting optical profilometry, and skin capacitance mapping. *BioMed Research International* 2013:913646.

37. Petit L., Fogouang L., Uhoda I., Smitz S., Piérard-Franchimont C., and Piérard G. E. 2003. Regional variability in mottled subclinical melanoderma in the elderly. *Experimental Gerontology* 38:327–31.

38. Piérard G. E., Hermanns-Lê T., Piérard S. L., Dewalque L., Charlier C., Piérard-Franchimont C., and Delvenne P. In vivo skin fluorescence imaging in young Caucasian adults with early malignant melanomas. *Clinical, Cosmetic and Investigational Dermatology* 7:225–30.

39. Maddodi N., Jayanthy A., and Setaluri V. 2012. Shining light on skin pigmentation: The darker and the brighter side of effects of UV radiation. *Photochemistry and Photobiology* 88:1075–82.

40. Ricci G., Patrizi A., Bendandi B., Menna G., Varotti E., and Masi M. 2004. Clinical effectiveness of a silk fabric in the treatment of atopic dermatitis. *The British Journal of Dermatology* 150:127–31.

41. Strese H., Kuck M., Benken R., Fluhr J. W., Schanzer S., Richter H., Meinke M. C. et al. 2013. Influence of finishing textile materials on the reduction of skin irritations. *Skin Research and Technology* 19:e409–16.

42. Rodriguez C., Calvin G., Lally C., and Lachapelle J. M. 1994. Skin effects associated with wearing fabrics washed with commercial laundry detergents. *Journal of Toxicology—Cutaneous and Ocular Toxicology* 13:39–45.

43. Seidenari S., Giusti F., Massone F., and Mantovani L. 2002. Sensitization to disperse dyes in a patch test population over a five-year period. *American Journal of Contact Dermatitis* 13:101–7.

44. Lazarov A., Cordoba M., Plosk N., and Abraham D. 2003. Atypical and unusual clinical manifestations of contact dermatitis to clothing (textile contact dermatitis): Case presentation and review of the literature. *Dermatology Online Journal* 9:1.

45. Matthies W. 2003. Irritant dermatitis to detergents in textiles. *Current Problems in Dermatology* 31: 123–38.

46. Gonzalez de Olano D., Subiza J. L., and Civantos E. 2009. Cutaneous allergy to cotton. *Annals of Allergy, Asthma & Immunology* 102:263–4.

47. Lensen G., Jungbauer F., Goncalo M., and Coenraads P. J. 2007. Airborne irritant contact dermatitis and conjunctivitis after occupational exposure to chlorothalonil in textiles. *Contact Dermatitis* 57:181–6.

48. de Groot A. C., Le Coz C. J., Lensen G. J., Flyvholm M. A., Maibach H. I., and Coenraads P. J. 2010. Formaldehyde-releasers: Relationship to formaldehyde contact allergy. Part 2. Formaldehyde-releasers in clothes: Durable press chemical finishes. *Contact Dermatitis* 63:1–9.

49. Reich H. C. and Warshaw E. M. 2010. Allergic contact dermatitis from formaldehyde textile resins. *Dermatitis: Contact, Atopic, Occupational, Drug* 21:65–76.

50. Davari P. and Maibach H. I. 2011. Contact urticaria to cosmetic and industrial dyes. *Clinical and Experimental Eermatology* 36:1–5.

51. Tognetti L., Giorgini S., and Lotti T. 2011. Prurigo-like eczema as an unsuspected presentation of textile dermatitis. *European Journal of Dermatology* 21:139–40.

52. Wong A., Ball N., and de Gannes G. 2011. Nonpruritic contact dermatitis from disperse blue dyes. *Dermatitis: Contact, Atopic, Occupational, Drug* 22:278–80.

53. Kiracofe E. A. and Zirwas M. J. 2012. Formaldehyde in textiles—What dermatologists need to know about the relationship to contact dermatitis: A review of the US Government Accountability Office's Report to Congressional Committees. *Journal of the American Academy of Dermatology* 67:313–4.

54. Wentworth A. B., Richardson D. M., and Davis M. D. 2012. Patch testing with textile allergens: The mayo clinic experience. *Dermatitis: Contact, Atopic, Occupational, Drug* 23:269–74.

55. Malinauskiene L., Bruze M., Ryberg K., Zimerson E., and Isaksson M. 2013. Contact allergy from disperse dyes in textiles: A review. *Contact Dermatitis* 68:65–75.

56. Narganes L. M., Sambucety P. S., Gonzalez I. R., Rivas M. O., and Prieto M. A. 2013. Lymphomatoid dermatitis caused by contact with textile dyes. *Contact Dermatitis* 68:62–4.

57. Aerts O., Duchateau N., Lambert J., and Bechtold T. 2014. Sodium metabisulfite in blue jeans: An unexpected cause of textile contact dermatitis. *Contact Dermatitis* 70:190–2.

58. Coman G., Blattner C. M., Blickenstaff N. R., Andersen R., and Maibach H. I. 2014. Textile allergic contact dermatitis: Current status. *Reviews on Environmental Health* 29:163–8.

59. Lisi P., Stingeni L., Cristaudo A., Foti C., Pigatto P., Gola M., Schena D., Corazza M., and Bianchi L. 2014. Clinical and epidemiological features of textile contact dermatitis: An Italian multicentre study. *Contact Dermatitis* 70:344–50.

60. Coman G., Blickenstaff N., Edwards A., and Maibach H. 2015. Dermatotoxicologic clinical solutions: Textile dye dermatitis patch testing. *Cutaneous and Ocular Toxicology* 34:68–71.

61. Slodownik D., Williams J., Tate B., Tam M., Cahill J., Frowen K., and Nixon R. 2011. Textile allergy—The Melbourne experience. *Contact Dermatitis* 65:38–42.

62. Van Comphaut I., Fumal I., Jacquemin D., Fissette J., and Piérard G. E. 1999. Skin barrier repair after burns. Electrometric evaluation using the passive sustainable hydration test. *Journal of Environmental Medicine* 1:47–50.

Section VI

Management

23

Dermatotoxicology and Sensitive Skin Syndrome

Golara Honari and Howard Maibach

Sensitive skin syndrome is a challenging condition, characterized by subjective cutaneous hypersensitivity and considerable impact on health-related quality of life. Affected individuals complain of itching, burning, and stinging sensations with exposure to many skin care products and/or environmental factors. While some biophysical alterations such as impaired barrier function and increased vascular reactivity have been observed, current evidence highlights a prominent role for increased sensory perception in the cutaneous nervous system and more needs to be learned about pathogenesis (1). Sensitive skin is classically a self-described condition, clinically diagnosed based on patient's history and symptoms. Many individuals have no underlying skin disease, but concomitant conditions such as AD, acne, rosacea, contact dermatitis, and other inflammatory dermatoses can be seen. Physicians and toxicologists must evaluate each patient for potential associated dermatoses. Despite challenges in developing a specific toxicology method for sensitive skin, it is important to pay attention to in vivo testing of products for these individuals. Objective measures such as erythema, desquamation, and inflammation as well as subjective measures such as burning, stinging, and itching should be tested while developing products for these subjects. It is important to differentiate patients with SSS from those affected by ACD (sensitized skin), ICD, photosensitivity, contact urticaria, and/or other inflammatory dermatoses. Hence, this chapter reviews toxicological methods to study the effect of environmental, physical, or chemical elements affecting skin in dermatoses that can share similar symptoms. These methods are not specific for sensitive skin.

Allergic Contact Dermatitis

ACD syndrome is caused by allergen specific T cell-mediated complex processes. Skin sensitization occurs when a susceptible individual is exposed to a chemical with the potential to sensitize. Reexposure to the same allergen in a sensitized person can mount a localized or widespread skin inflammation. ACD is a delayed-type hypersensitivity response composed of an induction (sensitization) phase and an effector (elicitation) phase (2).

Induction has multiple steps:

- Penetration of allergen into the skin and binding to skin components. An allergen needs to have certain physicochemical properties to be able to induce sensitivity. Most contact allergens are small, molecules with a molecular weight of less than 500 Da, and referred to as *hapten*. Larger molecules can hardly penetrate the SC and cannot act as allergens (3). At the same time, haptens are too small to be antigenic; they need to form a hapten–protein complex to activate antigen-presenting cells. Concept of protein/peptide haptenation is crucial to form immunogenic structures and is the focus of much research to develop predictive in vitro sensitization (4,5). Allergen in skin binds major histocompatibility complex (MHC) proteins, which are encoded by histocompatibility antigen genes and are present on epidermal antigen-presenting cells (Langerhans cells [LCs]) (4,6).
- The next step is the activation of LCs by haptens. LCs are responsible for the internalization and processing of the haptens. Allergen-induced production of inflammatory cytokines and multiprotein complexes, termed *inflammasomes*, induces the migration of the haptenized LC and dendritic cells (DCs) into the T cell-rich paracortical areas of regional lymph nodes (6,7).

- In the paracortical areas of the lymph node, naive T cells will recognize allergen–MHC molecule complexes to transform into allergen-specific T cells.
- The proliferation of allergen-specific T cells in the draining lymph node is supported by IL-1, released by the allergen-presenting cells and IL-2 released by activated T cells. IL-2 is a potent inducer of T cell proliferation (8).
- Systemic increase of effector-memory T cells. In the absence of further allergen contacts, their frequency in blood gradually decreases.

Effector phase starts upon reexposure to allergen, which leads to activation of effector memory T cells and release of multiple cytokines and chemokines, leading to more inflammatory response and clinical presentation of dermatitis.

It generally takes about 4 days to a few weeks to become sensitized, but elicitation can happen within 1 day up to a week.

Assessment of skin sensitization hazard of chemicals is an important component of the safety assessment of chemicals. In the absence of in vitro validated models, the predictive testing for skin sensitization potential currently has relied on animal testing. Skin sensitization testing, at least for cosmetic ingredients, has been banned in Europe. Animal testing with completed cosmetic products in European Union was prohibited in 2004; a testing ban for cosmetic ingredients was enforced in 2009, followed by a marketing ban as of March 2013 (9). These directives pose an urgent challenge for scientists in search of alternative methods. Currently validated methods to predict sensitizing potentials are mostly animal based. However, increasing understanding of the key steps of the sensitization process has led to the development of few in vitro predictive methods. In vitro assays such as direct peptide reactivity assay (DPRA) and the KeratinoSens™ have been validated for classifying a substance as a skin sensitizer. Formal validation of these assays is required before they can fully replace in vivo assays for hazard identification (10). Skin sensitization is an intrinsic property of a chemical substance and is referred to as a hazard; the likelihood that this hazard will be expressed is called *risk*. Risk is a function of hazard potency and exposure (risk = hazard × exposure). The likelihood of a particular person developing sensitivity is the function of his or her individual susceptibility (11).

Basic mechanisms of contact sensitivity, officially accepted animal models, and in vitro assays are reviewed here.

Predictive In Vitro Testing

Understanding the key biological mechanisms of the induction phase helps in designing in vitro test models. It is unlikely for a single alternative method to provide sufficient information to replace the in vivo models. Integrated data from different alternative testing and nontesting methods are required to address this end point (12).

The key steps for the adverse outcome pathway for skin sensitization include the following (12,13):

- Skin bioavailability: ability of a chemical to penetrate skin and reach the site of haptenation
- Haptenation: ability of a chemical to form covalent binding to skin proteins
- Release of proinflammatory signals by epidermal keratinocytes
- Activation and maturation of DCs
- Migration of DC from skin to the regional lymph nodes and presentation of the antigen to T cells
- Proliferation of memory T cells (lymphocytes capable of being stimulated and activated specifically by the haptenated protein)

Two assays have gained scientific validity by the European Centre for the Validation of Alternative Methods (ECVAM).

Direct Peptide Reactivity Assay

The DPRA is an in chemico assay which addresses the process of haptenation. Haptenation is the covalent binding of haptens to skin proteins and is considered the molecular initiating event of the skin sensitization. Haptenation is assessed by measuring the depletion of synthetic heptapeptides containing cysteine or lysine, after 24 hours of incubation with the test substance. The DPRA test method underwent European Union (EU) Reference Laboratory for Alternatives to Animal Testing (EURL ECVAM)-coordinated validation studies, and recommendations on this test were released in 2013 (14). The DPRA is designed for screening the sensitization potential of chemicals. Test chemicals are incubated for 24 hours with synthetic heptapeptides containing either cysteine (peptide/chemical ratio in the reaction mixture is 1:10) or lysine residues (peptide/chemical ratio in the reaction mixture is 1:50). Peptide depletion is measured by high-performance liquid chromatography with UV detection (15). Chemicals are classified into four reactivity categories based on average peptide depletion values for cysteine and lysine into minimal, low, moderate, and high reactivity (16). Sensitizing potency is assumed to correlate with the reactivity class. The accuracy of the DPRA for distinguishing sensitizers from nonsensitizers in 133 chemicals in relation to the local lymph node assay (LLNA) is reported to be 86% (87% sensitivity; 83% specificity) (17). A draft of the protocol by Organisation for Economic Cooperation and Development (OECD) is available for more details (18).

Keratinocyte-Based Antioxidant/Electrophile Response Element-Nrf2 Luciferase Reporter Gene Test Method (KeratinoSens)

The keratinocyte-based antioxidant/electrophile response element (ARE)-Nrf2 luciferase reporter gene test method addresses the activation of a key pathway in keratinocytes in response to potential sensitizers. The ARE-dependent pathway in keratinocytes is the second key step in skin sensitization. Nuclear factor erythroid 2-related factor 2 (Nrf2) is a transcription factor with a key role in promoting the expression of gene coding for cytoprotective proteins, following an electrophilic or oxidative stress. The activity of Nrf2 is primarily regulated by the cysteine-rich Kelch-like ECH-associated protein 1 (Keap1) sensor protein. Although other pathways may be involved in this regulation, the Keap1–Nrf2–ARE pathway is considered a major regulator of cytoprotective responses to oxidative and electrophilic stress. While the majority of skin sensitizers are electrophiles reacting with the nucleophilic centers in skin proteins, the activation of this pathway is a relevant measure of the skin sensitization potential of a chemical (19,20).

KeratinoSens in vitro test method is developed based on the mentioned mechanism earlier. It has gone through EURL ECVAM-coordinated validation studies, and recommendations on this test were released in February 2014 (19).

A recommended protocol is outlined here (20):

- Immortalized adherent cell line derived from HaCaT human keratinocytes transfected with a selectable plasmid (plasmid contains a luciferase gene under the transcriptional control of ARE). This allows quantitative measurements of luciferase gene induction, by using luminescence detection. Luciferase signal reflects the activation by sensitizers.
- Ninety-six-well plates are seeded. For each trial, three black well plates are seeded for the luciferase determination. One clear plate is seeded for the cytotoxicity determination. (Parallel cytotoxicity measurements are conducted to assess whether gene induction levels occur at subcytotoxic concentrations). One well remains blank in each plate with no cells and no treatment to assess the background values).
- After seeding, cells are grown for 24 hours in the 96-well plates. Then the medium is removed and replaced with fresh culture medium and the test chemicals and control substances.
- Test chemicals are serially diluted to make a range of doses. Each plate contains dilutions of the test articles and dilutions of solvent/control, and one well remains blank.
- Treated plates are incubated for 48 hours at 37°C in the presence of 5% CO_2 in the case of KeratinoSens.

- After the exposure time, cells in the triplicate plates for luminescence readings are rinsed with phosphate-buffered saline. A relevant lysis buffer is added to each well for 20 minutes at room temperature.
- Luciferase measurements: Luciferase is added to the cell lysates and plates placed in a luminometer, or the luminometer is programmed to add the luciferase substrate to each well and measure its activity.
- Cytotoxicity measurements: After 48 hours, the medium in the clear plate is replaced with fresh medium containing MTT (3-(4,5-dimethylthiazol-2-yl)-2,5-diphenyltetrazolium bromide) for 4 hours at 37°C in the presence of 5% CO_2, then the MTT medium is removed. Cell viability is measured by enzymatic conversion of the vital dye MTT (3-(4,5-dimethylthiazol-2-yl)-2,5-diphenyltetrazolium bromide), into a blue formazan salt that is quantitatively measured using a spectrometer.
- Results are calculated and reported in automated excel sheets, providing information on the following:
  - Maximal gene induction (Imax): Value observed at any concentration of the tested chemical and positive control is reported.
  - EC1.5 value: The concentration for which a gene induction is above the 1.5 threshold (50% enhanced gene activity).
  - Cell viability values: Cell viability reduced by 50% and 30% (IC50 and IC30 concentration values).
- Decision making: Potential skin sensitizers in the KeratinoSens test method are the following:
  - Chemicals with Imax significantly higher than 1.5-fold compared to the basal luciferase activity and the EC1.5 value are below 1000 μM in at least two out of the three repetitions.
  - At the lowest concentration with an EC value above 1.5, the cellular viability should be above 70%. Otherwise, the chemical is considered cytotoxic.
  - Compounds that only induce the gene activity at cytotoxic levels are considered nonsensitizing skin irritants.

Data obtained from KeratinoSens in relation to data from the LLNA have an accuracy of 77% (79% sensitivity and 72% specificity) for a set of 145 chemicals (21). More details are available on EURL ECVAM recommendations on the KeratinoSens assay for skin sensitization testing and OECD draft proposal on this assay (19,20).

EURL ECVAM is currently evaluating other mechanistically relevant test methods for reliability (transferability, within and between laboratory reproducibility) and their predictive capabilities for further use as part of integrated approaches for skin sensitization hazard assessment.

The human cell line activation test is currently under validation by ECVAM. This assay is an in vitro skin sensitization test, based on the augmentation of CD86 and CD54 expression in THP-1 cells after exposure to a potential sensitizer. Assay quantifies the induction of these markers, which are associated with DC maturation in vivo, on the surface of DC-like cell lines (22).

Predictive In Vivo Testing

Traditionally, guinea pigs have been the most commonly used test animals for sensitization studies. Buehler's occluded path test (without adjuvant) (23) and Magnusson and Kligman's guinea pig maximization test (using adjuvant) (24) have been used for years; both tests measure sensitization as well as elicitation reactions. Multiple variations have been developed (25), but the basic principles are similar and include: topical application and/or intradermal injection of test material to groups of animals, followed by a 1–2 week rest period and subsequent reexposure in an attempt to elicit the cutaneous hypersensitivity reactions. In some tests, an adjuvant is also administered to enhance (maximize) immune responses provoked by the test material.

Guinea Pig Maximization Test Method

A minimum of 10 animals used in the treatment group and at least 5 animals in the control group are used (or 20 test and 10 control animals). Induction is done initially on the skin of the shoulder region with three intradermal injections on day 0.

- 1:1 mixture of Freund's complete adjuvant (FCA)/water or saline
- Test substance (Appropriate concentrations may be determined from a pilot study using two or three animals)
- Test substance in a 1:1 mixture of FCA/water or saline

Control animals also receive three intradermal injections, but only the vehicle is used instead of the test substance. Five to seven days later, the skin is painted with 0.5 mL of 10% SLS in Vaseline, to create a local irritation; 24 hours later, the test substance is applied under occlusion for 48 hours.

The challenge is done on day 20–22 with reapplication of patches for 24 hours, and the results are assessed at 48 and 72 hours after the challenge. The Magnusson and Kligman grading scale is used for evaluation (0 = no visible change, 1 = discrete or patchy erythema, 2 = moderate and confluent erythema, 3 = intense erythema and swelling).

Buehler Test Method

A minimum of 20 animals in the treatment group and 10 animals in the control groups is used. The test material is applied on the skin of flank under occlusion for 6 hours, the vehicle is applied to the control group hair on the application, and sites are closely clipped. The same process is repeated a total of three times within 2 weeks and followed by 2 weeks of rest and then challenge. To challenge patches are again applied for 6 hours under occlusion and then evaluated at 24 and 56 hours after application. If necessary, a rechallenge is done by repeating the same procedure 1 week later.

Little advice is available on test substance concentration and vehicle selection on OECD guideline 406 (26). Due to multiple limitations of these assays including subjective assessment of the frequency of responses, it is not possible to assess sensitizing potencies of a chemical using this assay (11).

Local Lymph Node Assays

The LLNA, developed in 1992 (27), is based on an alternative strategy (25). LLNA studies the induction phase of skin sensitization; skin sensitizers are identified by their ability to provoke proliferative responses in the mouse local lymph node. The assay provides quantitative data suitable for dose-response assessment and requires lees number of animals compared to guinea pig tests. The original LLNA test guideline (OECD; TG 429) was adopted in 2002 and updated in 2010 (28). The assay is based on the fact that sensitizers induce a primary proliferation of lymphocytes in the lymph nodes draining the site of application. This proliferation is proportional to the dose applied and provides objective data on the sensitization potentials. Radioactive labeling with (^{3}H) thymidine is done to measure cell proliferation. A minimum of four animals is used per dose group, with a minimum of three concentrations of the test substance, plus a negative control group treated with the vehicle only, as well as a positive control, if appropriate. Later modifications of LLNA introduced two nonradioactive modifications, LLNA: DA (TG 442 A) (29), and LLNA: BrdU-ELISA (TG 442 B) (30) were validated. A reduced LLNA approach has been accepted, which could use up to 40% fewer animals. It can identify sensitizers but should not be used for hazard classification.

The protocol is as follows:

- A minimum of four animals is used per dose group (groups of four CBA/Ca female mice; 7–12 weeks of age) with a minimum of three concentrations of the test substance, plus a concurrent negative control group treated only with the vehicle for the test substance, and a positive control (concurrent or recent).

- Animals are treated topically on the dorsum of both ears with 25 µL of test material or with an equal volume of the vehicle; once a day for 3 days.
- Five days after the initial exposure, all mice will be injected with 20 µCi (7.4×10^5 Bq) of tritiated (3H)-methyl thymidine via the tail vein.
- Five hours later, all animals are humanely killed; draining of auricular lymph nodes is excised and processed.
- Cellular proliferation is determined by measuring incorporated radioactivity.
- When using nonradioactive modification to the LLNA:
  - LLNA: DA: Cellular proliferation is determined by the measurement of the (ATP) content by bioluminescence as an indicator of this proliferation (29).
  - LLNA:BrdU-ELISA: Cellular proliferation is determined by measuring 5-bromo-2-deoxyuridine (BrdU) content, an analog of thymidine. The BrdU content in deoxyribonucleic acid of lymphocytes is measured by enzyme linked immunosorbent assay (ELISA).
- Results are calculated based on the stimulation index (SI). The result is regarded positive when SI $\geq$ 3. However, the strength of the dose response, the statistical significance, and the consistency of the solvent/vehicle and positive control responses may also be used; details are available on OECD: TG 429 (28).

LLNA has generated data on sensitizing activities, including the potency of hundreds of chemicals (31,32). These databases form an essential resource for further development of in vitro predictive methods (33). Strategies for the replacement of animal testing are reviewed in more detail in EURL ECVAM publications (13).

Photoallergic Contact Dermatitis

Photoallergic reactions are immune-mediated reactions, which require presensitization with a photoreactive chemical. These reactions are typically delayed type (Gell and Coombs type IV reactions) and are often difficult to clinically differentiate from phototoxic reactions. Photoallergy occurs when certain photoreactive allergens in the skin absorb light and create an inflammatory response. These chemicals may be applied topically or diffuse into skin following systemic administration of a drug. Historically, an outbreak of photocontact dermatitis caused by an antibacterial, tetrachlorsalicylanilide, in the early 1960s (34–37), raised awareness about the need to perform photosensitivity testing on drugs and skin care products. Multiple agents are known to cause photoallergic reactions including topical antimicrobials, fragrances, sunscreen ingredients such as 6-methylcoumarin, benzophenone, nonsteroidal anti-inflammatory drugs, promethazine, benzocaine, and p-aminobenzoic acid.

Safety evaluation of products should include assessment of phototoxicity and photoallergenicity of drugs or topical products. Basic pathophysiology of photoallergic reactions and testing methods for the assessment of photoallergenic properties of chemicals are presented here. Photoallergens are haptens that require UV radiation to be able to bind carrier proteins and trigger allergic responses. While there is no validated predictive assay available to predict photoallergenicity, few in vitro and in vivo models have been developed for this purpose. The photoallergic potential of chemicals can be assessed by their potential to bind human serum albumin (HSA) following UV exposure. An adjunct histidine oxidation assay can be used to differentiate photoirritants and photoallergens. This chapter reviews the pathophysiology of photoallergic reactions and the few available toxicology methods.

Pathophysiology of Photoallergic Reactions

Photoallergic reactions are cell-mediated hypersensitivity processes requiring presensitization. Photoallergens are chemicals that absorb light and form reactive species that covalently bind proteins to transform into full allergens. A photoallergen/photohapten is basically a hapten that requires UV radiation for covalent coupling with a protein and forming a complete antigen (38–40). This feature has led to development of an in vitro assay to screen for photoallergens based on UV absorption spectrometry (41,42). A complete photoallergen can trigger a T cell-mediated immune response via interaction with LCs similar to a regular antigen. Photoirritants and photoallergens both form reactive species, but the chemical reactions are different, which might help to further differentiate photoallergens from phototoirritants (39,43).

Predictive In Vitro Testing

As mentioned earlier, a predictive method is lacking; currently available methods are reviewed.

- *UV absorption spectrometry*: Based on pathogeneses discussed earlier, photobinding, a well-accepted property of photoallergens, has founded the basis for UV absorption assays (41,43). In this assay, the test material is diluted in HSA. Two sets are used, one to irradiate with UV and one to keep in the dark as a control. After radiation, the unbound test chemical is separated from HSA by filtration. UV spectrometry is performed before and after separation. Photobinding leads to increased UV absorption. An increased absorbance of more than 5% of the dark control solution is considered significant (43).

- *Histidine oxidation assay*: Histidine is a substrate for singlet oxygen (39,44). The photooxidation of histidine has been used to screen for photoirritancy. Efficient histidine photooxidizers may be considered photoirritant rather than photoallergic. Although this is not always the case, this assay can be used as an adjunct to UV absorption to screen for photoallergens. Phototoxic chemical, creating singlet oxygen, can lower the concentration of histidine in the test solution. Basic principles include making preparations of histidine (1 mM) and the test material (at a concentration relevant to photobinding), in sets of two. One set is exposed to UV radiation, and subsequently, histidine concentration is measured before and after radiation, using modified Pauly reaction (43,45). Lovell and Jones (43) used histidine-binding assay to test the 30 chemicals used in the neutral red uptake (NRU) phototoxicity validation trial; six out of seven photoallergens were identified based on the fact that they absorbed light and showed less than 5% histidine loss. Photoirritants tend to have a higher ratio of histidine loss, but there are known photoirritants which do not cause histidine photooxidation.

Multiple investigators have proposed additional investigational methods and models (40,46,47), which include assessment of photoreactivity of compounds and their ability to produce ROS upon light exposure (48–50), as well as in vitro assays using human monocyte derived cells (51), human peripheral blood monocyte-derived DCs (52), and human skin epithelial-like cells (53).

Predictive In Vivo Testing

The basic principles of in vivo studies of photoallergenicity involve two steps: sensitization (induction) and elicitation. Sensitization is induced by repeated application of the test substance followed by exposure to UV radiation (UVA and UVB). To elicit a reaction, the test compound is applied and irradiated with UVA.

1. *Animal models*: The guinea pig is the most commonly accepted model and has been used to study photoallergy since the late 1960s (54).

     The method used by Gerberick and Ryan (55) is outlined here:
   a. Induction: Hartley strain albino guinea pigs are used.
      i. The test material is applied on the depilated nuchal area. Depending on the study design test material, the vehicle or empty chambers are used to apply the desired material under occlusion for about 2 hours. Hill Top Chamber® has been used for occlusion. On day 1, only four intradermal injections of 1:1 mixture of FCA/water outlined the four corners of a 2 × 2 cm area for the application of test substance.

      ii. Test materials and controls are applied three times a week for 2 weeks.

      iii. After each application of UVA, 10 J/cm^2 is delivered. Distance from the light source to the skin is about 6 in. The lumbar is covered with a foil during each irradiation.

      iv. Animals need to be depilated two to three times during the induction period.

  b. Challenge: After a 10–14 day rest period, the challenge is done.

      i. The lumbar region is depilated, and each animal will be tested either with the test material or the vehicle. Two chambers containing similar ingredients are placed on the left and right sides of the lumbar region for 2 hours.

      ii. After the removal of the patches, the test material is wiped with a moist soft cloth, and only one side is exposed to UVA 10 J/cm^2. The other side will be protected with aluminum foil shielding.

      iii. Test sites are evaluated at 24 and 48 hours and graded between 0 and 3. (0 = no reaction, 0.5 = slight patchy erythema, 1 = slight confluent or moderate patchy, 2 = moderate erythema, 3 = severe erythema).

      iv. A reaction that is more severe on the irradiated site compared to the photoprotected site indicates photocontactallergy. Similar responses on both sites indicate contact allergy.

2. *Human models*: The photomaximization procedure (56) is used to assess topical photocontact sensitizers. This test is basically formatted after the maximization test (57) developed to identify contact sensitizers. This method also includes two steps:

  a. Induction: Twenty-five consented healthy adults are enrolled in the study.

      i. The test agents are applied under occlusion for 24 hours, 2 times a week for 3 weeks.

      ii. Each application and removal is followed by UV radiation (UVA and UVB). Radiation dose is twice the individual's minimum erythema dose.

  b. Challenge: Rest period is 2 weeks, then the challenge is done.

      i. Test compounds are applied in duplicates for 24 hours under occlusion.

      ii. After the chambers are removed, only one set is irradiated with UVA 4 J/cm^2.

      iii. Skin response at each site is evaluated at 24, 48, and 72 hours. Results are graded from 0 to 5 (0 = no reaction, 1 = mild patchy erythema, 2 = papular reaction, moderate erythema, 3 = edema and severe erythema, 4= edema and papules, 5= deep erythema vesicular eruption).

      iv. A reaction that is more severe on the irradiated site compared to the photoprotected site indicates photocontactallergy. Similar responses on both sites indicate contact allergy.

Irritant Contact Dermatitis

Skin irritations are complex biological phenomena, ranging from acute reactions following immediate contact to chronic dermatitis (58,59). Chemicals can permeate through the skin via intercellular lipid, transcellularly with direct permeation through the cornified cells, by diffusion along the hair follicle and sweat glands, or through traumatized skin (60,61). Certain chemicals can cause severe tissue damage and necrosis, causing irreversible tissue damage; these are known as *corrosives*. On the other hand, *irritants* are substances that have reversible effects on the skin; *acute irritants* cause inflammation after a single application, while *cumulative irritants* trigger irritation with recurrent exposure (62). Repetitive exposures to substances with little intrinsic hazardous properties (such as water) are one of the leading causes of irritant dermatitis. Skin corrosion/irritation categories according to the United Nations Globally Harmonized System of Classification and Labeling of Chemicals (UN GHS) (63) are presented in Table 23.1. Optimal assessment of irritancy potential is best achieved when using the appropriate method for the irritation type.

TABLE 23.1

Skin Irritation/Corrosion Categories by the Globally Harmonized System of Classification and Labeling of Chemicals

Skin Corrosion Category 1			Skin Irritation Category 2	Mild Skin Irritation Category 3
Destruction of dermal tissue: Visible necrosis in at least one of three animals			Reversible adverse effects in dermal tissue	Reversible adverse effects in dermal tissue
Subcategory 1A Exposure: ≤3 minutes Observation: ≤1 hour	Subcategory 1B Exposure: >3 minutes to ≤1 hour Observation: ≤14 days	Subcategory 1C Exposure: >1 to ≤4 hours Observation: ≤14 days	Draize score: ≥2.3 to <4.0 or persistent inflammation until day 14 in at least two of three tested animals	Draize score: ≥1.5 to <2.3 in at least two of three tested animals

Source: OSHA, A guide to the globally harmonized system of classification and labelling of chemicals (GHS), accessed August 4, 2016, retrieved from https://www.osha.gov/dsg/hazcom/ghsguideoct05.pdf.

Human skin irritation is classically evaluated by visual and palpatory scorings, and more objective measures are obtained, using various methods and bioengineered devices. Attempts to conduct predictive testing for skin irritants should follow a stepwise algorithm and must be directed toward the specific aspect of irritation, which is under consideration. The main predictive methods to evaluate corrosive potency (potential to cause irreversible damage) and irritative potency (potential to cause reversible inflammatory effects) of substances on normal skin are reviewed here, including methods of in vitro testing validated by ECVAM to identify corrosives and differentiate them from noncorrosive substances as well as in vivo methods of corrosion/irritancy evaluation. The test guidelines published by OECD are internationally agreed methods used to identify and characterize hazardous properties of new and existing chemicals. These basic principles can be applied in the assessment of topical toxicity and the relative potency of hazardous chemicals.

Predictive In Vitro Testing

Corrosion Testing

The main principle of corrosion testing is based on the fact that corrosive chemicals damage the SC and barrier function. Three in vitro methods validated by ECVAM are outlined in the following. In addition to Guideline 431 (originally adopted in 2004) (64), two other in vitro test methods for testing of corrosivity have been validated and adopted as OECD Test Guidelines 430 (65) and 435 (66).

The assays that are currently validated for corrosion and irritation testing are listed in Table 23.2, and the methods are outlined in the following (67,68).

- *Transcutaneous electrical resistance (TER) test method*: TER test method utilizes excised rat skin and identifies corrosive materials by the ability to damage the barrier function, by measuring the reduction in TER.

  The test material (150 μL for liquids or sufficient amount of a solid to evenly cover the tested skin and 150 μL of deionized water added on the top) is applied for up to 24 hours to the epidermal surfaces of skin disks (three skin disks are used for each test and control substance) in a two-compartment test system. Skin disks function as the separation between the compartments. Measurements of electrical resistance is the primary end point; a reduction in the TER below a threshold level (5kΩ for rat) indicates corrosivity (69). Detailed guidelines are available at OECD Test Guideline 430: 2013 (65).

- *Membrane barrier test method for skin corrosion*: Membrane barrier test method for skin corrosion assay utilizes an artificial membrane designed to respond to corrosive substances and may be used to test solids, liquids (with the exception of aqueous materials with a pH between 4.5 and 8.5), and emulsions. The corrosive properties of a material are assessed based on the

TABLE 23.2

EURL-ECVAM-Validated In Vitro Test Methods for Skin Irritation/Corrosion Testing

Test Method Name	Corrosion Testing	Irritation Testing
TER	Distinguish between corrosive and noncorrosive chemicals of different physical forms	N/A
CORROSITEX™	Identification of corrosive properties for acids, bases, and their derivative	N/A
EpiSkin™	Human skin model	Human skin model
EpiDerm™ SIT (EPI-200)	Human skin model	Human skin model
Modified EpiDerm (EPI-200)	Human skin model	Human skin model
SkinEthic™ (RHE)	Human skin model	Human skin model

Source: Skin corrosion, accessed August 4, 2016, retrieved from https://eurl-ecvam.jrc.ec.europa.eu/validation-regulatory-acceptance/topical-toxicity/skin-corrosion; Skin irritation, accessed August 4, 2016, retrieved from https://eurl-ecvam.jrc.ec.europa.eu/validation-regulatory-acceptance/topical-toxicityskin-irritation#ecvam-validated-test-methods.

time required for the tested material to penetrate through this biobarrier (a proteinaceous gel, composed of protein, e.g., keratin, collagen, or mixtures of proteins) and a supporting filter membrane. The system is composed of a synthetic macromolecular biobarrier and a chemical detection system, which can detect a test substance. The tested material (500 μL of a liquid or 500 mg of a finely powdered solid) is evenly applied on the surface of the membrane barrier. Typically, four replicas are produced for each tested substance and its corresponding controls. Controls include a noncorrosive vehicle or solvent used with the test substance; a positive control, typically a chemical with intermediate corrosivity such as sodium hydroxide (GHS Corrosive subcategory 1B) (70); and a negative (noncorrosive) control substance, such as 10% citric acid or 6% propionic acid (66). Corrositex™ is a commercially available membrane barrier test, validated by ECVAM. Detailed guideline is available at OECD Test Guideline 435: 2006 (66).

- *Reconstructed human epidermis (RhE) test method*: RhE models are three-dimensional (3D) biostructures composed of cultured NHKs, which form a multilayered epidermis including SC. Assessments of skin corrosivity and/or irritancy via RhE models are based on the premise that corrosive substances penetrate through the SC and are toxic to the underlying cells. Corrosive chemicals are identified by their ability to decrease cell viability below defined threshold levels (64). Cell viability is measured by enzymatic conversion of a vital dye into a blue formazan salt that is quantitatively measured after extraction from tissues.

  Two or three replicates are used for each test chemical and for the controls in each experiment. Sufficient amount of test chemical should be applied to uniformly cover the epidermis surface; exposure times, incubation temperature, and applied chemical dose vary based on protocol details at OECD Test Guideline 431: 2013 (64). At the end of the exposure period, the test chemical is carefully washed from the epidermis surface with an aqueous buffer of 0.9% NaCl. Then the cell viability in RhE models is measured by the enzymatic conversion of the vital dye MTT [3-(4,5-Dimethylthiazol-2-yl)-2,5-diphenyltetrazolium bromide; Thiazolyl blue] into a blue formazan salt that is quantitatively measured after extraction from tissues. Cell viability values distinguishing corrosives from noncorrosives vary. EpiSkin™, Modified EpiDerm™, and SkinEthic™ test methods allow the subcategorization of corrosive substances into categories 1A, 1B, and 1C, in accordance with the UN GHS (70), but they are unable to distinguish between categories 1B and 1C (due to limited set of known category 1C chemicals) (64).

Irritation Testing

- *In vitro RhE test method*: Assessments of skin irritancy via RhE models are performed using basically the same test methods used to assess corrosivity but with different exposure protocols (64,71). Chemicals that lead to cell viability of ≤50% are considered irritants (for UN GHS

Category 2) (72), and those with cell viability >50% are considered nonirritants. Protocol details are available at OECD Test Guideline 439: 2013 (71).

Predictive In Vivo Testing

Acute Dermal Irritation/Corrosion Testing

The assessment of skin corrosivity involving laboratory animals was adopted in 1981 and revised in 1992 and 2002, OECD Test Guideline 404 (73). This method provides information on corrosive potentials of a liquid or solid. Preferred sequential testing strategy is to perform validated in vitro testing prior to this test. New substances are initially evaluated via in vitro testing. In vivo testing is used when data are insufficient on dermal corrosion/irritation potentials of existing substances.

The test is based on the evaluation of skin reactions to a single dose application of a test substance in an experimental animal. The degree of irritation/corrosion is scored at specified intervals for a complete evaluation of the effects. The duration of the study should be sufficient to evaluate the reversibility or irreversibility of the effects.

- *Initial test (in vivo dermal irritation/corrosion)*: In the in vivo dermal irritation/corrosion method, albino rabbit is the preferred animal. The fur of the dorsal area is removed by close clipping 24 hours prior to testing. The test substance is applied in a single dose to a small area of the skin (approximately 6 cm^2) of one animal and covered with a gauze patch and a nonirritating tape. The untreated skin areas serve as the control. Substances with a pH of less than 2.0 or more than 11.5 are suspected to be corrosive and should not be tested. The dose applied to the test site is 0.5 mL (liquid) or 0.5 g (solid), and covered with a gauze patch. The first patch is removed after 3 minutes. If no serious skin reaction is observed, a second patch will be placed on a different site for 1 hour. A third patch will be applied for 4 hours if the second patch is tolerated. After the removal of the third patch, the response is evaluated according to the grading in Table 23.3. Initial testing is done using one animal. The animals should be examined for signs of erythema and edema, immediately after patch removal, at 60 minutes and then at 24, 48, and 72 hours.

  If a corrosive effect is observed after any of the mentioned sequential exposures, the test is immediately terminated. The animal will be observed for 14 days.

TABLE 23.3

Grading of Dermal Responses (Draize Scale)

Erythema and Eschar Formation	
No erythema	0
Very slight erythema (barely perceptible)	1
Well-defined erythema	2
Moderate to severe erythema	3
Severe erythema (beef redness) to eschar formation	4
Edema Formation	
No edema	0
Very slight edema (barely perceptible)	1
Slight edema (edges of area well defined by definite raising)	2
Moderate edema (raised approximately 1 mm)	3
Severe edema (raised more than 1 mm and extending beyond area of exposure)	4

Source: OECD Test No. 404: Acute dermal irritation/corrosion, accessed August 4, 2016, retrieved from http://www.oecd-ilibrary.org/content/book/9789264070622-en; Patil, S. M., Patrick, E., and Maibach, H. I., Animal, human, and in vitro test methods for predicting skin irritation, in Marzulli, F. N., and Maibach, H. I., eds, *Dermatotoxicology Methods*, CRC Press, Boca Raton, Florida, 89–114, 1998.

Note: The primary irritation index (PII) is calculated by adding up the average of the erythema and edema values. PII < 2: mildly irritating; 2 < PII < 5: moderately irritating; PII > 5: severely irritating (require precautionary labeling).

- *Confirmatory test (in vivo dermal irritation)*: Confirmatory testing will be performed only in substances with no corrosive effect in initial testing. Two additional animals are tested, each with one patch of the test substance for 4 hours. The animals should be examined for signs of erythema and edema at 60 minutes, then at 24, 48, and 72 hours, and for 14 days. The substance is considered an irritant if inflammation persists by the end of this observation period. Additional animals may need to be used to clarify equivocal responses. Protocol details are available at OECD Test Guideline 404: 2002 (73).

The Draize Rabbit Skin Irritancy Test

The Draize rabbit skin, successfully used since the 1940s (74) and established as the basis for the methods mentioned earlier used in Test Guideline 404, involves the application of two semioccluded patches of an undiluted chemical to the shaved back of each animal (typically, three albino rabbits). Each material is tested on two 1 in. square sites on the same animal; one site is intact, and one is abraded in such a way that the SC is opened but no bleeding produced. Each test site is covered with two layers of 1 in. square surgical gauze secured in place with tape. Patches are removed 24 hours after the application, and the test sites are evaluated for erythema and edema using a prescribed scale with the degree of irritation scored for erythema (redness), eschar (scab formation), edema (swelling), and corrosive action at 24, 48, and 72 hours (Table 23.3) (62). Other animal assays assess cumulative irritation caused by some chemicals, which involve both exaggeration and repetition of exposures such as guinea pig immersion test or repeated patch test in a modified rabbit test (75). These tests are not required by regulatory agencies. However, in most instances, these methods have not gained widespread acceptance.

Currently, internationally accepted test methods for skin corrosion and irritation testing include the traditional in vivo animal test (based on Draize rabbit test) as well as in vitro test methods (discussed earlier). Animal testing for cosmetic products has been prohibited in Europe. Testing ban and marketing ban of cosmetic products, which were tested on animals, have been in effect since March 2013 (76).

Human Irritation Testing

Controlled studies with human volunteers have provided meaningful data, and their basic principles are discussed in the following. Predicative irritation assays in humans, using a small area of skin, can be done provided that systematic toxicity (from absorption) is low and informed consent is obtained. Although regulatory agencies do not routinely require testing in humans, human tests are sometimes preferred to animal tests. Test sites generally heal rapidly, within a week or so. More severe reactions should be periodically evaluated over a longer time to ensure resolution and determine inflammatory patterns. Some subjects may develop changes in pigmentation level at the test site following severe responses. Detailed consultation before consenting human subjects are extremely important.

Single-Application Irritation Patch Test

The single-application irritation patch test is used for the assessment of acute irritation potential and involves the application of 0.5 mL (0.5 g for solid test materials) on a 25 mm chamber (0.2 mL and 0.2 g have also been used) (77); solid test materials are moistened to the skin of human volunteers for up to 4 hours. New test materials may be applied for shorter periods (30 minutes to 1 hour), and if tolerated, the exposure time can progressively be increased to 4 hours. When testing new materials, the application of dilutions should be considered (78). Subjects should routinely be instructed to immediately remove patches if unusual discomfort occurs. Tested sites are assessed for the presence of irritation using a grading scale (Table 23.4) at 24, 48, and 72 hours after patch removal (77). Commercial patches, chambers, gauze squares, or cotton bandage material can be used, and patches are applied to either the upper back or the dorsal surface of the upper arm. Patches are secured with surgical tape without wrapping the trunk of the arm. For volatile materials, a relatively nonocclusive tape, such as Micropore® or Scanpore®, should be used (62). This test detects acute skin irritation hazard potential and should be

TABLE 23.4

Human Patch Test Grading Scales

Detailed Human Patch Test Grading Scale	
No apparent cutaneous involvement	0
Faint, barely perceptible erythema or slight dryness (glazed appearance)	½
Faint but definite erythema, no eruptions or broken skin *or* no erythema but definite dryness; may have epidermal fissuring	1
Well-defined erythema or faint erythema with definite dryness; may have epidural fissuring	1 ½
Moderate erythema, may have a *few* papules or deep fissures, moderate-to-severe erythema in the cracks	2
Moderate erythema with barely perceptible edema *or* severe erythema not involving a significant portion of the patch (halo effect around the edges); may have a few papules *or* moderate to severe erythema	2 ½
Severe erythema (beet red); may have generalized papules *or* moderate to severe erythema with slight edema (edges well defined by raising)	3
Moderate to severe erythema with moderate edema (confined to patch area) *or* moderate to severe erythema with isolated eschar formations or vesicles	3 ½
Generalized vesicles *or* eschar formation *or* moderate to severe erythema and/or edema extending beyond patch area	4
Simple Patch Test Grading Scale	
Negative, normal skin	0
Questionable erythema not covering entire area	±
Definite erythema	1
Erythema and induration	2
Vesiculation	3
Bullous reaction	4

Source: Hayes, B. B., Patrick, E., and Maibach, H. I., Dermatotoxicology, in Hayes, W., ed., *Principles and Methods of Toxicology*, fifth edition, CRC Press, Boca Raton, Florida, 1359, 2007; Patil, S. M., Patrick, E., and Maibach, H. I., Animal, human, and in vitro test methods for predicting skin irritation, in Marzulli, F. N., and Maibach, H. I., eds, *Dermatotoxicology Methods*, CRC Press, Boca Raton, Florida, 89–114, 1998.

used for hazard classification. It is not intended to predict other types of skin irritant dermatitis, such as cumulative irritant dermatitis (79).

Repeat-Application Cumulative Irritation Patch Test

The repeat-application cumulative irritation patch test assesses cumulative irritation. The early work of Marzulli and Maibach (75), Kligman and Wooding (80) and other investigators formed the basis of cumulative irritation assays (78,81). In the original assay, the test material was applied to a 25 mm² skin of the back via a saturated Webril™ or the skin surface was covered with a viscous material. Patches were removed after 24 hours, sites were evaluated, and a fresh set of patches were reapplied up to 21 days. Basic principles are similar to the single application, and many investigators have developed their version of it. Shorter study times have also been used in the evaluation of surfactants. Many investigators have developed their version (62,80). These methods do not always predict the safety of consumer products, which may be related to intrinsic differences in the reactivity of healthy skin versus damaged or sensitive skin (82).

Exaggerated Exposure Irritation Tests

Irritancy patch testing does not always correlate with the consumers' experience. Soaps are an example in which patch testing may overpredict the reaction in real life. Immersion testing and antecubital washing test, also known as *flex wash*, are examples of nonpatch irritancy techniques. Numerous versions of these tests have been used by investigators basically exposing the skin of consented human subjects to different concentrations of detergents for varied amounts of time; the end points are erythema and scaling (78,83,84).

Use of Bioengineering Devices

Multiple commercially available devices are used to measure the biophysical properties of skin. These measures provide objective data to be used in conjunction with the clinical evaluation of inflammatory responses (detailed discussion is in Chapter 1).

- TEWL measurments: TEWL reflects the integrity of the barrier function and can be determined by the use of evaporimeter (85).
- Laser Doppler velocimetry: Laser Doppler velocimetry has been used to quantify the increased blood flow to an inflamed tissue and can be used for the estimation of microcirculation (86).
- Squamometry: Squamometry is a noninvasive, protein-dependent, colorimetric evaluation of the SC and is a sensitive tool in the assessment of nonerythematous irritant dermatitis. An adhesive disk (D-SQUAME) is applied on the skin, and upon removal of the tape, superficial desquamating layer of the SC is harvested. Disks are subsequently stained, and the amount of dye found in the cells are quantified and scaled (87–89).

Phototoxicity

Phototoxicity (photoirritation) refers to tissue inflammation caused by the interaction of certain chemicals with light. Phototoxicity is a nonimmunological, dose-dependent phenomenon that happens when certain chemicals in the skin absorb light and create a pathological irritation. These chemicals may be applied topically or diffused into skin following systemic administration of a drug. The principle of photochemical activation (Grotthuss–Draper Law) states that light must be absorbed by a chromophore for a chemical reaction to happen. Therefore, the first step in the evaluation of the photosafety of a chemical is to have an absorption spectrum conducted. If a substance absorbs light within the range of UV and visible light (290–700 nm), reactive species can be generated, which can harm the tissue. Additional testing is required to assess the photosafety of a product that is intended for topical use or a systemic medication that diffuses to photoexposed skin (90). Validated testing methods for the assessment of phototoxic properties of chemicals are reviewed here.

General Considerations for Photoirritation Testing

Skin is optically heterogeneous, and via reflection, refraction, scattering, and absorption, it can modify the amount of radiation reaching deeper structures (91). These protective properties can be affected by the topical application of different products. Vehicles can decrease the amount of light reflected, scattered, or absorbed (92). They can also affect percutaneous absorption into the skin (92,93). Physical and chemical properties of vehicles can affect absorption, and photoproperties of applied medications, therefore testing of vehicles along with the medications is required by regulating agencies (94).

The approach to the initial evaluation of phototoxicological properties of a substance is summarized in Figure 23.1.

Predictive In Vitro Testing

Screening for UV and Visible Light Absorption

The initial assessment of the photosafety of substances starts by their ability to absorb UV/visible light (wavelengths between 290 and 700 nm). The ability of chemicals to absorb light is an intrinsic property of that specific chemical. To measure how strongly a chemical absorbs light in a given wavelength, molar extinction coefficient (MEC), also called *molar absorptivity*, is used. MEC is a constant for any given molecule under a specific set of conditions (e.g., solvent, temperature, wavelength) and reflects the efficiency with which a molecule can absorb a photon (typically expressed as liters $mol^{-1} \times cm^{-1}$) (95).

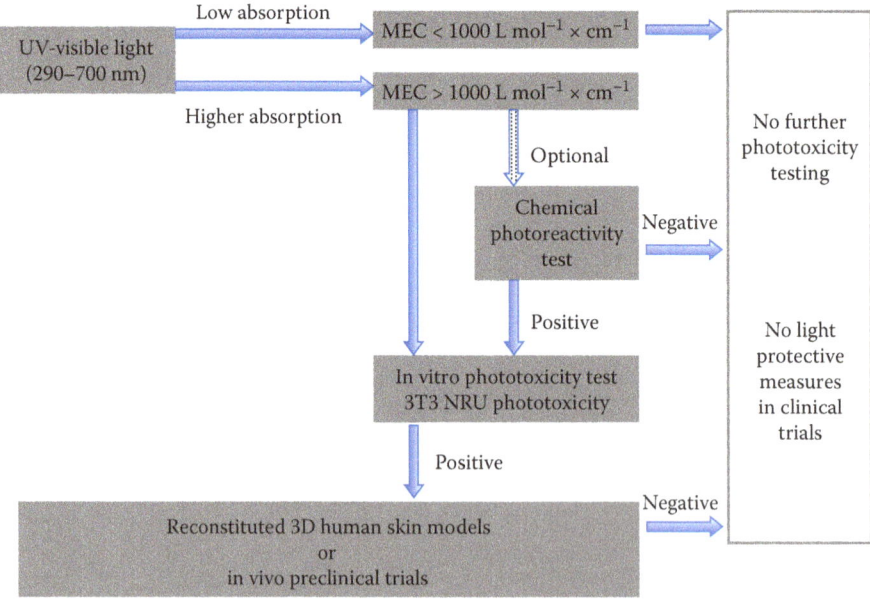

FIGURE 23.1 Outline of phototoxicity assessment strategies.

Photoreactivity Testing Using Chemical Assays

Phototoxicity refers to tissue inflammation caused by the interaction of light and a photoreactive chemical. A photoreactive chemical, at a sufficient tissue concentration, upon exposure to light can generate ROS, singlet oxygen, and/or superoxide. Therefore, ROS generation following visible light or UV exposure can indicate the potential phototoxicity of a chemical.

ROS assay is designed considering the principle mentioned earlier (44,49). This assay has high sensitivity and low specificity, creating many false positives; therefore, a positive result at any concentration would only point out the need for further assessment. On the other hand, the negative result on this assay, provided that the concentration of the test chemical is at least 200 μM, indicates a very low probability of phototoxicity and no further testing is required (94).

Phototoxicity Tests Using In Vitro Assays

1. *In vitro 3T3 NRU phototoxicity test (3T3-NRU-PT)*: In 3T3-NRU-PT, monolayer cell cultures of immortalized mouse fibroblast cell line Balb/c 3T3 are used to assess the cytotoxicity of a chemical in the presence or absence of a noncytotoxic dose of simulated solar light. Cytotoxicity is expressed as a concentration-dependent uptake of neutral red (NR) dye (3-amino-7-dimethylamino-2-methylphenazine hydrochloride) 24 hours after treatment with the test chemical and irradiation (90). NR is a weak cationic dye that penetrates cell membranes by nondiffusion and intracellularly accumulates in the lysosomes. In damaged cells, the alteration of the lysosomal membranes and their fragility by a phototoxic reaction lead to decreased uptake and binding of NR is considered one sequential process. On this bases, viable, damaged, or dead cells can be distinguished. The concentration of test materials resulting in 50% reduction in NR uptake (means that cell viability is reduced by 50%) is called IC_{50} and is used to evaluate results.

   The protocol follows the following steps (full details are available on Test Guideline 432: 2004) (90).

   • A permanent mouse fibroblast cell line, Balb/c 3T3, is used.
   • To test one chemical, two sets of 96-well plates will be seeded with 1×10^4 cells per well and incubated for 24 hours (37°C; 5% CO_2 in air). Both sets will go through the entire test

procedure under identical conditions except that one plate is irradiated and one plate is kept in the dark.

- On the second day, the test chemicals are added to wells. The test chemicals are dissolved in a physiologically buffered solution, free of protein and light-absorbing components. Dilution series will be added to wells.

- The highest concentration should be physiological, not exceeding 1000 µg/mL, and osmolality should not exceed 10 mM. A geometric dilution series of eight test substance concentrations including a negative control or solvent are added to the wells for 1 hour (37°C; 5% CO_2 in air). A known phototoxic chemical (Chlorpromazine) is added to each well as a positive control.

- One set of the wells is exposed to 5 J/cm^2 in the UVA range for 50 minutes, while the other set is kept in dark.

- All wells are subsequently rinsed with phosphate-buffered saline and incubated in a culture medium over night (37°C; 5% CO_2 in air).

- On the third day, the NR in the medium is added to each well (100 µL of 50 µg/mL solution) for 3 hours.

- The wells are subsequently washed, and the optical density of the NR extract at 540 nm is measured in a spectrophotometer.

- Data will be evaluated by calculating a photo irritation factor (PIF) or mean photo effect.

- The interpretation of data is based on the values mentioned earlier as well as comparison of results between photo-exposed and photo-protected sets.

The PIF is calculated based on the results of the NR uptake by comparing the IC_{50} with and without irradiation (PIF = IC_{50} without irradiation/IC_{50} with irradiation). MPE may also be calculated for the interpretation of results (90,96).

This test does not assess the phototoxic potency of a chemical and is not designed to evaluate the photogenotoxicity, photoallergy, or photocarcinogenicity of a substance.

The 3T3-NRU-PT assay-gained regulatory acceptance in all EU Member States in 2000 and in the OECD Member States in 2004 as Test Guideline 432. Based on the original OECD test guidelines (Test Guidelines 432: 2004) (90), chemicals with MEC of 10 L mol^{-1} × cm^{-1} were considered unlikely to be photoreactive and additional phototoxicity testing was not required for such products. Later on, the threshold was increased to 1000 L mol^{-1} × cm^{-1} (94,97). In the Step 4 version of the International Committee on Harmonization Expert Working Group in 2013, a reduction of the maximum test concentration from 1000 to 100 µg/mL is suggested (98). Further in vitro testing is required for substances with higher MEC.

Test Guideline 432 is widely used in the chemical and cosmetics industries and is considered a reliable predictive of acute phototoxicity effects in animals and humans in vivo (90).

Disadvantages of this assay include the following:

- Only substances soluble in water can be tested.

- In vivo and in vitro results do not always correlate since bioavailability and biokinetics cannot be modeled.

- This assay can only use irradiation in the UVA and visible range; UVB wavelengths are excluded considering their cytotoxicity to Balb/c 3T3 cells. Considering that the majority of phototoxic reactions involve UVA, this limitation is accepted.

2. *Reconstituted 3D human skin models*: RhE models are 3D biostructures composed of cultured NHKs, which form a multilayered epidermis including the SC. Assessments of skin phototoxicity via RhE models are based on the premise that a phototoxic chemical after exposure to light will damage cells and can be identified by their ability to lower cell viability. Then cell viability in RhE models is measured by the enzymatic conversion of the vital dye MTT [3-(4,5-dimethylthiazol-2-yl)-2,5-diphenyltetrazolium bromide; thiazolyl blue], into a blue formazan salt that is quantitatively measured after extraction from tissues. Few 3D models have been

used for in vitro phototoxicity testing including EpiDerm, EpiSkin, and SkinEthic (99). EpiDerm underwent prevalidation studies founded by the ECVAM in 1999 and was found to generate good results. However, these models are costly, not appropriate for screening, and may not be able to accurately predict safe, nonphototoxic concentrations of tested materials (100–102).

A recommended protocol is outlined here (102):

- 3D RhE models are used in 6 well plates; two sets of wells.
- Test material, positive or negative control, is applied directly on the tissue surface of the cultured tissue and incubated overnight (20 µL of the test material or an adjusted dose based on the properties of the test material).
- On the second day, the test material is rinsed off using buffered saline solution and one set of wells is irradiated using UVA solar simulator for 60 minutes, delivering a total of 6 J/cm^2.
- After irradiation, the tissues are rinsed with saline and incubated again overnight in a fresh medium.
- On the third day, the cultures are transferred to 24 well plates containing 0.3 mL of MTT (1 mg/mL solution) and incubated for 3 hours.
- Subsequently, tissues are rinsed and transferred to an isopropanol solution. Isopropanol helps extract the formazan from the tissues leading to the deep blue/purple color.
- Extracts are transferred to 96 well plates, and absorption at 570 nm is measured in a spectrophotometer.
- Results are calculated based on the percentage of MTT reduction compared to control-treated cultures.
- Phototoxic potential is predicted by >30% increase in cell toxicity in photoexposed cultured tissues.

These models have a structure similar to in vivo epidermis and contain both viable primary skin cells and skin barrier. The variety of chemicals, including complex mixtures, can be tested on 3D skin models. The barrier function of the SC can lead to more relevant results and less false-positive reactions compared to highly sensitive monolayer cells. The higher concentration of tested materials (compared to monolayer cells) can be used; therefore, it is more relevant to in vivo usage (102). Despite the advantages of 3D models over the monolayer cells used in 3T3-NRU-PT models, these models are more permeable compared to human skin and lack the dermal component.

Predictive In Vivo Testing

In vivo testing has been carried out in multiple lab animals, including rabbits, mice, guinea pigs, and swine. However, animal tests may create results not correlating to human testing. Maibach et al. (103) as well as Kaidbey and Kligman (104) proposed human phototoxicity testing. Human testing with the approval of institutional review boards and after obtaining informed consent can be performed. Since theoretically almost any individual can develop phototoxic reaction, given sufficient exposure, these tests can be conclusive in a small number of volunteers. These reactions usually resolve quickly after the removal of stimuli (105).

Phototoxicity testing in humans:

- Ten consented healthy adults are enrolled.
- Two sets of test products and relevant controls (typically the vehicle) are applied on each side of the back skin, under occlusion for 6 hours. Commercially available patch test chambers about 12 mm in diameter are used. Additional control is done by the application of one empty chamber on each side.
- Patches are removed after 6 hours, and only one side is radiated with UVA 20 J/cm^2. A solar simulator or a xenon arc lamp can be used as a source of radiation. Appropriate filtration with a Schott WG 345 filter blocks the erythemogenic UVC and UVB ranges. Longer wavelengths

such as visible light and infrared are filtered using coated dichromic mirror, water filter, and UG11 filters.

- Skin assessment is done immediately after radiation and at 24- and 48-hour intervals. Reactions are graded and compared between radiated and unradiated sides. Reactions are graded from 0 to 5 (0 = no reaction, 1 = mild erythema ± scaling, 2 = moderate to strong erythema, 3 = moderate to strong erythema with a papular response, 4 = 3 + edema, 5 = vesicular eruption).

Reactions that are more prominent on the irradiated side indicate phototoxicity, while reactions that are equal on both sides refer to a nonphototoxic irritation (105).

Contact Urticaria

Contact urticaria syndrome is a group of heterogeneous inflammatory reactions, happening within minutes after exposure to the offending agent. Underlying mechanisms are mainly immunological or nonimmunological; however, certain chemicals such as ammonium persulfate, parabens, and ethylene diamine induce contact urticaria via unknown mechanisms (106–108). Immunological and nonimmunological contact urticarias have been studied using multiple in vivo models, but no predictive testing method has been established. The testing methods are limited to in vivo models. The majority of animal tests have investigated mechanistic aspects of nonimmunological contact urticaria, rather than establishing predictive models. Test models established in the assessment of nonimmunological and immunological contact urticarial are reviewed.

Pathogenesis of Nonimmunological Contact Urticaria

Nonimmunological contact urticaria (NICU) occurs in the absence of prior sensitization to a substance. Reactions typically remain localized to the area of contact and may present as sensory reactions such as stinging, burning, or itching to transient erythema or typical hives. The underlying mechanisms are not fully understood, but reactions are possibly caused by the release of inflammatory mediators induced by the causative agent. The causative agents via the release of inflammatory mediators can either directly or indirectly affect flow and or permeability of dermal vessels creating some of the clinical reactions. Multiple mediators and pathways are proposed and studied, including prostaglandins, histamine, mast cell activation, and neurogenic inflammation, yet much remains unknown about pathogenesis (107,109,110).

The intensity of NICU varies with the concentration of the offending agent, and is also affected by properties affecting skin penetration including site of exposure (111–114).

Benzoic acid, cinnamic acid, cinnamic aldehyde, methyl nicotinate, or dimethyl sulfoxide are well-known urticants. Antihistamines do not inhibit immediate reactions to these substances, indicating that histamine is not a key mediator (115,116). However, topical application of nonsteroidal anti-inflammatory gels significantly reduced erythema or edema induced by theses urticants, suggesting that NICU is partially or extensively mediated by prostaglandins (117). The role of sensory nerves and UV light and the molecular structure of urticants have also been studied in the development of NICU (118–121). Cinnamal is a major component of Myroxylon pereirae resin; both can cause nonimmunological immediate contact reactions (122). An almost equal rate of immediate reaction to fragrance mix and Myroxylon pereirae in patients with either negative or positive patch test to these substances is reported, suggesting entirely separate mechanisms involved in immediate and delayed reactions (123).

Animal Test Models for Nonimmunological Contact Urticaria

Animal test methods are being used to identify urticogenic agents and at times to investigate the pathogenesis. The guinea pig ear swelling test is the best animal test available for screening NICU (124,125). The guinea pig ear lobe resembles human skin in many respects, including the morphology and timing of the reactions. Concentrations of the eliciting substances also correlate with concentrations affecting human skin.

Protocol involves the baseline measurement of ear thickness with a micrometer immediately prior to open topical application of the test material followed by subsequent measurements at short periods of up to 1–2 hours. A positive reaction in the guinea pig ear lobe comprises erythema and edema. The quantification of the edema by measuring the change in ear thickness is an accurate, quick, and reproducible method. The maximal response is 100% increase in ear thickness, and it appears 40–50 minutes after the application, depending on the vehicle (121,124).

The tachyphylaxis phenomenon is a decrease in reactivity to a nonimmunological urticant after reapplication the following days. The length of the refractory period is about 4 days for methyl nicotinate, 8 days for diethyl fumarate and cinnamic aldehyde, and 16 days for benzoic acid, cinnamic acid, and dimethylsulfoxide (126).

Human Test Models for Nonimmunological Contact Urticaria

The transient nature of NICU and its minor effects make human testing a reasonable option.

1. *Open application test*: Test substances are typically applied on the skin of the upper back, extensor upper arm, or forearm.
    a. Testing one substance at a time: 0.1 mL of the test substance is spread on a 3 × 3 cm area of the skin.
    b. Testing more than one substance at the same time: 0.01 mL of the test substance is applied on 1 × 1 cm area of the skin.

    There are marked differences between skin sites in the reactivity to the putative urticogenic agents. Petrolatum and water are the most commonly used vehicles (127), but alcohol vehicles and added propylene glycol may enhance test sensitivity (128,129). The test sites are evaluated at 20, 40, and 60 minutes in order to see the maximal response. In visual grading, scores for the erythema and edema components of the reaction (+ weak, ++ moderate, +++ strong) have been used (110,129), but objective measurements are preferred (130). Colorimetric, spectrophotometric measurements, and laser Doppler flowmetry can be used to assess erythema and blood flow. The test is usually performed on healthy appearing skin, but when used as a diagnostic test, it may be useful to test suspected agents on previously affected skin areas or slightly irritated skin. Repeated open tests on the same test site may be needed to detect weak immediate irritant reactions (131).

2. *Chamber test*: In a chamber test, substances are applied in small aluminum chambers (Finn chamber, Epitest, Hyrylä, Finland) and fixed to the skin with porous acrylic tape similar to methods used for routine patch testing for contact allergy. The occlusion time is 15 minutes, and the test is read at 20, 40, and 60 minutes. The occlusion enhances percutaneous penetration and may increase the sensitivity of the test. An advantage of the chamber test is that a smaller skin area is needed than in the open test (132).

    Practical issues to consider in testing for NICU:
    a. Concentration of an agent may be difficult to define; hence, dilution series are recommended. They make it possible to determine the threshold irritant concentration for that particular patient and skin area.
    b. It is critical that a suitable panel of control subjects is tested to assess specificity of the diagnostic test.
    c. Oral and topical nonsteroidal anti-inflammatories may lead to false-negative results that can last up to 3 days (117,133,134).
    d. Tanned skin may also cause false-negative reactions, which can last up to 2–3 weeks (119,135).

Pathogenesis of Immunological Contact Urticaria

Immunological contact urticaria (ICU) is far less common than NICU and requires presensitization. It is typically a type-1 hypersensitivity reaction requiring immunoglobulin E (Ige)-mediated response to a substance, most commonly a protein or a protein–hapten complex. These IgE antibodies react with IgE receptors on mast cells, eosinophils, basophils, and LCs among other cell types. Upon penetration of an allergen to skin and interaction with IgE complexes, the degranulation of the involved cells occurs and multiple mediators such as histamine, proteases, proteoglycans, and exoglycosidases are released from cells, leading to wheal and flare response. Additionally, the synthesis of leukotrienes, prostaglandins, and platelet-activating factors also occurs as a result of the IgE–allergen interaction and leads to vascular permeability. Extracutaneous and anaphylactoid reactions may happen in the case of massive release of these mediators in highly sensitized individuals (136). Long-standing antigen exposures as well as interactions of IgE with LCs can mediate eczematous reactions. LCs present antigens to type 2 T helper cells and induce a delayed type hypersensitivity reaction (137). Individuals with AD are at a higher risk of developing ICU (138,139). Compared to NICU, ICU more commonly occurs on damaged skin (140). More details on the pathogenesis of ICU and reactions with mixed or unknown mechanisms are available earlier in this chapter.

Animal Test Models for Immunological Contact Urticaria

Predictive models for ICU are less developed compared to NICU. Animal models have been more focused on pathogenesis rather than prediction. The guinea pig can be sensitized to a variety of chemicals that have been reported as ICU and proteins. The sensitization process and techniques vary when evaluating the chemicals potential in skin sensitization tests, such as the guinea pig maximization test or examining the relative ability of proteins to behave as potential respiratory allergens (24,141,142). In all these procedures, once animals have been sensitized, intradermal challenges can be used to elicit an immediate hypersensitivity response in the skin. Increased vascular permeability can be visualized in the test animals if the Evans Blue dye is injected prior to the challenge. The reaction can be assessed in 20 minutes following the intradermal injection by measuring the diameter and intensity of blueness. It is not certain whether these data would predict ICU in humans.

Mouse has been proposed as a possible model of chemically induced ICU. On the basis of the work with trimellitic anhydride (a chemical capable of causing both immediate and delayed types of hypersensitivity), an approach that involves the topical application of the test chemical to Balb/c strain mice, followed by epicutaneous challenge on the ear, after 1 week, has been suggested (39). Measuring the amount of ear swelling over a 2-hour course assesses urticarial reactions (112,143). These tests have low specificity and do not provide reliable predictive information.

Human Testing for Immunological Contact Urticaria

Human testing is only done for diagnostic purposes in clinical situations. The main methods involve skin testing with the suspected substance and serological assays for specific IgE antibodies. While simple open application of a putative allergen may be sufficient, the closed patch test or skin prick test (SPT) may be necessary to elicit a reaction. In cases where a chemical hapten is the putative allergen, it is necessary to conjugate it to a protein prior to testing. Commonly, the protein selected is HSA. Guidelines on the preparation of suitable hapten–protein conjugates are available (144).

In patients with clinical history of severe skin reactions, testing with serial dilutions of the putative allergen should be performed. Serologic tests are helpful diagnostic tools in patients with a history of anaphylactic-type reactions. IgE testing has been conducted using the radioallergosorbent test, originally described over 30 years ago, and is a valuable tool in identification of many immunological urticants (145).

Skin Tests for Immediate Hypersensitivity Reactions

1. *SPT*: SPT is the standard method for detecting clinically significant IgE-mediated allergy. Numerous allergens are commercially available. Test materials can also be made on an individual basis if not available commercially. Testing is done typically on the skin of the back or arm. Drops (5–10 nL) of the test material are placed 3–5 cm apart and pricked with a special prick test lancet. Histamine dihydrochloride, 10 mg/mL, and the base solution serve as positive

and negative controls. After puncturing the skin, drops are removed using a soft tissue. The results are read after 15–20 minutes by measuring the size of the wheal produced around the piercing. The longest diameter and the diameter perpendicular to it are measured. Positive results are those that are at least 3 mm, or half the size of the wheal created by histamine. Erythema without edema is not considered positive and is not clinically relevant. When testing with nonstandard materials, it is important to test healthy controls to differentiate irritative from immunological reactions. Prick by prick is a modification of SPT, in which the tested material, usually fresh foodstuff, is pricked and the skin is immediately pricked using the same lancet. Prick by prick test carries a potential risk of infection particularly if fresh meat, poultry, fish, etc., are tested (146,147).

2. *Intradermal test*: Intradermal tests are used in the clinical assessment of patients with suspected allergies and negative SPT. The test is technically more involved compared to SPT, and its use is limited. A sterile solution of diluted allergen (50–100 μL) is injected intradermally, using a 25-gauge needle. Intradermal injections of histamine (50–100 μL) and normal saline serve as positive and negative controls. The correct way to inject the allergens would create a small papule. The injection sites will be evaluated within 20–30 minutes, and while a standard reading method is lacking, a wheal-and-flare reaction is considered positive if the largest diameter of the wheal is at least twice the diameter of the initial papule created by the injection (148).

3. *Scratch test*: The scratch test can be used when standard allergens are not available. In this method, superficial scratches about 5 mm long are made on the skin of the back or arm, using a blood lancet or a venipuncture needle. Scratches should not lead to bleeding, and the lancet is not puncturing the skin; hence, there is less potential risk of infection and/or unwanted reactions compared to SPT when testing food items such as meat, fruits, vegetables, flours, and spices. Allergens are applied for 5–10 minutes on the scratch sites, which are 3–5 cm apart, then wiped with a soft tissue. Fresh food is applied as is, and dry allergens are mixed with normal saline. Most allergens triggering immediate responses are water soluble (149). Histamine dihydrochloride, 10 mg/mL, and the base solution serve as positive and negative controls. Results are read 15–20 minutes after application. Similar to SPT, only the reactions with erythema and edema are considered for reading, and the longest diameter perpendicular to the scratch is measured and compared to histamine reactions. Reactions equal to or greater than that from histamine are considered positive and clinically relevant. It is difficult to distinguish nonimmunological and immunological reactions based on this method, and results should be interpreted with caution. The scratch-chamber test is a modification of scratch test when the scratched skin is covered with the allergen and an 8 or 12 mm Finn chamber. The remainder of the test method and reading results is similar to the scratch test (150).

4. *Chamber test*: Test materials are placed into a Finn chamber, and if dry, they are moistened with normal saline and applied on the intact skin of the back or arm. The chambers are left in place for 15 minutes, and then, the readings are done at short intervals up to 60 minutes. A wheal-and-flare reaction is regarded as positive, and erythema without edema is unlikely to be positive.

5. *Open application test*: The open application test can be used in the evaluation of ICU or NICU. Although a standardized procedure is lacking, a proposed procedure is discussed earlier in the evaluation of NICU. This test can be used when there is high clinical suspicion, and careful approach is taken to avoid systemic reactions. The rub test is a modified open application test, in which the test substance is gently rubbed on the intact healthy skin or on slightly affected skin.

6. *Skin application food test* (SAFT): In SAFT, the direct penetration of the allergen into skin is avoided. A solid piece of food or 0.8 mL of a liquid food is placed on a 4 cm^2 gauze and taped to the skin of the back for 10–30 minutes. The test can also be performed using patch test Finn chambers. Reactions are scored as +, erythema; ++, erythema and edema; and +++, erythema and edema within the area of chamber or beyond application site; only 3+ reactions are considered positive (151).

To date, no reliable method is established to predict potential immunological or nonimmunological urticants. Testing methods for immediate contact reactions are mostly used in clinical settings. Further understanding of mechanisms involved in the pathogenesis of contact urticaria syndrome is critical for the development of reliable predictive tests.

Conclusion

SSS is a condition clinically diagnosed based on symptoms and history. A step-by-step evaluation of potential concomitant dermatoses is critical in the evaluation of these patients. While there are no specific dermatotoxicologic test methods available for sensitive skin, all the conditions mentioned earlier and other inflammatory dermatoses such as rosacea, acne, and connective tissue disease need to be considered and ruled out.

REFERENCES

1. Misery L, Loser K, Stander S. Sensitive skin. *J Eur Acad Dermatol Venereol.* 2016;30 Suppl 1:2–8.
2. Saint-Mezard P, Krasteva M, Chavagnac C et al. Afferent and efferent phases of allergic contact dermatitis (ACD) can be induced after a single skin contact with haptens: Evidence using a mouse model of primary ACD. *J Invest Dermatol.* 2003;120(4):641–647.
3. Bos JD, Meinardi MM. The 500 dalton rule for the skin penetration of chemical compounds and drugs. *Exp Dermatol.* 2000;9(3):165–169.
4. Gerberick F, Aleksic M, Basketter D et al. Chemical reactivity measurement and the predicitve identification of skin sensitisers: The report and recommendations of ECVAM workshop 64. *Altern Lab Anim.* 2008;36(2):215–242.
5. Mutschler J, Gimenez-Arnau E, Foertsch L et al. Mechanistic assessment of peptide reactivity assay to predict skin allergens with kathon CG isothiazolinones. *Toxicol In Vitro.* 2009;23(3):439–446.
6. Rustemeyer T, van Hoogstraten IM, von Blomberg ME et al. Mechanisms of allergic contact dermatitis. In: Rustemeyer T, Elsner P, John SM, Maibach HI, eds. *Kanerva's Occupational Dermatology.* Second ed. Berlin; New York: Springer; 2012:113–146.
7. Iversen L, Johansen C. Inflammasomes and inflammatory caspases in skin inflammation. *Expert Rev Mol Diagn.* 2008;8(6):697–705.
8. Hoyer KK, Dooms H, Barron L et al. Interleukin-2 in the development and control of inflammatory disease. *Immunol Rev.* 2008;226:19–28.
9. Commission of the European Communities. Timetables for the phasing-out of animal testing in the framework of the 7th amendment to the cosmetics directive (Council directive 76/768/EEC). Accessed August 1, 2016. Retrieved from http://ec.europa.eu/consumers/sectors/cosmetics/files/doc/antest/sec _2004_1210_en.pdf.
10. Basketter D, Alepee N, Casati S et al. Skin sensitisation—Moving forward with non-animal testing strategies for regulatory purposes in the EU. *Regul Toxicol Pharmacol.* 2013;67(3):531–535.
11. Basketter DA. Skin immunology and sensitisation. In: Chilcott RP, Price S, eds. *Principles and Practice of Skin Toxicology.* Singapore: John Wiley & Sons Inc; 2008:151–168.
12. Adler S, Basketter D, Creton S et al. Alternative (non-animal) methods for cosmetics testing: Current status and future prospects—2010. *Arch Toxicol.* 2011;85(5):367–485.
13. Casati S, Worth A, Amcoff P, Whelan M. EURL ECVAM strategy for replacement of animal testing for skin sensitisation hazard identification and classification. *Joint Research Centre—Institute for Health and Consumer Protection* [EUR 25816]. 2013;2014(3/12).
14. OECD in chemico skin sensitisation: Direct peptide reactivity assay (DPRA). Accessed August 4, 2016. Retrieved from http://www.oecd.org/chemicalsafety/testing/Draft_DPRA_TG_final_15May 2014.pdf.
15. Gerberick GF, Vassallo JD, Bailey RE, Chaney JG, Morrall SW, Lepoittevin JP. Development of a peptide reactivity assay for screening contact allergens. *Toxicol Sci.* 2004;81(2):332–343.
16. Gerberick GF, Vassallo JD, Foertsch LM et al. Quantification of chemical peptide reactivity for screening contact allergens: A classification tree model approach. *Toxicol Sci.* 2007;97(2):417–427.

17. EURL ECVAM November 2013. Direct peptide reactivity assay (DPRA) for skin sensitisation testing. August 1, 2016. Retrieved from http://ihcp.jrc.ec.europa.eu/our_labs/eurl-ecvam/eurl-ecvam-recommendations /files-dpra/EURL_ECVAM_Recommendation_DPRA_2013.pdf.

18. OECD. In vitro skin sensitization: Direct peptide reactivity assay (DPRA). August 1, 2016. Retrieved from http://www.oecd.org/env/ehs/testing/OECD_draft%20TG_DPRA_13Nov2013.pdf.

19. EURL ECVAM February 2014. Recommendations on KeratinoSens™ assay for skin sensitisation testing. August 1, 2016. Retrieved from http://ihcp.jrc.ec.europa.eu/our_labs/eurl-ecvam/eurl-ecvam-recommendations /file-kerati/JRC_SPR_Keratinosens_Rec_17_02_2014.pdf.

20. OECD. In vitro skin sensitization: Keratinocyte-based ARE-Nrf2 luciferase reporter gene test method— Draft proposal for new test guidelines. August 1, 2016. Retrieved from http://www.oecd.org/env/ehs /testing/OECD_DraftTG_Keratinosens_11Nov2013%20(2).pdf.

21. Natsch A, Ryan CA, Foertsch L et al. A dataset on 145 chemicals tested in alternative assays for skin sensitization undergoing prevalidation. *J Appl Toxicol.* 2013;33(11):1337–1352.

22. Nukada Y, Ashikaga T, Miyazawa M et al. Prediction of skin sensitization potency of chemicals by human cell line activation test (h-CLAT) and an attempt at classifying skin sensitization potency. *Toxicol In Vitro.* 2012;26(7):1150–1160.

23. Buehler EV. Delayed contact hypersensitivity in the guinea pig. *Arch Dermatol.* 1965;91:171–177.

24. Magnusson B, Kligman AM. The identification of contact allergens by animal assay: The guinea pig maximization test. *J Invest Dermatol.* 1969;52(3):268–276.

25. Andersen KE, Maibach HI. Guinea pig sensitization assays: An overview. *Curr Probl Dermatol.* 1985;14:263–290.

26. OECD 406–1992. OECD guidelines for testing of chemicals—Skin sensitization. August 1, 2016. Retrieved from http://www.oecd-ilibrary.org/docserver/download/9740601e.pdf?expires=1399005722 &id=id&accname=guest&checksum=027E7128FE5A93D1A13C55AEE77CA663.

27. Kimber I, Basketter DA. The murine local lymph node assay: A commentary on collaborative studies and new directions. *Food Chem Toxicol.* 1992;30(2):165–169.

28. OECD Test No. 429:2010. Skin sensitization: Local lymph node assay. August 1, 2016. Retrieved from http://www.oecd-ilibrary.org/docserver/download/9742901e.pdf?expires=1399005906&id=id&accname =guest&checksum=BB7913F89FDD9557CF6B48F7CC797929.

29. OECD Test No. 442A–2010. Skin sensitization: Local lymph node assay: DA. August 1, 2016. Retrieved from http://www.oecd-ilibrary.org/environment/test-no-442a-skin-sensitization_9789264090972-en ;jsessionid=2fn99d9jfq3qk.x-oecd-live-01.

30. OECD Test No. 442B–2010. Skin sensitization: Local lymph node assay: BrdU-ELISA. August 1, 2016. Retrieved from http://www.oecd-ilibrary.org/docserver/download/9744211e.pdf?expires=1399006436 &id=id&accname=guest&checksum=0FDBA3F39C7D0628DCA57BFCA8763844.

31. Gerberick GF, Ryan CA, Kern PS et al. Compilation of historical local lymph node data for evaluation of skin sensitization alternative methods. *Dermatitis.* 2005;16(4):157–202.

32. Kern PS, Gerberick GF, Ryan CA et al. Local lymph node data for the evaluation of skin sensitization alternatives: A second compilation. *Dermatitis.* 2010;21(1):8–32.

33. Basketter DA, Gerberick GF, Kimber I. The local lymph node assay in 2014. *Dermatitis.* 2014; 25(2):49–50.

34. Wilkinson DS. Photodermatitis due to tetrachlorsalicylanilide. *Br J Dermatol.* 1961;73:213–219.

35. Wilkinson DS. Two cases of photodermatitis due to tetrachlorsalicylanilide (TCSA). *Proc R Soc Med.* 1961;54:817–818.

36. Wells GC, Harman RR. Two cases of photodermatitis due to tetrachlorsalicylanilide. *Proc R Soc Med.* 1961;54:819.

37. Calnan CD. Photodermatitis due to tetrachlorsalicylanilide. *Proc R Soc Med.* 1961;54:819–820.

38. Moser J, Hye A, Lovell WW et al. Mechanisms of drug photobinding to proteins: Photobinding of suprofen to human serum albumin. *Toxicol In Vitro.* 2001;15(4–5):333–337.

39. Lovell WW. A scheme for in vitro screening of substances for photoallergenic potential. *Toxicol In Vitro.* 1993;7(1):95–102.

40. Tokura Y. Immune responses to photohaptens: Implications for the mechanisms of photosensitivity to exogenous agents. *J Dermatol Sci.* 2000;23 Suppl 1:S6–9.

41. Barratt MD, Brown KR. Photochemical binding of photoallergens to human serum albumin: A simple in vitro method for screening potential photoallergens. *Toxicol Lett.* 1985;24(1):1–6.

42. Pendlington RU, Barratt MD. Photochemical binding of photoallergens to human serum albumin: A simple in vitro method for screening potential photoallergens. *Toxicol In Vitro.* 1990;4(4–5):307–310.

43. Lovell WW, Jones PA. Evaluation of mechanistic in vitro tests for the discrimination of photoallergic and photoirritant potential. *Altern Lab Anim.* 2000;28(5):707–724.

44. Onoue S, Hosoi K, Wakuri S et al. Establishment and intra-/inter-laboratory validation of a standard protocol of reactive oxygen species assay for chemical photosafety evaluation. *J Appl Toxicol.* 2013;33(11):1241–1250.

45. Johnson BE, Walker EM, Hetherington AM. In vitro models for cutaneous phototoxicity. In: Marks R, Plewig G, eds. *Skin Models.* Berlin Heidelberg: Springer-Verlag; 1986:264–281.

46. Neumann NJ, Blotz A, Wasinska-Kempka G et al. Evaluation of phototoxic and photoallergic potentials of 13 compounds by different in vitro and in vivo methods. *J Photochem Photobiol B.* 2005;79(1):25–34.

47. Kurita M, Shimauchi T, Kobayashi M et al. Induction of keratinocyte apoptosis by photosensitizing chemicals plus UVA. *J Dermatol Sci.* 2007;45(2):105–112.

48. Onoue S, Tsuda Y. Analytical studies on the prediction of photosensitive/phototoxic potential of pharmaceutical substances. *Pharm Res.* 2006;23(1):156–164.

49. Onoue S, Kawamura K, Igarashi N et al. Reactive oxygen species assay-based risk assessment of drug-induced phototoxicity: Classification criteria and application to drug candidates. *J Pharm Biomed Anal.* 2008;47(4–5):967–972.

50. Onoue S, Hosoi K, Wakuri S et al. Establishment and intra-/inter-laboratory validation of a standard protocol of reactive oxygen species assay for chemical photosafety evaluation. *J Appl Toxicol.* 2013;33(11):1241–1250.

51. Hoya M, Hirota M, Suzuki M et al. Development of an in vitro photosensitization assay using human monocyte-derived cells. *Toxicol In Vitro.* 2009;23(5):911–918.

52. Karschuk N, Tepe Y, Gerlach S et al. A novel in vitro method for the detection and characterization of photosensitizers. *PLoS One.* 2010;5(12):e15221.

53. Galbiati V, Bianchi S, Martinez V et al. NCTC 2544 and IL-18 production: A tool for the in vitro identification of photoallergens. *Toxicol In Vitro.* 2014;28(1):13–17.

54. Harber LC, Targovnik SE, Baer RL. Studies on contact photosensitivity to hexachlorophene and trichlorocarbanilide in guinea pigs and man. *J Invest Dermatol.* 1968;51(5):373–377.

55. Gerberick GF, Ryan CA. Contact photoallergy testing of sunscreens in guinea pigs. *Contact Dermat.* 1989;20(4):251–259.

56. Kaidbey KH, Kligman AM. Photomaximization test for identifying photoallergic contact sensitizers. *Contact Dermat.* 1980;6(3):161–169.

57. Kligman AM. The identification of contact allergens by human assay: III. The maximization test: A procedure for screening and rating contact sensitizers. *J Invest Dermatol.* 1966;47(5):393–409.

58. Malten KE, den Arend JA. Irritant contact dermatitis: Traumiterative and cumulative impairment by cosmetics, climate, and other daily loads. *Derm Beruf Umwelt.* 1985;33(4):125–132.

59. Chew A, Maibach HI. Ten genotypes of irritant contact dermatitis. In: Chew A, Maibach HI, eds. *Irritant Dermatitis.* Berlin: Springer; 2006:5.

60. Moser K, Kriwet K, Naik A et al. Passive skin penetration enhancement and its quantification in vitro. *Eur J Pharm Biopharm.* 2001;52(2):103–112.

61. Elias PM. The epidermal permeability barrier: From the early days at Harvard to emerging concepts. *J Invest Dermatol.* 2004;122(2):xxxvi–xxxix.

62. Hayes BB, Patrick E, Maibach HI. Dermatotoxicology. In: Hayes W, ed. *Principles and Methods of Toxicology.* Fifth ed. Boca Raton, FL: CRC Press; 2007:1359.

63. OSHA. A guide to the globally harmonized system of classification and labelling of chemicals (GHS). Accessed August 4, 2016. Retrieved from https://www.osha.gov/dsg/hazcom/ghsguideoct05.pdf.

64. OECD 431–2013. In vitro skin corrosion: Reconstructed human epidermis (RHE) test method. Accessed August 1, 2016. Retrieved from http://www.oecd.org/env/ehs/testing/Draft_Revised_TG%20 431_Clean_22_Oct_2013.pdf.

65. OECD 430–2004. In vitro skin corrosion: Transcutaneous electrical resistance test (TER): OECD guidelines for the testing of chemicals, section 4. Paris: OECD Publishing. Accessed August 1, 2016. Retrieved from http://www.oecd-ilibrary.org/content/book/9789264071124-en.

66. OECD 435–2006. OECD guideline for the testing of chemicals: In vitro membrane barrier test method for skin corrosion—435. Accessed August 1, 2016. Retrieved http://www.oecd-ilibrary.org/environment /test-no-435-in-vitro-membrane-barrier-test-method-for-skin-corrosion_9789264067318-en.

67. Skin corrosion. Accessed August 4, 2016. Retrieved from https://eurl-ecvam.jrc.ec.europa.eu/validation -regulatory-acceptance/topical-toxicity/skin-corrosion.

68. Skin irritation. Accessed August 4, 2016. Retrieved from https://eurl-ecvam.jrc.ec.europa.eu/validation -regulatory-acceptance/topical-toxicity/skin-irritation#ecvam-validated-test-methods.

69. Oliver GJA, Pemberton MA, Rhodes C. An in vitro skin corrosivity test—Modifications and validation. *Food Chem Toxicol*. 1986;24(6–7):507–12.

70. OSHA. A guide to the globally harmonized system of classification and labelling of chemicals (GHS). Accessed August 4, 2016. Retrieved from https://www.osha.gov/dsg/hazcom/ghs.html.

71. OECD 439–2013. OECD guidelines for the testing of chemicals: In vitro skin irritation: Reconstructed human epidermis test method—439. Accessed August 4, 2016. Retrieved from http://ntp.niehs.nih.gov /iccvam/SuppDocs/FedDocs/OECD/OECD-TG439-2013-508.pdf.

72. United Nations Globally Harmonized System of Classification and Labeling of Chemicals. Health hazards—Part 3. Accessed August 4, 2016. Retrieved from http://www.unece.org/fileadmin/DAM /trans/danger/publi/ghs/ghs_rev03/English/03e_part3.pdf.

73. OECD Test No. 404: Acute dermal irritation/corrosion. Accessed August 4, 2016. Retrieved from http:// www.oecd-ilibrary.org/content/book/9789264070622-en.

74. Draize JH, Woodard G, Calvery HO. Methods for the study of irritation and toxicity of substances applied topically to the skin and mucous membranes. *J Pharmacol Exp Ther*. 1944;82:377.

75. Marzulli FN, Maibach HI. The rabbit as a model for evaluating skin irritants: A comparison of results obtained on animals and man using repeated skin exposures. *Food Cosmet Toxicol*. 1975;13(5):533–540.

76. Joint Research Centre the European Commission's In-House Science Service. Advancing safety assess- ment without animals: EURL ECVAM. Accessed August 4, 2016. Retrieved from http://ihcp.jrc.ec .europa.eu/our_labs/eurl-ecvam/clip-dec-13/eurl-ecvam-script-Dec-2013.pdf.

77. Basketter DA, York M, McFadden JP et al. Determination of skin irritation potential in the human 4-h patch test. *Contact Dermat*. 2004;51(1):1–4.

78. Patil SM, Patrick E, Maibach HI. Animal, human, and in vitro test methods for predicting skin irrita- tion. In: Marzulli FN, Maibach HI, eds. *Dermatotoxicology Methods*. Boca Raton, FL: CRC Press; 1998:89–114.

79. Jirova D, Basketter D, Liebsch M et al. Comparison of human skin irritation patch test data with in vitro skin irritation assays and animal data. *Contact Dermat*. 2010;62(2):109–116.

80. Kligman AM, Wooding WM. A method for the measurement and evaluation of irritants on human skin. *J Invest Dermatol*. 1967;49(1):78–94.

81. Philips L, Steinberg M, Maibach HI. A comparison of rabbit and human skin response to certain irri- tants. *Toxicol Appl Pharmacol*. 1972;21(3):369–82.

82. Frosch PJ, Kligman AM. The soap chamber test: A new method for assessing the irritancy of soaps. *J Am Acad Dermatol*. 1979;1(1):35–41.

83. Kooyman DJ, Snyder FM. Tests for the mildness of soaps. *Arch Dermatol Syph*. 1942;46:846–855.

84. Gabard B, Chatelain E, Bieli E et al. Surfactant irritation: In vitro corneosurfametry and in vivo bioen- gineering. *Skin Res Technol*. 2001;7(1):49–55.

85. Laudanska H, Reduta T, Szmitkowska D. Evaluation of skin barrier function in allergic contact der- matitis and atopic dermatitis using method of the continuous TEWL measurement. *Rocz Akad Med Bialymst*. 2003;48:123–127.

86. Bircher A, de Boer EM, Agner T et al. Guidelines for measurement of cutaneous blood flow by laser Doppler flowmetry: A report from the standardization group of the European Society of Contact Dermatitis. *Contact Dermat*. 1994;30(2):65–72.

87. Hendrix SW, Miller KH, Youket TE et al. Optimization of the skin multiple analyte profile bioana- lytical method for determination of skin biomarkers from D-squame tape samples. *Skin Res Technol*. 2007;13(3):330–342.

88. Black D, Boyer J, Lagarde JM. Image analysis of skin scaling using D-squame samplers: Comparison with clinical scoring and use for assessing moisturizer efficacy. *Int J Cosmet Sci*. 2006; 28(1):35–44.

89. Serup J, Winther A, Blichmann C. A simple method for the study of scale pattern and effects of a moisturizer—Qualitative and quantitative evaluation by D-squame tape compared with parameters of epidermal hydration. *Clin Exp Dermatol*. 1989;14(4):277–282.

90. OECD. *Test no. 432:* In vitro 3T3 NRU phototoxicity test. Paris: OECD; 2004.
91. Kornhauser A, Wamer WG, Lambert LA. Cellular and molecular events following ultraviolet irradiation of skin. In: Marzulli FN, Maibach HI, eds. *Dermatotoxicology.* Fifth ed. Washington, DC: Taylor & Francis; 1996:189–230.
92. Anderson RR, Parrish JA. The optics of human skin. *J Invest Dermatol.* 1981;77:13–19.
93. Marzulli FN, Maibach HI. Photoirritation (phototoxicity, phototoxic dermatitis). In: Marzulli FN, Maibach HI, eds. *Dermatotoxicology.* Fifth ed. Washington DC: Taylor & Francis; 1996:231–237.
94. FDA. Guidance for industry photosafety testing. Accessed January 8, 2016. Retrieved from http://www.fda.gov/downloads/drugs/guidancecomplianceregulatoryinformation/guidances/ucm337572.pdf.
95. International Committee on Harmonization. Guidance on photosafety evaluation of pharmaceuticals S10—Step 2 version dated 13 November, 2012. Accessed August 4, 2016. Retrieved from http://www.fda.gov/downloads/Drugs/GuidanceComplianceRegulatoryInformation/Guidances/UCM337572.pdf.
96. Spielmann H, Balls M, Dupuis J et al. The international EU/COLIPA in vitro phototoxicity validation study: Results of phase II (blind trial): Part 1: The 3T3 NRU phototoxicity test. *Toxicol In Vitro.* 1998;12(3):305–327.
97. Henry B, Foti C, Alsante K. Can light absorption and photostability data be used to assess the photosafety risks in patients for a new drug molecule? *J Photochem Photobiol B.* 2009;96(1):57–62.
98. Ceridono M, Tellner P, Bauer D et al. The 3T3 neutral red uptake phototoxicity test: Practical experience and implications for phototoxicity testing—The report of an ECVAM-EFPIA workshop. *Regul Toxicol Pharmacol.* 2012;63(3):480–488.
99. Netzlaff F, Lehr CM, Wertz PW et al. The human epidermis models EpiSkin, SkinEthic and EpiDerm: An evaluation of morphology and their suitability for testing phototoxicity, irritancy, corrosivity, and substance transport. *Eur J Pharm Biopharm.* 2005;60(2):167–178.
100. Kejlova K, Jirova D, Bendova H et al. Phototoxicity of bergamot oil assessed by in vitro techniques in combination with human patch tests. *Toxicol In Vitro.* 2007;21(7):1298–1303.
101. Liebsch M, Traue D, Barrabas C et al. Prevalidation of the EpiDerm phototoxicity test. In: Clark D, Lisansky S, Macmillan R, eds. *Alternatives to Animal Testing II: Proceedings of the Second International Scientific Conference Organised by the European Cosmetic Industry.* Brussels/Newbury: CPL Press. 1999:160–166.
102. Jones P. In vitro phototoxicity assays. In: Chilcott RP, Price S, eds. *Skin Toxicology.* England: John Wiley & Sons, Ltd; 2008:169–183.
103. Maibach HI, Sams WM, Epstein JH. Screening for drug toxicity by wavelengths greater than 3100A. *Arch Dermatol 1967.* 1967;95:12–15.
104. Kaidbey KH, Kligman AM. Identification of topical photosensitizing agents in humans. *J Invest Dermatol.* 1978;70(3):149–51.
105. Pearse AD, Anstey A. Clinical aspects of phototoxicity. In: Chilcott RP, Price S, eds. *Skin Toxicology.* London: Wiley; 2008:245–257.
106. Harvell J, Bason M, Maibach HI. Contact urticaria and its mechanisms. *Food Chem Toxicol.* 1994; 32(2):103–12.
107. Amin S, Tanglertsampan C, Maibach HI. Contact urticaria syndrome: 1997. *Am J Contact Dermat.* 1997;8(1):15–19.
108. Konstantinou GN, Grattan CE. Food contact hypersensitivity syndrome: The mucosal contact urticaria paradigm. *Clin Exp Dermatol.* 2008;33(4):383–389.
109. Von Krogh G, Maibach HI. The contact urticaria syndrome. *Semin Dermatol.* 1982;1:59–66.
110. Amin S, Lahti A, Maibach HI. Contact urticaria and the contact urticaria syndrome (immediate contact reactions). In: Zhai H, Wilhelm KP, Maibach HI, eds. *Dermatotoxicology.* Seventh ed. 2008: 525–536.
111. Zhai H, Zheng Y, Fautz R et al. Reactions of non-immunologic contact urticaria on scalp, face, and back. *Skin Res Technol.* 2012;18(4):436–441.
112. Lauerma AI, Maibach HI. Animal models for immunologic contact urticaria and nonimmunologic contact urticaria. In: Maibach HI, ed. *Toxicology of Skin.* Philadelphia, PA: Taylor & Francis; 2001:252–254.
113. Basketter D, Gerberick F, Kimber I et al. *Toxicology of Contact Dermatitis.* Chichester, UK: John Wiley & Sons; 1999.

114. Marrakchi S, Maibach HI. Functional map and age-related differences in the human face: Nonimmunologic contact urticaria induced by hexyl nicotinate. *Contact Dermat.* 2006;55(1):15–19.

115. Lahti A. Terfenadine does not inhibit non-immunologic contact urticaria. *Contact Dermat.* 1987;16(4): 220–223.

116. Lahti A, McDonald DM, Tammi R et al. Pharmacological studies on nonimmunologic contact urticaria in guinea pigs. *Arch Dermatol Res.* 1986;279(1):44–49.

117. Lahti A, Vaananen A, Kokkonen EL et al. Acetylsalicylic acid inhibits non-immunologic contact urticaria. *Contact Dermat.* 1987;16(3):133–135.

118. Gollhausen R, Kligman AM. Human assay for identifying substances which induce non-allergic contact urticaria: The NICU-test. *Contact Dermat.* 1985;13(2):98–106.

119. Larmi E, Lahti A, Hannuksela M. Effect of ultraviolet B on nonimmunologic contact reactions induced by dimethyl sulphoxide, phenol and sodium lauryl sulphate. *Photodermatol.* 1989;6(6):258–262.

120. Larmi E, Lahti A, Hannuksela M. Effects of infra-red and neodymium yttrium aluminium garnet laser irradiation on non-immunologic immediate contact reactions to benzoic acid and methyl nicotinate. *Derm Beruf Umwelt.* 1989;37(6):210–214.

121. Basketter D, Lahti A. Immediate contact reactions. In: Johansen JD, Frosch PJ, Lepoittevin JP, eds. *Contact Dermatitis.* Fifth ed. Berlin Heidelberg: Springer; 2011:137–153.

122. Safford RJ, Basketter DA, Allenby CF et al. Immediate contact reactions to chemicals in the fragrance mix and a study of the quenching action of eugenol. *Br J Dermatol.* 1990;123(5):595–606.

123. Tanaka S, Matsumoto Y, Dlova N et al. Immediate contact reactions to fragrance mix constituents and myroxylon pereirae resin. *Contact Dermat.* 2004;51(1):20–21.

124. Lahti A, Maibach HI. An animal model for nonimmunologic contact urticaria. *Toxicol Appl Pharmacol.* 1984;76(2):219–224.

125. Lahti A, Maibach HI. Species specificity of nonimmunologic contact urticaria: Guinea pig, rat, and mouse. *J Am Acad Dermatol.* 1985;13(1):66–69.

126. Lahti A, Maibach HI. Long refractory period after one application of nonimmunologic contact urticaria agents to the guinea pig ear. *J Am Acad Dermatol.* 1985;13(4):585–589.

127. Lahti A. Immediate contact reactions. In: Rycroft RJ, Menne T, Frosch PJ, eds. *Textbook of Contact Dermatitis.* Berlin Heidelberg; New York: Springer; 1995:62–74.

128. Lahti A, Kopola H, Harila A et al. Assessment of skin erythema by eye, laser Doppler flowmeter, spectroradiometer, two-channel erythema meter and minolta chroma meter. *Arch Dermatol Res.* 1993;285(5):278–282.

129. Ylipieti S, Lahti A. Effect of the vehicle on non-immunologic immediate contact reactions. *Contact Dermat.* 1989;21(2):105–106.

130. Lahti A, Poutiainen AM, Hannuksela M. Alcohol vehicles in tests for non-immunological immediate contact reactions. *Contact Dermat.* 1993;29(1):22–25.

131. Hannuksela A, Niinimaki A, Hannuksela M. Size of the test area does not affect the result of the repeated open application test. *Contact Dermat.* 1993;28(5):299–300.

132. Hannuksela M. Skin tests for immediate hypersensitivity. In: Rycroft RJ, Menne T, Frosch PJ, eds. *Textbook of Contact Dermatitis.* Berlin Heidelberg; New York,: Springer; 1995:287–292.

133. Johansson J, Lahti A. Topical non-steroidal anti-inflammatory drugs inhibit non-immunologic immediate contact reactions. *Contact Dermat.* 1988;19(3):161–165.

134. Kujala T, Lahti A. Duration of inhibition of non-immunologic immediate contact reactions by acetyl-salicylic acid. *Contact Dermat.* 1989;21(1):60–61.

135. Larmi E. Systemic effect of ultraviolet irradiation on non-immunologic immediate contact reactions to benzoic acid and methyl nicotinate. *Acta Derm Venereol.* 1989;69(4):296–301.

136. Hannuksela M. Mechanisms in contact urticaria. *Clin Dermatol.* 1997;15(4):619–622.

137. Najem N, Hull D. Langerhans cells in delayed skin reactions to inhalant allergens in atopic dermatitis—An electron microscopic study. *Clin Exp Dermatol.* 1989;14(3):218–222.

138. Nicholson PJ, Llewellyn D, English JS. Guidelines development group: Evidence-based guidelines for the prevention, identification and management of occupational contact dermatitis and urticaria. *Contact Dermat.* 2010;63(4):177–186.

139. Bourrain JL. Occupational contact urticaria. *Clin Rev Allergy Immunol.* 2006;30(1):39–46.

140. Amaro C, Goossens A. Immunological occupational contact urticaria and contact dermatitis from proteins: A review. *Contact Dermat.* 2008;58(2):67–75.
141. Blaikie L, Morrow T, Wilson AP et al. A two-centre study for the evaluation and validation of an animal model for the assessment of the potential of small molecular weight chemicals to cause respiratory allergy. *Toxicology.* 1995;96(1):37–50.
142. Sarlo K, Fletcher ER, Gaines WG et al. Respiratory allergenicity of detergent enzymes in the guinea pig intratracheal test: Association with sensitization of occupationally exposed individuals. *Fundam Appl Toxicol.* 1997;39(1):44–52.
143. Lauerma AI, Fenn B, Maibach HI. Trimellitic anhydride-sensitive mouse as an animal model for contact urticaria. *J Appl Toxicol.* 1997;17(6):357–360.
144. Bernstein DI, Zeiss CR. Guidelines for preparation and characterization of chemical-protein conjugate antigens: Report of the subcommittee on preparation and characterization of low molecular weight antigens. *J Allergy Clin Immunol.* 1989;84(5 Pt 2):820–822.
145. Wide L. A RAST neutralization test for detection of blocking antibodies in serum after hyposensitization. *Int Arch Allergy Appl Immunol.* 1976;52(1–4):219–226.
146. Rance F, Juchet A, Bremont F, Dutau G. Correlations between skin prick tests using commercial extracts and fresh foods, specific IgE, and food challenges. *Allergy.* 1997;52(10):1031–1035.
147. Heinzerling L, Mari A, Bergmann KC et al. The skin prick test—European standards. *Clin Transl Allergy.* 2013;3(1):3–7022–3–3.
148. Bindslev-Jensen C. Skin tests for immediate hypersensitivity In: Johansen JD, Frosch PJ, Lepoittevin JP, eds. *Contact Dermatitis.* Fifth ed. Berlin Heidelberg: Springer; 2011:511–517.
149. Abou Chakra OR, Sutra JP, Poncet P et al. Key role of water-insoluble allergens of pollen cytoplasmic granules in biased allergic response in a rat model. *World Allergy Organ J.* 2011;4(1):4–12.
150. Niinimaki A. Scratch-chamber tests in food handler dermatitis. *Contact Dermat.* 1987;16(1):11–20.
151. Oranje AP. Skin provocation test (SAFT) based on contact urticaria: A marker of dermal food allergy. *Curr Probl Dermatol.* 1991;20:228–231.

24

Formulations for Sensitive Skin

Golara Honari and Howard Maibach

Sensitive skin is a prevalent condition affection up to half of women and a third of men in some western societies (1–5). Unpleasant sensations of itching, burning, and stinging with exposure to various skin care products and/or environmental factors are experienced by affected individuals. The pathophysiological mechanisms are not yet fully elucidated; however, some biophysical and biochemical alterations such as impaired barrier function, smaller corneocytes, increased vascular reactivity, and decreased SC ceramides have been observed (6–10). Current evidence highlights a prominent role for increased sensory perception in the cutaneous nervous system (11). This chapter reviews the general considerations in formulations suitable for sensitive skin as well as targeted formulations based on our current understanding of involved pathomechanisms.

General Considerations

Sensitive skin is also known as *reactive skin*, *hyperreactive skin*, *intolerant skin*, and *irritable skin*. It is important to differentiate sensitive skin from sensitized skin, affected by specific allergens. Sensitive skin is very common, and as mentioned earlier, up to 50% of women in western countries and Japan complain of associated symptoms (5,12,13). Skin phenotype is not associated with the symptoms, but cultural conducts might affect the self-reported prevalence; large surveys from China report complaints in about 15% of women (14).

The high prevalence of sensitive skin creates challenges for patients, physicians, and the cosmetic industry. Product formulations for sensitive skin are somewhat challenging considering the lack of validated dermatotoxicological testing specific for sensitive skin. Recent surveys of more than 28,000 American adults showed that about 11% use skin care products directed toward sensitive skin (15). This highlights another challenging fact, which is lack of a standard definition for consumer products marketed for sensitive skin. Regulatory and marketing measures are exceedingly important topics that are beyond the scope of this chapter.

In addition to the considerations mentioned earlier, it is best to develop basic formulations with few ingredients to minimize the risk of overreaction. Specifically, avoid using ingredients with the potential to induce irritation or sensitivity such as glycolic acid, lactic acid, propylene glycol, fragrances, herbal or essential oil extracts, and lanolin (16). Alcohol-based formulations should also be avoided. Skin cleansers should preferably be nonfoaming, with a neutral PH, and contain no exfoliates. Physical sunscreens are generally better tolerated than chemical sunscreens. In general, shorter ingredient lists composed of elements with less potential to cause active sensitization and or irritation are favored. Key features can be summarized as follows:

- Short list of ingredients
- Avoiding sensitizers and irritants
- Increase hydration and TEWL
- Enhance barrier repair and function
- Active intervention such as anti-inflammatory and neuromodulatory ingredients may be considered

Better understanding of the underlying pathomechanisms has helped with active targeted therapies, reviewed in the following.

Barrier-Enhancing Products

Some patients with sensitive skin have altered skin barrier function, decreased amount of lipids, and smaller corneocytes, affecting barrier stability (7,8,10,17), leading to increases (TEWL and decreased skin tolerance threshold (18,19). It has been shown that individuals with sensitive skin are more likely to react to an irritant patch test and have a higher risk of developing contact allergies up to five times more compared to controls (3,6,20). Therefore, using barrier-enhancing skin care products free of irritant and potential allergens is an integral part of management.

SC lipids are essential in establishing barrier hemostatic function.

Topical application of lipids can improve barrier repair and reduce TEWL. Physiological and non-physiological lipids enhance barrier function in different ways.

Main SC lipids include ceramides, cholesterol, and free fatty acids. Upon exogenous application, these lipids quickly travel through the SC to the nucleated epidermis and will be incorporated into the lamellar bodies (21,22). Lamellar bodies are secretory structures derived from the trans-Golgi network. They secrete their contents, including lipids (glucosylceramides, sphingomyelin, phospholipids, and cholesterol) into the upper layers of the epidermis and are crucial to SC homeostasis and barrier function (23).

Therefore, the composition of topically applied physiological lipids can affect the formation of normal and abnormal lamellar bodies and their subsequent function.

It has been shown that optimal benefit in barrier repair is achieved when equimolar mixtures of physiological lipids are used in topical products (24). Yang et al. (25) showed that the equimolar ratio of ceramides, cholesterol, and fatty acids (either the essential fatty acid, linoleic acid, or the nonessential fatty acids, palmitic or stearic acids) allows normal repair and accelerated barrier repair up to threefolds with the application of optimal lipid mixtures. The topical application of a lipid mixture of (cholesterol, ceramide palmitate, and linoleate 4.3:2.3:1:1.08) has been shown to accelerate barrier repair following extensive disruption of the barrier by acetone (25). The application of only one or two of these lipids to distressed skin can delay barrier recovery (24).

Nonphysiological lipids such as petrolatum and mineral oil can enhance barrier repair by forming bulk hydrophobic phase in the SC interstices (24,26–28).

The goals mentioned earlier apply when developing cleansers for sensitive skin. Attempts should be made to maintain the integrity of barrier function and skin surface lipids as well as SC hydration and surface pH. Ongoing research is being done to further advance formulations that are more appropriate for sensitive skin (16,29–31).

Neuromodulatory and Anti-Inflammatory Pharmacological Interventions

Increased sensory perception is a prominent part of sensitive skin. Unmyelinated sensory C fibers have a primary role in nociceptive sensations in the skin and are associated with sensitive skin symptoms. It is conceivable that the cutaneous nervous system is also involved in the perception of unpleasant sensations triggered by environmental exposures such as rapid temperature changes. Increased sensation can potentially be associated with increased neuronal stimulation due to insufficient barrier function (11,32). However, many patients with sensitive skin do not express biophysical or biochemical changes in their epidermis. Many patients with AD experience similar symptoms, while earlier studies suggested increased density of peripheral nerves in the patients with AD compared to controls; however, other studies do not confirm this (33,34). Tsutsumi et al. (35) showed normal epidermal nerve density in both patients with or without atopic dermatitis. Buhe et al. (36) recently showed that the number of peptidergic C fibers, which are involved in the perception of pain, temperature, and itching, were especially decreased in individuals with sensitive skin compared to controls, suggesting that this subtype of nerve endings may undergo degeneration following contact with environmental factors. Specific nociceptive channels on these nerve endings, such as TRP channels, could be overstimulated, leading to the release of neuropeptides including calcitonin gene-related peptide (CGRP) (36). Epidermal TRP channels are expressed on cutaneous nerve endings and are known to promote the release of neuropeptides, inducing cutaneous neurogenic inflammation (11,32,36). Neurotransmitters including SP, CGRP, and vasoactive intestinal peptide may induce neurogenic inflammation with vasodilation and mast cell degranulation. Neurogenic inflammation mediated through protease-activated receptor 2 (PAR2) has been the subject of studies as a potential attributing factor. PAR2 is a receptor expressed on keratinocytes, endothelial cells, and afferent nerve fibers and can be activated by proteases such as tryptase and kallikrein during inflammation (37,38). PAR2 activation leads to the release of inflammatory neuropeptides such as CGRP and SP and is suspected to be involved in a histamine-independent itch-signaling pathway (36,39,40). Activated PAR2 also promotes inflammatory hyperalgesia via TRPV1, which is thought to have a role in skin hyperreactivity (32,41). PAR2 also increases the expression of cell adhesion molecules on keratinocytes, via the activation of nuclear factor κB (NFκB) promoting inflammatory responses (42,43). Acid-sensing ion channels (ASICs) are voltage-insensitive cation channels responding to extracellular acidification highly expressed on sensory nerves and might also be involved in neurogenic inflammation (44). Buhe et al. (36) did not find significant difference in PAR2, TRPV1, NFκB, or ASIC-1 expression between individuals with or without sensitive skin, but additional studies in larger cohorts are warranted (36).

As mentioned earlier, TRPV1 is a key integrator of itch sensation (32). TPRV1 is a nonselective cation channel and a thermoreceptor activated by temperatures of up to 42°C and is a receptor for capsaicin (45). TRPV3 and TRPA1 have also been identified as nociceptive receptors (46–48).

Considering TRPs as biological targets, their antagonists can be developed to actively control symptoms associated with sensitive skin. Targeting TRPV1 has led to the development of *trans-4-tert*-butylcyclohexanol, which is a selective antagonist of this receptor. In vivo and in vitro studies have shown that *trans-4-tert*-butylcyclohexanol reduces skin reactivity to capsaicin (49–51).

The topical application of 4-t-butylcyclohexanol along with the potent anti-inflammatory licochalcone has proven beneficial as effective active ingredients for the treatment of sensitive skin. The topical application of these compounds resulted in an immediate relief from symptoms such as erythema and stinging (52–54).

Genetic Modification

Kim et al. (55,56) described the dysfunction of muscle contraction, carbohydrate, and lipid metabolism, as well as the downregulation of adiponectin (ADIPOQ) gene in patients with sensitive skin compared to controls. ADIPOQ is an adipocyte-derived adipokine with antiapoptotic, anti-inflammatory, and antioxidative activities. It is also involved in the regulation of muscle phenotypes and functions (57,58). Decreased expression of ADIPOQ was accompanied by decreased levels of phospho-AMP-activated protein kinase, decreased synthesis of ATP, and lower pH leading to abnormal muscle contraction and skin sensitivity (55,56). It is not clear whether ADIPOQ is genetic or acquired, but further understanding of involved factors may open possibilities for novel therapeutic agents targeting ADIPOQ stimulation in sensitive skin (56,59).

Role of Microbiome

The human skin is colonized by up to one billion microorganisms per square centimeter including bacteria, fungi, viruses, and mites (11). These microorganisms can provide protection against diseases by secreting antimicrobial peptides or free fatty acids to prevent the colonization of the skin by pathogens, thereby ensuring epithelial health. In vitro studies have shown that the incubation of nerve cells with lysates of a probiotic strain called *Bifidobacterium longum* significantly inhibited capsaicin-induced CGRP release by neurons (60). Also, the in vivo application of a cream containing *Bifidobacterium longum* extract (10%) twice a day for 2 months led to a significant decrease in skin sensitivity in the study group compared to controls (60).

Conclusion

Sensitive skin is a common condition posing challenges for patients, dermatologists, and the industry. Despite the lack of standard guidelines for sensitive skin formulations, general considerations mentioned earlier should be implemented to provide nonirritating and nonsensitizing skin care products. The ongoing advances in the understanding of the pathophysiology of sensitive skin provide promising developments in the care of these individuals. Active therapeutic interventions are rapidly developing, and the developments of novel targeted therapies seem promising.

REFERENCES

1. Farage MA. How do perceptions of sensitive skin differ at different anatomical sites? An epidemiological study. *Clin Exp Dermatol.* 2009;34(8):e521–30.
2. Misery L, Myon E, Martin N et al. Sensitive skin in France: An epidemiological approach. *Ann Dermatol Venereol.* 2005;132(5):425–429.
3. Willis CM, Shaw S, De Lacharriere O et al. Sensitive skin: An epidemiological study. *Br J Dermatol.* 2001;145(2):258–263.
4. Guinot C, Malvy D, Mauger E et al. Self-reported skin sensitivity in a general adult population in France: Data of the SU.VI.MAX cohort. *J Eur Acad Dermatol Venereol.* 2006;20(4):380–390.
5. Misery L, Sibaud V, Merial-Kieny C et al. Sensitive skin in the American population: Prevalence, clinical data, and role of the dermatologist. *Int J Dermatol.* 2011;50(8):961–967.
6. Roussaki-Schulze AV, Zafiriou E, Nikoulis D et al. Objective biophysical findings in patients with sensitive skin. *Drugs Exp Clin Res.* 2005;31 Suppl:17–24.
7. Raj N, Voegeli R, Rawlings AV et al. A fundamental investigation into aspects of the physiology and biochemistry of the stratum corneum in subjects with sensitive skin. *Int J Cosmet Sci.* 2016. doi: 10.1111/ics.12334.
8. Pinto P, Rosado C, Parreirao C et al. Is there any barrier impairment in sensitive skin?: A quantitative analysis of sensitive skin by mathematical modeling of transepidermal water loss desorption curves. *Skin Res Technol.* 2011;17(2):181–185.
9. Richters RJ, Uzunbajakava NE, Falcone D et al. Clinical, biophysical and immunohistochemical analysis of skin reactions to acute skin barrier disruption—A comparative trial between participants with sensitive skin and those with nonsensitive skin. *Br J Dermatol.* 2016;174(5):1126–1133.
10. Cho HJ, Chung BY, Lee HB et al. Quantitative study of stratum corneum ceramides contents in patients with sensitive skin. *J Dermatol.* 2012;39(3):295–300.
11. Misery L, Loser K, Stander S. Sensitive skin. *J Eur Acad Dermatol Venereol.* 2016;30 Suppl 1:2–8.
12. Kamide R, Misery L, Perez-Cullell N et al. Sensitive skin evaluation in the Japanese population. *J Dermatol.* 2013;40(3):177–181.
13. Misery L, Boussetta S, Nocera T et al. Sensitive skin in Europe. *J Eur Acad Dermatol Venereol.* 2009;23(4):376–381.
14. Xu F, Yan S, Wu M et al. Self-declared sensitive skin in China: A community-based study in three top metropolises. *J Eur Acad Dermatol Venereol.* 2013;27(3):370–375.
15. Experian. Market intelligence. *Cosmetics and Toiletries.* 2016;131(4):44.
16. Heinicke IR, Adams DH, Barnes TM et al. Evaluation of a topical treatment for the relief of sensitive skin. *Clin Cosmet Investig Dermatol.* 2015;8:405–412.
17. Cua AB, Wilhelm KP, Maibach HI. Cutaneous sodium lauryl sulphate irritation potential: Age and regional variability. *Br J Dermatol.* 1990;123(5):607–613.
18. Branco N, Lee I, Zhai H et al. Long-term repetitive sodium lauryl sulfate-induced irritation of the skin: An in vivo study. *Contact Dermatitis.* 2005;53(5):278–284.
19. Misery L, Jean-Decoster C, Mery S et al. A new ten-item questionnaire for assessing sensitive skin: The sensitive scale-10. *Acta Derm Venereol.* 2014;94(6):635–639.
20. Farage MA. Self-reported immunological and familial links in individuals who perceive they have sensitive skin. *Br J Dermatol.* 2008;159(1):237–238.
21. Mao-Qiang M, Feingold KR, Jain M et al. Extracellular processing of phospholipids is required for permeability barrier homeostasis. *J Lipid Res.* 1995;36(9):1925–1935.

22. Man MQ, Feingold KR, Elias PM. Exogenous lipids influence permeability barrier recovery in acetone-treated murine skin. *Arch Dermatol.* 1993;129(6):728–738.

23. Raymond AA, Gonzalez de Peredo A, Stella A et al. Lamellar bodies of human epidermis: Proteomics characterization by high throughput mass spectrometry and possible involvement of CLIP-170 in their trafficking/secretion. *Mol Cell Proteomics.* 2008;7(11):2151–2175.

24. Mao-Qiang M, Feingold KR, Thornfeldt CR et al. Optimization of physiological lipid mixtures for barrier repair. *J Invest Dermatol.* 1996;106(5):1096–1101.

25. Yang L, Mao-Qiang M, Taljebini M et al. Topical stratum corneum lipids accelerate barrier repair after tape stripping, solvent treatment and some but not all types of detergent treatment. *Br J Dermatol.* 1995;133(5):679–685.

26. Ghadially R, Halkier-Sorensen L, Elias PM. Effects of petrolatum on stratum corneum structure and function. *J Am Acad Dermatol.* 1992;26(3 Pt 2):387–396.

27. Rawlings AV, Lombard KJ. A review on the extensive skin benefits of mineral oil. *Int J Cosmet Sci.* 2012;34(6):511–518.

28. Mao-Qiang M, Brown BE, Wu-Pong S et al. Exogenous nonphysiologic vs physiologic lipids: Divergent mechanisms for correction of permeability barrier dysfunction. *Arch Dermatol.* 1995;131(7):809–816.

29. Jeong S, Lee SH, Park BD et al. Erratum to comparison of the efficacy of atopalm((R)) multi-lamellar emulsion cream and physiogel((R)) intensive cream in improving epidermal permeability barrier in sensitive skin. *Dermatol Ther (Heidelb).* 2016;6(1):57-016-0103-z.

30. Jeong S, Lee SH, Park BD et al. Comparison of the efficacy of atopalm((R)) multi-lamellar emulsion cream and physiogel((R)) intensive cream in improving epidermal permeability barrier in sensitive skin. *Dermatol Ther (Heidelb).* 2016;6(1):47–56.

31. Fan L, He C, Jiang L et al. Brief analysis of causes of sensitive skin and advances in evaluation of anti-allergic activity of cosmetic products. *Int J Cosmet Sci.* 2016;38(2):120–127.

32. Stander S, Schneider SW, Weishaupt C et al. Putative neuronal mechanisms of sensitive skin. *Exp Dermatol.* 2009;18(5):417–423.

33. Urashima R, Mihara M. Cutaneous nerves in atopic dermatitis: A histological, immunohistochemical and electron microscopic study. *Virchows Arch.* 1998;432(4):363–370.

34. Sugiura H, Omoto M, Hirota Y et al. Density and fine structure of peripheral nerves in various skin lesions of atopic dermatitis. *Arch Dermatol Res.* 1997;289(3):125–131.

35. Tsutsumi M, Kitahata H, Fukuda M et al. Numerical and comparative three-dimensional structural analysis of peripheral nerve fibres in epidermis of patients with atopic dermatitis. *Br J Dermatol.* 2016;174(1):191–194.

36. Buhe V, Vie K, Guere C et al. Pathophysiological study of sensitive skin. *Acta Derm Venereol.* 2016;96(3):314–318.

37. Steinhoff M, Corvera CU, Thoma MS et al. Proteinase-activated receptor-2 in human skin: Tissue distribution and activation of keratinocytes by mast cell tryptase. *Exp Dermatol.* 1999;8(4):282–294.

38. Molino M, Barnathan ES, Numerof R et al. Interactions of mast cell tryptase with thrombin receptors and PAR-2. *J Biol Chem.* 1997;272(7):4043–4049.

39. Shimada SG, Shimada KA, Collins JG. Scratching behavior in mice induced by the proteinase-activated receptor-2 agonist, SLIGRL-NH2. *Eur J Pharmacol.* 2006;530(3):281–283.

40. Steinhoff M, Vergnolle N, Young SH et al. Agonists of proteinase-activated receptor 2 induce inflammation by a neurogenic mechanism. *Nat Med.* 2000;6(2):151–158.

41. Amadesi S, Nie J, Vergnolle N et al. Protease-activated receptor 2 sensitizes the capsaicin receptor transient receptor potential vanilloid receptor 1 to induce hyperalgesia. *J Neurosci.* 2004;24(18):4300–4312.

42. Buddenkotte J, Stroh C, Engels IH et al. Agonists of proteinase-activated receptor-2 stimulate upregulation of intercellular cell adhesion molecule-1 in primary human keratinocytes via activation of NF-kappa B. *J Invest Dermatol.* 2005;124(1):38–45.

43. Steinhoff M, Buddenkotte J, Shpacovitch V et al. Proteinase-activated receptors: Transducers of proteinase-mediated signaling in inflammation and immune response. *Endocr Rev.* 2005;26(1):1–43.

44. Chen CC, Wong CW. Neurosensory mechanotransduction through acid-sensing ion channels. *J Cell Mol Med.* 2013;17(3):337–349.

45. Caterina MJ, Schumacher MA, Tominaga M et al. The capsaicin receptor: A heat-activated ion channel in the pain pathway. *Nature.* 1997;389(6653):816–824.

46. Steinhoff M, Biro T. A TR(I)P to pruritus research: Role of TRPV3 in inflammation and itch. *J Invest Dermatol*. 2009;129(3):531–535.

47. Wilson SR, Nelson AM, Batia L et al. The ion channel TRPA1 is required for chronic itch. *J Neurosci*. 2013;33(22):9283–9294.

48. Anand U, Otto WR, Facer P et al. TRPA1 receptor localisation in the human peripheral nervous system and functional studies in cultured human and rat sensory neurons. *Neurosci Lett*. 2008;438(2):221–227.

49. Pereira U, Boulais N, Lebonvallet N et al. Development of an in vitro coculture of primary sensitive pig neurons and keratinocytes for the study of cutaneous neurogenic inflammation. *Exp Dermatol*. 2010;19(10):931–935.

50. Kueper T, Krohn M, Haustedt LO et al. Inhibition of TRPV1 for the treatment of sensitive skin. *Exp Dermatol*. 2010;19(11):980–986.

51. Costa A, Eberlin S, Polettini AJ et al. Neuromodulatory and anti-inflammatory ingredient for sensitive skin: In vitro assessment. *Inflamm Allergy Drug Targets*. 2014;13(3):191–198.

52. Sulzberger M, Worthmann AC, Holtzmann U et al. Effective treatment for sensitive skin: 4-t-Butylcyclohexanol and licochalcone A. *J Eur Acad Dermatol Venereol*. 2016;30 Suppl 1:9–17.

53. Schoelermann AM, Jung KA, Buck B et al. Comparison of skin calming effects of cosmetic products containing 4-t-butylcyclohexanol or acetyl dipeptide-1 cetyl ester on capsaicin-induced facial stinging in volunteers with sensitive skin. *J Eur Acad Dermatol Venereol*. 2016;30 Suppl 1:18–20.

54. Schoelermann AM, Weber TM, Arrowitz C et al. Skin compatibility and efficacy of a cosmetic skin care regimen with licochalcone A and 4-t-butylcyclohexanol in patients with rosacea subtype I. *J Eur Acad Dermatol Venereol*. 2016;30 Suppl 1:21–27.

55. Kim EJ, Lee DH, Kim YK et al. Decreased ATP synthesis and lower pH may lead to abnormal muscle contraction and skin sensitivity in human skin. *J Dermatol Sci*. 2014;76(3):214–221.

56. Kim EJ, Lee DH, Kim YK et al. Adiponectin deficiency contributes to sensitivity in human skin. *J Invest Dermatol*. 2015;135(9):2331–2334.

57. Goldstein BJ, Scalia R. Adiponectin: A novel adipokine linking adipocytes and vascular function. *J Clin Endocrinol Metab*. 2004;89(6):2563–2568.

58. Krause MP, Liu Y, Vu V et al. Adiponectin is expressed by skeletal muscle fibers and influences muscle phenotype and function. *Am J Physiol Cell Physiol*. 2008;295(1):C203–12.

59. Kim EJ, Lee DH, Kim YK et al. Decreased expression of activin A receptor 1C may result in Ca(2+)-induced aberrant skin hypersensitivity. *Exp Dermatol*. 2016;25(5):402–404.

60. Gueniche A, Bastien P, Ovigne JM et al. Bifidobacterium longum lysate, a new ingredient for reactive skin. *Exp Dermatol*. 2010;19(8):e1–8.

25

Treatments for Sensitive Skin

Martina Kerscher and Heike Buntrock

Introduction

Sensitive skin is a complex dermatological condition, which has become an important challenge for dermatologists as well as a relevant topic for researchers and the cosmetic industry. Approximately, 50% of women and 40% of men classify themselves as having sensitive skin (1). This is confirmed by the results of a study, which revealed the presence of sensitive skin condition in 44% of subjects (2). While Willis et al. (3) and Misery et al. (4) showed that women are significantly more concerned than men (51% vs. 38%), a survey of practicing dermatologists revealed sensitive skin as an increasingly common condition also in men. Most of the dermatologists noticed an increase in male patients reporting sensitive facial skin over the past 5 years (5).

Patients with sensitive skin complain of abnormal sensory symptoms such as itching, burning, pricking, stinging, even pain as well as stretching sensations of the skin. These symptoms are often associated with redness, dryness, or impaired hydration of the affected skin (1,6), although obvious physical signs of skin irritation are frequently absent (7–9). The phenomenon of sensitive skin is typically accompanied by high skin reactivity to cosmetics and various environmental factors (4). Therefore, the prevalence of sensitive skin seems to be particularly high in the industrialized countries (3,10,11) and may be triggered by hypersensitivity to a range of stimuli including stress, environmental causes (e.g., cold, wind, sun, pollution), and increased use of cosmetic products (10,12). In most cases of sensitive skin, the cause remains unclear respectively endogenous or exogenous factors such as allergic contact dermatitis (ACD), toxic irritant dermatitis, or contact urticaria can be diagnosed only in a few patients (9). Not least for this reason, sensitive skin discomfort proves to have considerable impact on patient quality of life (1).

Sensitive Skin Patient

According to Draelos (13), typically patients with sensitive skin are female, well educated, well spoken, and unhappy. They frequently apply new cosmetics, but after the persistence of irritation, they consult a dermatologist with a blacklist of ingredients or with a number of unsuitable products. Usually, several physicians have already been consulted without an effective treatment solution. As the management of sensitive skin is always difficult for both the dermatologist and the patient, the development of a good physician–patient relation is important. Patients with sensitive skin should be fully informed on the characteristics of sensitive skin as well as the possible treatment options and therapeutic measures that should be undertaken with patience and tenacity. Due to the high degree of suffering or everyday psychological stimuli (stress, emotion), some patients could benefit from psychological or even psychiatric help (8,9,13).

Management of Sensitive Skin

Unfortunately, there is no simple treatment routine for managing sensitive skin. To find a regimen of facial skin care products that does not cause discomfort, it is necessary to plan a reasonable, appropriate, and well-timed procedure. The detailed protocol is time consuming, but allows a methodical step-by-step evaluation of the complex and multifactorial syndrome. While this hyperreactivity can be genetic and triggered or aggravated by different factors such as climate, food, or hormones (8), numerous patients may induce this condition by using skin care products, cosmetics, or cosmeceuticals that degrade the SC barrier (9,13). As a defective barrier function is an important component of sensitive skin, barrier repair is always an important issue (10,14). Therefore, skin care products with a pH of 5–5.5, which do not interfere with the physiological pH, are particularly suitable for patients with sensitive skin. In selected cases, the skin should rest from insult for at least 2 weeks.

Detailed Examination and Treatment Procedure

- After the exclusion of possible exogenous and endogenous factors, *all* topical skin care products, cosmetics, and cosmeceuticals (e.g., makeup, rouge, cleanser, face cream, or eye contour cream) as well as topical medications (e.g., containing benzoyl peroxide, tretinoin, glycolic acid) or cosmetic procedures (e.g., peeling, waxing, heat exposure, massage) should be discontinued.
- After 2 weeks, the patient should be evaluated for the first time, periodically thereafter.
  - Examination if underlying dermatoses are present (e.g., seborrheic dermatitis, eczema, psoriasis, acne, rosacea, perioral dermatitis [PD])
  - Assessment of skin physiology by biophysical measurements (e.g., corneometry, evapometry, sebumetry, pH value)
  - Implementation of LAST (10% aqueous solution of lactic acid) for assessment of skin neurosensitivity
  - Evaluation of patient's mental status
  - Performing patch and photopatch test if clinically indicated, just to exclude ACD or photoallergic contact dermatitis
- After the improvement of the abnormal sensory symptoms, which often might take 6–12 months (15), well-tolerated products without potentially irritating ingredients can be individually reintroduced into everyday use. In order to define exactly which products are easily tolerated, the patient should add one facial product every 2 weeks (15), starting with the least problematic. Draelos (13) recommends one facial cosmetic of low-allergenic potential per week in the following order: lipstick, face powder, powder blush. To integrate new products into a skin care regimen, individual testing could be performed by applying new products nightly, for at least five nights, to a 2 cm area lateral to the eye (13).
- The management of a patient diary (treatment and complaint) can be useful. Positive and negative results should be analyzed by the dermatologist.
- Finally, the dermatologist should provide an effective treatment solution through product selection and usage guidelines, which include products or ingredients to avoid and those suitable for continued use (Figure 25.1).

Due to lack of patient compliance, this step-by-step method is not promising in all cases. For some female patients, it is not possible to discontinue all their cosmetics and use only products which they consider inappropriate. They will hesitate to follow dermatologist's recommendations (13), and they will again fall into a cycle, in which they will use an increasing number of skin type-inadequate products,

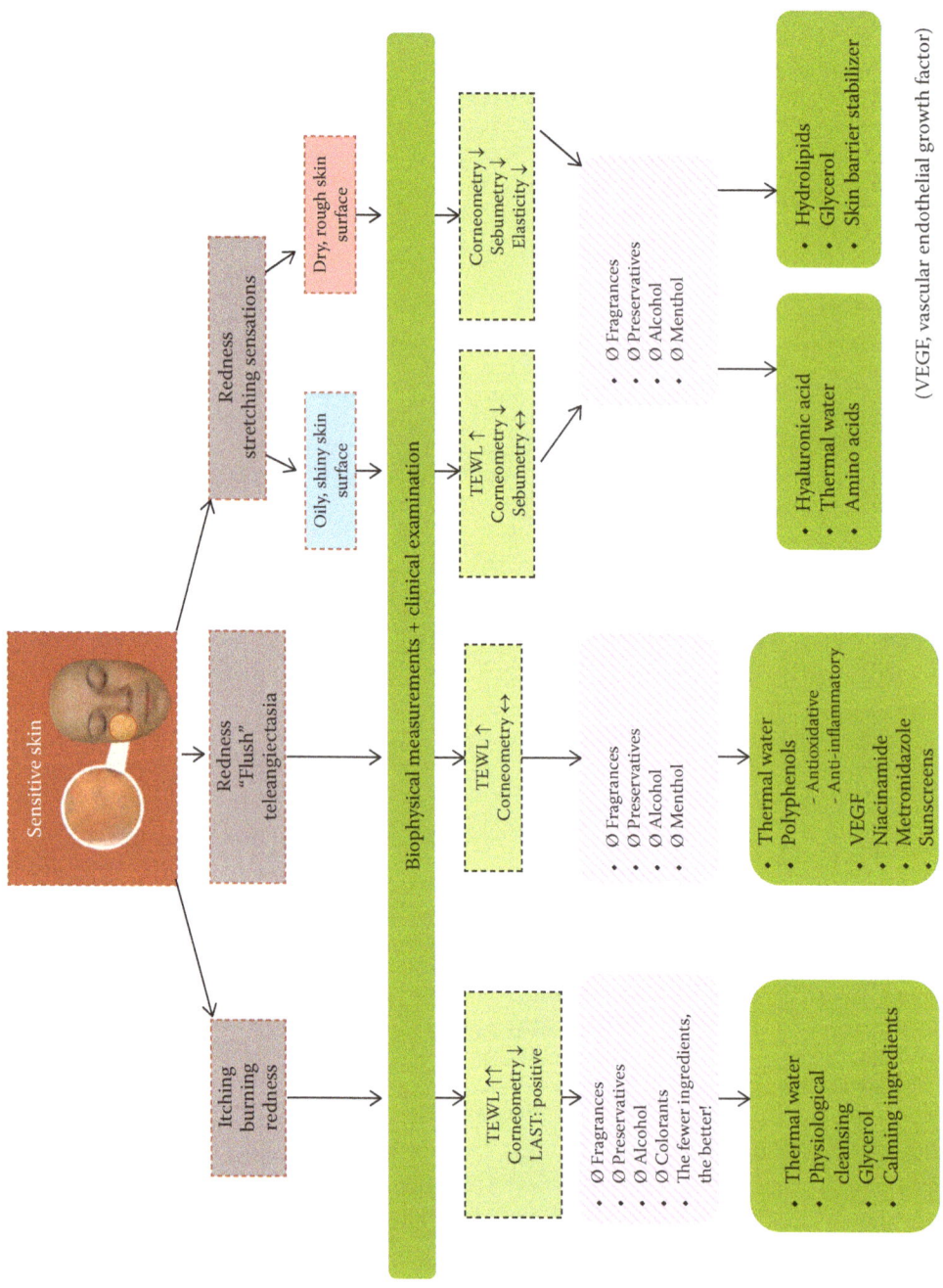

FIGURE 25.1 Treatment algorithm for sensitive skin.

thus resulting in a hypersensitive skin. Draelos (13) believes that such patients become topical corticosteroid dependent. Unfortunately, they use corticosteroids to minimize their abnormal sensory symptoms while continuing to use the offending products (13).

Skin Care Products

Numerous skin care products are now available especially for sensitive skin; frequently, they are labeled *hypoallergenic*. Labeling a product as *hypoallergenic* implies that it is based on a special formulation, is gentle and safe for skin, and causes less allergic reaction. But the fact that there are no standardized guidelines for sensitive skin, formulations are associated with the problem that there is no specific labeling available. Nowadays, sensitive skin care is an enormous commercial market totaling to many billions annually. Although the majority of manufacturers create high quality products for those with sensitive skin, clinical testing in patients with sensitive skin should be mandatory for hypoallergenic products (13,16).

Basically, potentially irritating or drying substances (Table 25.1) and procedures (Table 25.2) should be avoided or used sparingly. Patients with sensitive skin should use only a few and simple formulated products with a minimum of ingredients or, if possible, not more than 10–15 ingredients. The fewer ingredients, the better! Even chemical sunscreens, which are often added to conventional day creams, should not be used for sensitive skin. They should be replaced by physical UV filters such as titanium dioxide or zinc oxide. Sunscreen gels, waterproof UV products, and filters with very high sun protection factors should principally be avoided by people claiming about sensitive skin. Moreover, a careful examination of the ingredients is of importance. Nevertheless, if a product application is responsible for discomfort (e.g., redness, burning, and stinging), its use should immediately be discontinued. Mostly, removing the irritant greatly reduces the skin reaction. In addition, cool (not cold) wet compresses or thermal water spray can soothe the affected skin. Applying further skin care products, even hypoallergenic products, may aggravate the reaction.

Regarding skin cleansing, an intact skin barrier function is essential for a healthy skin. Therefore, excessive washing of the skin, especially with low-pH exfoliative or abrasive substances as well as with alkaline soaps, should be avoided. Instead, mild cleansing products (intended for sensitive skin) should be used. They should be fragrance free, nonfoaming, and not alcohol based. Synthetic detergent cleansers (syndets) should be preferred because they provide an optimum skin cleansing while minimizing barrier damage. Lipid-free cleansers cleansing without water (nonrinsing cleaning lotions) and leaving a thin moisturizing film on the skin might also be a really good solution. They can be used for people whose skin is extremely dry as well as sensitive. Cleansing masks, peelings, or implements such as a sponge, cotton wool, or brushing machines should be avoided as they are mostly too rough for sensitive skin. Finally, cleaned facial skin should be thoroughly dried by gently patting with a paper tissue.

After cleansing, sensitive skin needs to be moisturized (26,27). Moisturizers should preferably be oil-in-water emulsions, which contain occlusive agents and moisture-retaining substances to increase the hydration of the SC. They should protect the skin barrier by respectively minimizing skin barrier damage. Thus, they not only serve as lipid-replenishing, rehydrating, and smoothing skin care, but also maintain the skin's health.

While moisturizers as well as thermal water spray can be applied several times a day, cosmetics should be used sparingly. Cosmetics selection guidelines for patients with sensitive skin are defined in Table 25.3.

Depending on abnormal sensory symptoms and the particular degree of specific clinical signs of sensitive skin, individual treatment concepts, which have both a preventive and reparative character, can be developed (Figure 25.1).

TABLE 25.1

Important Contact Allergens in Skin Care Products and Skin Cleansers

Fragrances	Most common causes of contact dermatitis from cosmetics and skin care products are complex mixtures of more than 2000 potential allergens such as the following:
	• Oak moss (Evernia prunastri)
	• Isoeugenol
	• Eugenol
	• Cinnamal (cinnamic aldehyde)
	• Geraniol
	• Hydroxycitronellal (laurine)
	• Cynamyl alcohol (cinnamic alcohol)
	• Cinnamic aldehyde (alpha-amyl cinnamic aldehyde)
	• Hydroxyisohexyl 3-cyclohexene carboxaldehyde
	• Coumarin
	• Citral
	• Citronellol
	• Farnesol
	• Alpha-hexyl-cinnamal
	• Limonene
	• Myroxylon pereira (balsam of Peru) (17–21)
Preservatives	Second most common cause of contact dermatitis from cosmetics and skin care products
	• Formaldehyde
	• Methylchloroisothiazolinone
	• 2-Bromo-2-nitropropane-1,3-diol
	• Parabens (methyl, ethyl, propyl, butyl, isobutyl, and isopropyl paraben)
	• Quaternium-15
	• Imidazolidinyl urea
	• Dimethyl-dimethyl hydantoin
	• Thimerosal (22)
Hair dyes and hair bleaches	Third most common ingredient to cause contact dermatitis
	• p-Phenylenediamine
	• Aminophenol
	• Resorcinol
	• Toluene-2,5-diamine
	• Ammonium persulfate
	• Hydrogen peroxide
	• Glycerylthioglycolate (23,24)
Sunscreens	• 4-Aminobenzoic acid
	• 4-*Tert*-butyl-4′-methoxy-dibenzoylmethane (Parsol 1789)
	• 3-(4-Methylbenzylidene)-DL-camphor (Eusolex 6300)
	• 2-Hydroxy-4-methoxy-benzophenone (Eusolex 4360)
	• 4-Isopropyl-dibenzoylmethane (Eusolex 8020) (25)
Antioxidants	• Butylated hydroxyanisole
	• Butylated hydroxytoluene
Ointment bases	• Lanolin
	• Amerchol
	• Propylene glycol
	• Polyethylene glycol
Emulsifier and washing-active substances	• Cetyl alkohol
	• Cetostearyl alcohol
	• Glyceryl stearate
	• SLS
Botanicals and other substances	• Propolis
	• Panthenol (vitamin B)
	• Rosin (colophony)
	• Camomile
	• Tea tree oil
	• Cocamide diethanolamine (cocamide DEA)
	• Azo- and anthraquinone dyes (19)

TABLE 25.2

Potentially Irritating or Drying Cosmetic Procedures

Heat	Hot steam, heating masks
Cold	Extremely cold compresses, eye cooling pads
Cleansing	Overcleansing, low-pH products, soaps, alcohol-based products
Exfoliation	Low-pH alpha hydroxy acids or glycolic acid
Friction	Massage, peeling, dermabrasion, roll-off treatments, sponges, brushing, and suction
Masks	Overdrying masks, heating masks
Oil treatments	Essential oils, aroma therapy
Hair removal	Epilation, depilation (e.g., waxing)

TABLE 25.3

Cosmetics Selection and Usage Guidelines

Use the smallest possible number of cosmetics.

Use cosmetics designed for sensitive, intolerant, or hypoallergenic skin.

Carefully examine the list of ingredients to avoid those of a previous allergic or irritant reaction.

Use preservative and fragrance-free, noncomedogenic cosmetics (without chemical sunscreen agents).

Use powder cosmetics instead of cream-based products (e.g., powder rouge, bronzing powder).

Hypoallergenic makeup should moisturize the skin, act as corrective, and must be easy to apply.

Mix the corrective foundation with a suitable moisturizer and apply it by gently tapping with the fingers.

Liquid foundations should base on silicone derivatives (e.g., cyclomethicone, dimethicone).

Eyeliner and mascara should be black.

Avoid waterproof cosmetics.

Avoid nail polishes.

Clean brushes after each use.

Spraying thermal water all over the face after applying makeup will make it last longer while softening, moisturizing, and protecting the skin.

Store cosmetics in a cool, dry place. and do not leave them uncovered.

Avoid cosmetics beyond its expiration date.

Note: See the review by Draelos (13) for further detail.

General Recommendations

Sometimes, some simple recommendations and tips can help patients with sensitive skin:

- Use as few topical skin care products, cosmetics, and cosmeceuticals as possible.
- Apply products designed for sensitive or hypersensitive skin.
- The fewer the number of ingredients, the better (<15)!
- Avoid soaps, preservatives, alcohol-based, perfumed, or mentholated products.
- Generally, avoid products or procedures known to irritate skin.
- Store skin care products, cosmetics, and cosmeceuticals in a cool, dry, and dark place. Do not leave them uncovered (in contact with the air), and avoid them beyond its expiration date.
- Look for sterile, airtight tubes or pump dispensers to keep preservative-free products sterile throughout the entire use. Hermetic packaging protects the product from contact with air and hands.
- Nevertheless, wash hands before handling skin care products, cosmetics, and cosmeceuticals.
- Avoid hot or long bathing as well as taking hot and/or cold showers.
- Avoid all sources of skin friction (e.g., massage, tight clothes, jewelry).

- Avoid extreme temperature changes, sun exposure, heat (e.g., sauna, hot water, fireplaces), cold (e.g., eye cooling pads, extremely cold compresses, air condition), and wind.
- Avoid overcleansing the skin.
- Thoroughly dry the skin.

Novel Approaches for Treatment of Sensitive Skin

Although the prevalence of sensitive skin is rising, only a few studies have been published reporting on the effectiveness of topical products to relieve the symptoms of sensitive skin. To date, most studies concentrate on individual ingredients, but not on combinations of active ingredients to treat sensitive skin. Some promising studies are discussed in the following.

In general, the clinical benefits of a daily facial skin care regimen of mild cleansing and moisturizing with products designed for sensitive skin could be shown in a study by Hawkins et al. (28). In this study, 95 subjects with self-assessed sensitive facial skin, who had dry, itchy, as well as easily irritated skin with a history of reactions to cosmetic products, were included. Subjects were given a mild, self-foaming facial cleanser, sensitive skin day lotion or cream (depending on the form they normally used), and a sensitive skin night cream to use at home in place of the products that they would normally use. After 3 weeks of facial product application, changes in skin hydration, skin dryness, and skin sensitivity were evaluated by expert visual assessment and patient self-assessment as well as LAST and instrumental measurements. The results reported significant improvements in overall skin health and a demonstrable decrease in the sensitivity of facial skin, as evidenced in the LAST results, which showed a significant decrease in the mean group cumulative stinging score (28).

More recent studies investigate new active ingredients such as *trans*-4-tert-butylcyclohexanol, pimecrolimus 1%, and bacterial lysate to treat or prevent abnormal sensory symptoms.

While the human thermoreceptor hTRPV1 was previously identified to contribute to sensitive skin, although facilitating neurogenic inflammation, skin sensitivity toward capsaicin (natural activator of TRPV1) could also be shown to correlate with sensitive skin (29–31). Furthermore, in a screening campaign, the selective antagonist *trans*-4-tert-butylcyclohexanol was identified, which is able to inhibit capsaicin-induced hTRPV1 activation. In a clinical study, 30 women applied an oil/water emulsion containing 31.6 ppm capsaicin, and results showed that 0.4% of this inhibitor significantly reduces capsaicin-induced burning ($p < .0001$) in vivo. According to Kueper et al. (32), *trans*-4-tert-butylcyclohexanol has the potential as a novel bioactive for the treatment of sensitive skin.

For many years, pimecrolimus 1% cream has been approved as an effective, noncorticosteroid, anti-inflammatory treatment for atopic dermatitis (AD) (33,34); now, it has been proven effective in patients with sensitive skin and its underlying mechanism. In 32 patients with sensitive skin, the severity of pruritus and burning sensations was significantly decreased after using topical 1% pimecrolimus cream. A positive capsaicin-like response was seen in 63% of patients and 19% of patients showed a positive camphor-like response on application sites. A negative capsaicin-like response and/or negative camphor-like response were present in 18.8% of the patients. Authors concluded that pimecrolimus may rapidly inhibit or alleviate the itch or burning sensation of patients with sensitive skin. Also, the therapeutic effect of pimecrolimus seems to be relevant to the mechanisms that activate or sensitize TRPV1 and desensitizes TRPV1 in the skin sensory afferents (35). However, this treatment option is only on prescription and for patients suffering from severe symptoms.

Since clinical trials suggest that probiotic supplementation might be beneficial to the skin, Guéniche et al. hypothesized that a probiotic lysate, *Bifidobacterium longum* sp. extract, applied to the skin could be able to improve sensitive skin. First in vitro and then in a randomized, double-blind, placebo-controlled trial, authors demonstrated that this specific bacterial extract has a beneficial effect on reactive skin. Sixty-six female volunteers with reactive skin applied either the cream with bacterial extract at 10% or the control to their faces, arms, and legs twice a day for 2 months. The efficacy was assessed by clinical and self-assessment scores and LAST, and skin barrier recovery was evaluated by measuring TEWL following barrier disruption by tape stripping. Results demonstrated that volunteers who applied the cream with bacterial extract had a significant decrease in skin dryness after 29 days as well as a significant decrease in skin sensitivity at the end of treatment. Moreover, the treatment led to an increased skin resistance against physical and chemical aggressions compared to the control, such as noticed by the significantly increased number of strippings required to disrupt the skin barrier function. Authors speculate that this specific bacterial extract may decrease skin sensitivity by reducing neuron reactivity and neuron accessibility. New active ingredients, based on a bacteria lysate, could be developed to treat or prevent symptoms of sensitive skin (36).

According to recent studies, moisturizing and antiirritant ingredients such as thermal water can be used to relieve the sensations of sensitive skin on the face. Thermal waters have been used for years both as an active ingredient and in aerosol form, with very good results in patients with sensitive skin. A current review has led to a better understanding of the mechanisms of action of thermal spring waters, summarizing their protective action against both the short-term and long-term deleterious effects of radical oxygen species induced by, for example, UV exposure (antioxidant, immunomodulating, and anticarcinogenic effects) and reporting an anti-inflammatory and anti-irritant potential. These results justify the use of thermal spring waters as an active ingredient in topical formulations for sensitive skin (37).

Finally, a multicenter, clinical pilot study investigated in 94 patients with a history of contact allergy the tolerance of a sterile cleanser and a sterile moisturizer, both free of emulsifiers, preservatives, and fragrances. The results showed a significant improvement of all objective signs of irritated skin and suggest that adequately formulated cosmeceuticals might reduce sensitive skin, with clinical improvement of dryness, erythema, and stinging (38).

Summary

Sensitive skin, a common skin condition and an increasing challenge for dermatologists, can be characterized by discomfort without visible irritation or by obvious symptoms such as dryness, erythema, itching, burning, pricking, stinging, pain, and stretching sensations of the skin when exposed to a variety of physical (e.g., cold, wind, sun, friction), chemical (e.g., cosmetics ingredients, pollution), or psychological stimuli (e.g., stress, emotion). Even though in many patients this hyperreactivity is genetic, numerous exogenous and endogenous factors can trigger or aggravate this multifactorial syndrome. Moreover, patients with irritated skin increase their risk of developing contact allergic reactions, and on the other hand, patients with contact allergies complain about abnormal sensory symptoms of sensitive skin.

In recent years, the number of so-called hypoallergenic or hypersensitive skin care products to soothe and improve various signs of sensitive skin has tremendously increased. But the fact that there are no standard guidelines for sensitive skin formulations contributes to the complexity of treating patients with sensitive skin. In order to facilitate the use of the mentioned topical skin care products, cosmetics, and cosmeceuticals in everyday dermatological routine, the classification of patients into different skin conditions can be helpful. To aid screening according to the individual sensitive skin conditions, the *treatment algorithm for sensitive skin* was developed, which can help in providing a targeted individual treatment plan for each patient (Figure 25.1). Basically, patients with sensitive skin should use only a few and simple formulated products. Gentle cleansing and moisturizing products (intended for sensitive skin) can be used, but they should be fragrance free, nonfoaming, and not alcohol based. The smaller the number of topical skin care products, cosmetics, and cosmeceuticals as well as their ingredients, the better. Potentially irritating or drying substances and procedures should be avoided or used sparingly.

A frequent problem in the confirmation or comparison of efficacy of cosmeceutical products is still a lack of controlled, evidence-based studies. Important parameters for the quality of cosmetics and cosmeceuticals are evidence-based in vivo and in vitro efficacy as well as scientifically proven wanted and unwanted effects.

REFERENCES

1. Misery L, Myon E, Martin N et al. Sensitive skin: Psychological effects and seasonal changes. *J Eur Acad Dermatol Venereol* 2007; 21(5): 620–628.

2. Williams S, Krüger N, Keschawarzi M et al. Prevalence of "greasy," "dry," "normal" and "sensitive" skin in Germany. *41th Meeting of the German Society of Dermatology, JDDG 2005, Dresden, Germany* (Poster).

3. Willis CM, Shaw S, De Lacharrière O et al. Sensitive skin: An epidemiological study. *Br J Dermatol* 2001; 145(2): 258–263.

4. Misery L, Sibaud V, Merial-Kieny C et al. Sensitive skin in the American population: Prevalence, clinical data, and role of the dermatologist. *Int J Dermatol* 2011; 50(8): 961–967.

5. Vanoosthuyze K, Zupkosky PJ, Buckley K. Survey of practicing dermatologists on the prevalence of sensitive skin in men. *Int J Cosmet Sci* 2013; 35(4): 388–393.

6. Berardesca E, Farage M, Maibach H. Sensitive skin: An overview. *Int J Cosmet Sci* 2013; 35(1): 2–8.

7. Seidenari S, Francomano M, Mantovani L. Baseline biophysical parameters in subjects with sensitive skin. *Contact Derm* 1998; 38(6): 311–315.

8. Pons-Guiraud A. Sensitive skin: A complex and multifactorial syndrome. *J Cosmet Dermatol* 2004; 3(3): 145–148.

9. Kerscher M. Principles of treatment and protection for sensitive skin. *Hautarzt* 2011; 62(12): 906–913.

10. Richters R, Falcone D, Uzunbajakava N et al. What is sensitive skin? A systematic literature review of objective measurements. *Skin Pharmacol Physiol* 2015; 28(2): 75–83.

11. Jourdain R, de Lacharrière O, Bastien P et al. Ethnic variations in self-perceived sensitive skin: Epidemiological survey. *Contact Dermat* 2002; 46(3): 162–169.

12. Farage MA, Maibach HI. Sensitive skin: Closing in on a physiological cause. *Contact Dermat* 2010; 62(3): 137–149.

13. Draelos ZD. Cosmetic selection in the sensitive-skin patient. *Dermatol Ther* 2001; 14(3): 194–199.

14. Farage MA, Katsarou A, Maibach HI. Sensory, clinical and physiological factors in sensitive skin: A review. *Contact Dermat* 2006; 55(1): 1–14.

15. Amin S, Engasser P, Maibach HI. Sensitive skin: What is it? In: *Textbook of Cosmetic Dermatology*, second edn (Baran R, Maibach HI, eds). London: Martin Dunitz, 1998: 343–349.

16. Kligman AM, Sadiq I, Zhen Y et al. Experimental studies on the nature of sensitive skin. *Skin Res Technol* 2006; 12(4): 217–222.

17. Nardelli A, Drieghe J, Claes L et al. Fragrance allergens in "specific" cosmetic products. *Contact Dermat* 2011; 64(4): 212–219.

18. Heisterberg MV, Menné T, Johansen JD. Contact allergy to the 26 specific fragrance ingredients to be declared on cosmetic products in accordance with the EU cosmetics directive. *Contact Dermat* 2011; 65(5): 266–275.

19. Warshaw EM, Belsito DV, Taylor JS et al. North American Contact Dermatitis Group patch test results: 2009 to 2010. *Dermatitis* 2013; 24(2): 50–59.

20. Krautheim A, Uter W, Frosch P et al. Patch testing with fragrance mix II: Results of the IVDK 2005-2008. *Contact Dermat* 2010; 63(5): 262–269.

21. Thyssen JP, Linneberg A, Menné T et al. The prevalence and morbidity of sensitization to fragrance mix I in the general population. *Br J Dermatol* 2009; 161(1): 95–101.

22. Timm-Knudson VL, Johnson JS, Ortiz KJ et al. Allergic contact dermatitis to preservatives. *Dermatol Nurs* 2006; 18(2): 130–136.

23. Krasteva M, Bons B, Ryan C et al. Consumer allergy to oxidative hair coloring products: Epidemiologic data in the literature. *Dermatitis* 2009; 20(3): 123–141.

24. Hasan T, Rantanen T, Alanko K et al. Patch test reactions to cosmetic allergens in 1995–1997 and 2000–2002 in Finland—A multicentre study. *Contact Dermat* 2005; 53(1): 40–45.

25. Schauder S. Lichtkrank durch Lichtschutz. Photoallergische Kontaktekzeme durch UV-Filter in Sonnenschutzmitteln und Kosmetika Dt Ärzteb 1995; 92(28/29): A-2008–2009.

26. Cheong WK. Gentle cleansing and moisturizing for patients with atopic dermatitis and sensitive skin. *Am J Clin Dermatol* 2009; 10: 113–117.

27. Lebwohl M, Herrmann LG. Impaired skin barrier function in dermatologic disease and repair with moisturization. *Cutis* 2005; 76(6): 7–12.

28. Hawkins SS, Subramanyan K, Liu D et al. Cleansing, moisturizing, and sun-protection regimens for normal skin, self-perceived sensitive skin, and dermatologist-assessed sensitive skin. *Dermatol Ther* 2004; 17: 163–168.

29. Aubdool AA, Brain SD. Neurovascular aspects of skin neurogenic inflammation. *J Invest Derm Symp P* 2011; 15(1): 33–39.

30. Chuang HH, Prescott ED, Kong H et al. Bradykinin and nerve growth factor release the capsaicin receptor from PtdIns(4,5)P2-mediated inhibition. *Nature* 2001; 411(6840): 957–962.
31. Ständer S, Schneider SW, Weishaupt C et al. Putative neuronal mechanisms of sensitive skin. *Exp Dermatol* 2009; 18(5): 417–423.
32. Kueper T, Krohn M, Haustedt LO et al. Inhibition of TRPV1 for the treatment of sensitive skin. *Exp Dermatol* 2010; 19(11): 980–986.
33. Luger T, De Raeve L, Gelmetti C et al. Recommendations for pimecrolimus 1% cream in the treatment of mild-to-moderate atopic dermatitis: From medical needs to a new treatment algorithm. *Eur J Dermatol* 2013; 23(6): 758–766.
34. Werfel T. Topical use of pimecrolimus in atopic dermatitis: Update on the safety and efficacy. *J Dtsch Dermatol Ges* 2009; 7(9): 739–742.
35. Xie Z, Lan Y. Effectiveness of pimecrolimus cream for women patients with sensitive skin and its underlying mechanism. *Zhongguo Yi Xue Ke Xue Yuan Xue Bao* 2012; 34(4): 375–378.
36. Guéniche A, Bastien P, Ovigne JM et al. Bifidobacterium longum lysate, a new ingredient for reactive skin. *Exp Dermatol* 2010; 19(8): E1–8.
37. Seite S. Thermal waters as cosmeceuticals: La Roche-Posay thermal spring water example. *Clin Cosmet Investig Dermatol* 2013; 623–628.
38. Vie K, Pons-Guiraud A, Dupuy P et al. Tolerance profile of a sterile moisturizer and moisturizing cleanser in irritated and sensitive skin. *Am J Contact Dermat* 2000; 11(3): 161–164.

Index

Page numbers followed by f and t indicate figures and tables, respectively.